COMPLEMENTARY THERAPIES FOR THE BODY, MIND AND SOUL

Edited by **Marcelo Saad**

Complementary Therapies for the Body, Mind and Soul
http://dx.doi.org/10.5772/59418
Edited by Marcelo Saad

Contributors

Seyed Ahmad Emami, Behjat Javadi, Milad Iranshahy, Shin Takayama, Shuqing Ding, Sheng Liu, Marcelo Saad, Roberta De Medeiros, Yu-Chiang Hung, Wen-Long Hu, Chun-Ting Liu, Mohammad Reza Vaez Mahdavi, Mohamad Reza Vaez Mahdavi, Okjin Kim, Sunhwa Hong, Hyun-A Lee, Yung-Ho Chung, Si-Jong Lee, Xing-Tai Li, Haixue Kuang, Jia Zhao, Ping-Chung Leung, Yasuyo Hijikata

Published by InTech
Janeza Trdine 9, 51000 Rijeka, Croatia

Publishing Process Manager Iva Lipovic
Technical Editor InTech DTP team
Cover InTech Design team

First published August, 2015
Printed in Croatia

Additional hard copies can be obtained from orders@intechopen.com

Complementary Therapies for the Body, Mind and Soul, Edited by Marcelo Saad
p. cm.
ISBN 978-953-51-2158-9

For EU product safety concerns:
IN TECH d.o.o., Prolaz Marije Krucifikse Kozulić 3, 51000 Rijeka, Croatia,
info@intechopen.com or visit our website at intechopen.com.

Meet the editor

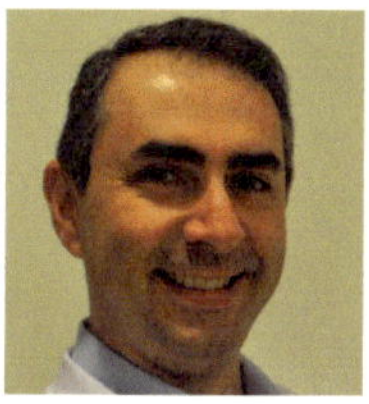

Marcelo Saad graduated in Medicine from the Federal University of Sao Paulo, Brazil, from where he also received his MSc and PhD in Rehabilitation Sciences. As medical specialties, he is board certified both in Physiatry (Physical Rehabilitation) and Acupuncture. Currently, he is President of the Medical Spiritist Association of S. Paulo and Director Member at the Medical College of Acupuncture of S. Paulo. Besides his work as a physician, he develops activities in scientific publication, is on the editorial boards of some medical journals, delivers technical lectures, and participates in scholar tasks. His fields of interest are acupuncture, rehabilitation, complementary therapies, and spirituality in health.

Contents

Preface

The most widespread term for non-orthodox treatments is "Complementary and Alternative Medicine" (CAM). The National Center for Complementary and Alternative Medicine, agency of the US National Institutes of Health, defines CAM as a group of diverse medical and healthcare interventions, practices, products, or disciplines that are not generally considered part of conventional medicine [1]. A critique of this term involves the inconsistency in gathering under the same term the words "Complementary" and "Alternative." The first word refers to a method that can be joined together with the conventional medicine, whereas the last word is associated to something used instead of it. For the purposes of the present book, the editors prefer the term Complementary Therapies (CT), which refers to the therapeutic practices that have been studied and have the potential to complement the orthodox therapeutic approach.

Defining CT is difficult, because the field is very broad and constantly changing. Generally, they are understood as the practices, products, or health systems that are outside the realm of conventional medicine, used to treat disease, or to promote health and well-being.

These therapies fulfill unmet needs at conventional treatment and diversify the conceptual framework of medicine. Modern medicine achieved amazing progresses but, in recent years, many patients have shown dissatisfaction with conventional medicine due to its mostly technical approach, the morbidity by side effects of the treatment, the high costs associated, and absence of cure for some diseases. In this scenario, there is a growing interest of patients about CT worldwide [2], as these practices also are increasingly being offered in renowned health services.

An approach oriented for a broader meaning of healing should combine in a coordinated way treatments from conventional medicine and complementary therapies. Modernly, this is achieved by the "Integrative Medicine" approach. This is aligned to the concept of patient-centered healthcare, which is the comprehensive provision of what an individual needs particularly. However, it is a challenge to provide ethical, medically responsible counseling and provision of CT that respects and acknowledges the patient's values. The boundaries between CT and conventional medicine are not absolute, as the scientific knowledge advances. The body of evidence on the efficacy and safety of different types of CT is dynamic and requires constant updating by health professionals.

CT may be classified in different paradigms of health and illness [3]. The body paradigm encompasses CT that work through biologic mechanisms, targeting biologic factors as the primary determinants of health. The mind paradigm extends the body paradigm to include factors such as stress, psychological coping styles, and social supports as primary determinants of health and disease. The spirit paradigm assumes that one or more transcendental aspects or personalities existing outside the limitations of the material universe can influence health and disease.

The title of this book includes the words body, mind, and soul. The body and the mind (and their reciprocal relations) have been extensively studied scientifically. What about the soul? One can view the soul from scientific, theological, and philosophical perspectives [4–7]. The soul is frequently associated to a brain product, so a component of mind. But we could understand the soul as the transpersonal spirit, the ethereal and immaterial essence of the individual, what constitutes the individuality. Thus, the soul is different from mind, understood as the awareness (consciousness), memory, emotion, and cognition (intellect). However, there are still undefined interfaces among them, such as coping styles, mystical experiences, and phenomena such as near-death experiences.

About the chapters

On the BODY section, Yu-Chiang Hung et al. reviewed the Chinese vision to the treatment of atherosclerosis-related diseases. The association of traditional herbs, acupuncture, kinesiotherapy, and meditation is welcome, as they could support the control of such chronic condition, associated with high morbidity and mortality rates. Shuqing Ding et al. bring us more than 20 years of clinical and research practice about the role of acupuncture in chronic functional constipation, besides all the theoretic bases for treatment with Western and Eastern medicines. Hijikata Yasuyo has brought 35 years of experience with patients in severe complex conditions treated successfully with Kampo and/or TCM. Mohammad Reza VaezMahdavi et al. described attitudes and opinions of Iranian traditional medicine regarding low back pain, based on the therapeutic theory in Iranian traditional medicine. Milad Iranshahy et al. discussed the approach of Islamic traditional medicine to treat cancer, linking it to the current knowledge about cytotoxic and antitumor activities of the medicinal plants used.

On the MIND section, Takayama Shin shared this amazing experience about the traditional Japanese medicine Kampo. May this text inspire other people for the usage of their regional traditional medicines, either in moments of catastrophe or on a regular basis. Okjin Kim et al. wrote about the therapies based on animal-assisted intervention, discoursing about definition, history, benefits, and the utility in rehabilitation and psychotherapy. Ping-chung Leung explored the common components in the fundamental practices of both Indian Yoga and Chinese Qigong, such as stretching of muscles, tendons, and ligaments; controlled breathing; and meditation. Liu Sheng explored the role of acupuncture in the treatment of drug addiction, reassuring the importance of this technique in confronting this so terrible evil.

On the SOUL section, Marcelo Saad et al. exposed a possibility to conciliate the scattered data about distant healing techniques and at the same time overcome their apparent contradictions. And Xing-Tai Li proposed a scientific hypothesis relating the Chinese concepts of Qi (or Chi) energy and the Western concepts of mitochondrial bioenergy. The book emphasizes the cited CT within the context of integrative medicine, and their role in healing and wellness, as enhancement to conventional treatment. We hope you find in the present work the sincere desire to collaborate with the dissemination of knowledge. May this book be useful and pleasant to you.

Marcelo Saad
Medical Spiritist Association of S. Paulo, S. Paulo, Brazil
Medical College of Acupuncture of S. Paulo, Brazil

References

[1] Anonymous - National Center for Complementary and Alternative Medicine. Exploring the Science of Complementary and Alternative Medicine - Third Strategic Plan 2011–2015. NIH Publication No. 11-7643. USA, February 2011.

[2] Saad M. Preface. In Saad M, de Medeiros R (eds.) Complementary Therapies for the Contemporary Healthcare (ISBN 978-953-51-0801-6). InTech, 2012. DOI: 10.5772/3307.

[3] Tataryn DJ. Paradigms of health and disease: A framework for classifying and understanding complementary and alternative medicine. Journal of Alternative and Complementary Medicine. 2002;8(6):877-892.

[4] Perakis CR. What About the Soul? Academic Medicine. 2013;88(10):1521.

[5] Dolan B. Soul searching: A brief history of the mind/body debate in the neurosciences. Neurosurgical Focus. 2007;23(1):E2.

[6] Santoro G, Wood MD, Merlo L, et al. The anatomic location of the soul from the heart, through the brain, to the whole body, and beyond: A journey through Western history, science, and philosophy. Neurosurgery. 2009;65(4):633-643.

[7] Walach H. Mind – Body – Spirituality. Mind & Matter. 2007;5(2):215-240.

Section 1

Body

Chapter 1

Complementary Therapy with Traditional Chinese Medicine for Treating Atherosclerosis-Related Diseases

Yu-Chiang Hung, Chun-Ting Liu and Wen-Long Hu

Additional information is available at the end of the chapter

Abstract

Atherosclerosis-related diseases are the leading cause of morbidity or mortality in the world. They result in serious outcomes such as sudden cardiac death, unstable angina pectoris, acute myocardial infarction, stroke, or intermittent claudication due to vessel obliteration or plaque rupture with subsequent thrombosis. There are some limitations with standard treatments such as antiplatelet drugs, angiotensin-converting enzyme inhibitors, beta-blockers, coronary artery bypass surgery, and percutaneous transluminal coronary angioplasty. Therefore, complementary and alternative medicine is necessary for medication. Traditional Chinese medicine is the main complementary therapy used in the Chinese community. This article aims to explore complementary therapy with traditional Chinese medication for atherosclerosis-related diseases. There is some scientific evidence to support that traditional Chinese medicine could treat atherosclerosis and its associated conditions. Acupuncture through needling on ST36, ST40, PC6, or BL15 could alleviate atherosclerosis-related cardiovascular diseases. *Tai chi* and meditation have beneficial effects for mental and physical health. In addition, extracts or compounds of single Chinese herbs such as *Salvia miltiorrhiza, Panax notoginseng, Ginkgo biloba, Curcuma longa, Crataegus pinnatifida, Paeonia lactiflora, Prunella vulgaris, Polygonum multiflorum, Coptis chinensis,* and red yeast rice also could treat atherosclerosis-related diseases through their endothelial protective, antioxidative, anti-inflammatory, inhibiting of smooth muscle cells proliferation, and lipid-lowering effects. In accordance with evidence-based medicine, well-designed and conducted clinical studies such as randomized control clinical trials will be necessary in the future.

Keywords: atherosclerosis, complementary medicine, traditional Chinese medicine

1. Introduction

Atherosclerosis is the most common type of arteriosclerosis. It is a disease of the arteries characterized by the deposition of fatty plaques on their inner walls, which hardens or narrows medium to large blood vessels, especially the aorta, coronary arteries, and cerebral arteries [1]. Atherosclerosis-related diseases often lead to serious outcomes such as sudden cardiac death, unstable angina pectoris, acute myocardial infarction, stroke, and intermittent claudication due to vessel obliteration or plaque rupture with subsequent thrombosis [1,2]. Epidemiological studies indicate that, because of the adoption of Western lifestyle, the prevalence of atherosclerosis is increasing all over the world and will likely reach epidemic proportions in the coming decades [2]. The earliest visible lesion in the development of atherosclerosis is the fatty streak. It consists of aggregates of foam cells (i.e., lipoprotein-loaded macrophages) in the subendothelial space. Fatty streaks may also include T cells, aggregated platelets, and smooth muscle cells. A fatty streak is the precursor lesion of an atheroma that may become an atheromatous plaque [2]. In response to plaque growth, the arterial wall can remodel itself by increasing its external diameter to accommodate the plaque without narrowing the lumen. Thrombosis is the last stage in the disease process that is responsible for clinically observable adverse events mentioned previously.

Traditional Chinese medicine (TCM), especially herbal medicine, has been used for the treatment of cardiovascular diseases for hundreds of years, as documented in the *Yellow Emperor's Inner Canon* (*Huangdi Neijing*) and the *Essential Prescriptions from the Golden Cabinet* (*Jin Gui Yao Lue*). In Taiwan, Chinese herbal medicine is commonly used as complementary and alternative therapy for the treatment of cardiovascular-related diseases such as hypertension, dyslipidemia, and stroke. Thus, studies of the medicines used for the prevention and treatment of atherosclerosis have received much attention in the recent years. The cellular and molecular details regarding the underlying efficacious mechanisms of Chinese herbal medicine in treating atherosclerosis have just begun to be understood. Therefore, the purpose of this article is to present a brief description of the mechanisms of atherogenesis and to summarize the recent research results regarding the mechanisms of antiatherogenic Chinese herbal compounds commonly used in clinical practice. Other interventions of TCM such as acupuncture, *tai chi* and meditation will also be briefly discussed.

2. Pathology and risk factors of atherosclerosis

The pathology of atherosclerosis is a progressive process with increasing age that is related to some risk factors such as hypertension, hyperlipidemia, diabetes mellitus, obesity, and cigarette smoking [1]. Atherosclerosis begins with damage to the endothelium, which results in endothelial vasodilator dysfunction. The endothelium subsequently cannot modulate tone, growth, hemostasis, and inflammation throughout the circulatory system. Injured endothelial cells (EC) produce cell surface adhesion molecules such as vascular cell adhesion molecule-1 (VCAM-1), and thereby cause monocytes and T-lymphocytes to adhere to the endothelium and migrate beneath it [1,2]. Circulating monocytes and T-lymphocytes provoke an inflammatory response. The tight junctions between EC loosen and increase the permeability to lipids, especially low-density lipoprotein (LDL). Once the oxidation of LDL has crossed the damaged endothelium into the intima, monocytes differentiate into macrophages and begin to take up oxidized LDL [1]. Macrophages bite and retain the lipid, and then become foam cells. The fatty streak consisting of lipid-containing foam cells in the arterial wall can evolve into atherosclerotic plaques or atheromas [1]. In addition, T-lymphocytes secrete cytokines that induce vascular smooth muscle cells to migrate from the media to the intima and proliferate shortly thereafter [1]. Over time, a growing lesion consisting of lipid and smooth muscle cells invade and narrow the lumen of the artery. Other extracellular matrix (ECM) components such as collagen, elastin, glycoprotein, and proteoglycans give tensile strength and viscoelasticity to the arterial wall. Increasing the synthesis of ECM components such as matrix metalloproteinases (MMPs) contributes significantly to ECM destruction, which renders the plaque more prone to rupture [1]. Once a plaque ruptures, it can trigger an acute thrombosis or embolism by activating platelets. It may finally lead to myocardial infarction, stroke, and even death.

3. Conventional treatment of atherosclerosis

Atherosclerosis treatment usually begins with lifestyle changes such as a low cholesterol diet, regular exercise, and quitting smoking. Depending on the severity of the disease, a person may be prescribed oral medication such as antiplatelets, angiotensin-converting enzyme (ACE) inhibitors, or beta-blockers. In patients with advanced disease, certain medical procedures such as percutaneous transluminal coronary angioplasty or coronary artery bypass surgery may be necessary.

4. Status and purpose

Conventional medical costs paid by patients or by the Bureau of National Health Insurance (Taipei, Taiwan) are expensive. The caregiver burden on the patients' families and government has increased yearly. In addition, conventional therapies for atherosclerosis-related diseases have some limitations such as statin-induced rhabdomyolysis or hepatitis, and antiplatelet agent-related gastrointestinal bleeding or peptic ulcer. Complementary and alternative therapy is another option for atherosclerosis medication. Traditional Chinese medicine is the primary complementary therapy used in the Chinese community. The aim of this paper is to explore complementary therapy with traditional Chinese medication for treating atherosclerosis-related diseases.

5. Atherosclerosis corresponds to blood stasis syndrome

According to TCM theory, obstructed circulation of blood results in blood stasis syndrome (Xue Yu), which is an important pattern of slowing or retardation of the blood circulation. The main symptoms may include stabbing pain with a fixed position, tenderness, local purpura, lumps, dark-purple lips and finger nails, a blue-purple tongue, and a thready or hesitant pulse. Blood stasis syndrome in TCM corresponds to atherosclerosis in modern Western medicine. Both blood stasis syndrome and atherosclerosis are the predevelopment or initial stage of ischemic heart disease, myocardial infarction, or stroke (Figure 1). With early treatment by medication, the progression of cardiovascular or cerebral vascular disease will not worsen.

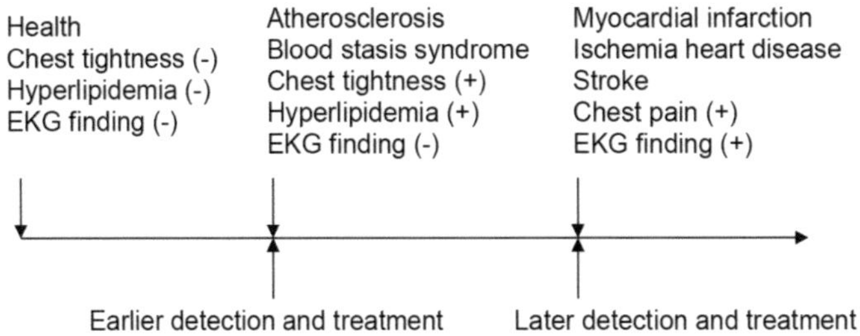

Figure 1. Progression from health to cardiovascular or cerebrovascular disease. EKG, electrocardiogram.

6. Atherosclerosis-related cardiovascular or cerebral vascular diseases

Table 1 shows atherosclerosis-related cardiovascular or cerebrovascular diseases. Atherosclerosis can cause embolism, thrombosis, ischemia, infarction, stenosis, or occlusion of the arteries. Some Chinese herbs can promote blood circulation or remove blood stasis and may be useful for treating atherosclerosis-related diseases.

ICD-9-CM	Diseases
4140	Coronary atherosclerosis
4400	Atherosclerosis of the aorta
4149	Chronic ischemic heart disease, unspecified
4148	Other specified forms of chronic ischemic heart disease
4118	Other acute and subacute forms of ischemic heart disease
410	Acute myocardial infarction
4110	Postmyocardial infarction syndrome
412	Old myocardial infarction
4297	Other certain sequelae of myocardial infarction, not elsewhere classified
444	Arterial embolism and thrombosis
4292	Cardiovascular disease, unspecified
433	Occlusion and stenosis of precerebral arteries
434	Occlusion of cerebral arteries

ICD-9-CM, *International Classification of Diseases, 9th Revision, Clinical Modification* (US Centers for Disease Control and Prevention (CDC), Salt Lake City, Utah; 1996).

Table 1. Atherosclerosis-related cardiovascular or cerebrovascular diseases

7. Chinese single herbs and atherosclerosis-related diseases

7.1. Effect of herbal extracts/compounds on the initiation of an atherosclerotic lesion

Several strategies exist for the treatment of atherosclerosis and associated diseases such as risk factor modification, antioxidation, anti-inflammation, and antiplatelet accumulation. Hypercholesterolemia, a primary risk factor that leads to atherosclerosis, is associated with the development and progression of atherosclerosis. Hypercholesterolemia and endothelial injury lead to the infiltration of LDL particles into the subendothelial space. Lowering cholesterol can provide the initial blockade [2].

The 10 traditional Chinese herbs commonly used in clinical practice that reportedly reduce the production of LDL and/or oxidative LDL are *Salvia miltiorrhiza* [3], *Panax notoginseng* [4], *Ginkgo biloba* [5], *Curcuma longa* [6], *Crataegus pinnatifida* [7], *Paeonia lactiflora* [8], *Prunella vulgaris* [9], *Polygonum multiflorum* [10], *Coptis chinensis* [11,12], and red yeast rice [13]. Single compounds or crude extracts isolated from *Salvia miltiorrhiza* [3], *Ginkgo biloba* [14], *Prunella vulgaris* [9], *Polygonum multiflorum* [15], and red yeast rice [16] restore epithelial function by regulating the endothelial nitric oxide synthase/nitric oxide (eNOS/NO) pathway. Oxidized low-density lipoprotein (ox-LDL) in the absence of high-density lipoprotein (HDL) can stimulate EC activation and subsequent expression of adhesion molecules such as the vascular cell adhesion molecule (VCAM-1) and the intercellular adhesion molecule (ICAM-1) [17]. These adhesion molecules recruit circulating macrophages and T-lymphocytes into the subintima; this action is mediated by macrophage chemoattractant protein-1 (MCP-1) [17].

As Table 2 shows, single compounds and/or herbal extracts from these 10 TCM herbs inhibit the expression of adhesion molecules (i.e., VCAM-1 and ICAM-1). Among them, *Salvia miltiorrhiza* [3], *Panax notoginseng* [4], and *Coptis chinensis* [18] can downregulate the expression of MCP-1. Furthermore, ox-LDL can stimulate macrophages and T-lymphocytes to produce inflammatory cytokines such as interleukin-1-beta (IL-1β) and tumor necrosis factor alpha (TNF-α) in the vessel wall, which further activate EC and promote vascular smooth muscle cell (VSMC) proliferation and migration [1]. *Salvia miltiorrhiza* [3], *Curcuma longa* [19], *Paeonia lactiflora* [8], and *Coptis chinensis* [18] suppress the expression of TNF-α. Nuclear factor kappa B (NF-κB) can regulate the expression of multiple inflammatory cytokines such as MCP and cell adhesion molecules (e.g., ICAM-1 and VCAM-1) so as to affect the atherogenic process. Most of the 10 TCM herbs can block the NF-κB pathway involved in the inflammatory process (Table 2).

7.2. Effect of herbal extracts/compounds on the propagation of an atherosclerotic lesion

Stimulated by inflammatory cytokines such as interleukin-1α (IL-1α) and TNF-α, VSMCs propagate and migrate from the media to the intima and produce collagen, which forms the substance of the fibrous cap of the mature lesion [1,20]. Signaling interactions between CD40- and CD40L-expressing cells result in the formation of matrix metalloproteinases (MMPs), which degrade collagens and the thin fibrous cap and lead to the formation of vulnerable plaques and rupture [20]. Among the 10 TCM herbs, *Salvia miltiorrhiza* [3] and *Panax notogin-*

Herb/ interventions	eNOS/ NO	LDL/ox-LDL	VCAM-1	ICAM-1	MMP-9/2	CD40	MCP-1	NF-κB	TNF-α
Salvia miltiorrhiza	↑ [3]	↓ [3]	↓ [3]	↓ [3]	↓ [3]	↓ [3]	↓ [3]	↓ [3]	↓ [3]
Panax notoginseng		↓ [4]	↓ [38]	↓ [38]	↓ [21]	↓ [21]	↓ [4]	↓ [4]	
Ginkgo biloba	↑ [14]	↓ [5]	↓ [39]	↓ [39]	↓ [22]			↓ [40]	
Curcuma longa		↓ [41]	↓ [6]	↓ [6]	↓ [19,23]			↓ [23]	↓ [19]
Crataegus pinnatifida		↓ [7]	↓ [24]	↓ [24]	↓ [24]				
Paeonia lactiflora		↓ [8]	↓ [42]	↓ [43]				↓ [43]	↓ [8]
Prunella vulgaris	↑ [9]	↓ [9]	↓ [38]	↓ [38]				↓ [38]	
Polygonum multiflorum	↑ [15]	↓ [10]	↓ [39]	↓ [39]					
Coptis chinensis		↓ [11, 12]	↓ [40]	↓ [40]	↓ [25]		↓ [18]	↓ [25]	↓ [18]
Red yeast rice	↑ [16]	↓ [13]	↓ [41]	↓ [42]	↓ [26]			↓ [26, 41]	
Acupuncture	↑ [38]	↓ [39]		↓ [39]	↓ [41]		↓ [39]		↓ [40]
Tai chi/yoga		↓ [42,43]							

The up arrow (↑) indicates increased expression; the down arrow (↓) indicates decreased expression.

eNOS, endothelial nitric oxide synthase; ICAM-1, intercellular adhesion molecule; LDL, low-density lipoprotein; MCP-1, macrophage chemoattractant protein; MMP-9, matrix metalloproteinase-9; NF-κB, nuclear factor-kappaB; NO, nitric oxide; ox-LDL, oxidized low-density lipoprotein; TNF-α, tumor necrosis factor alpha; VCAM-1, vascular cell adhesion molecule-1.

Table 2. Multiple signaling molecules involved in atherosclerosis and regulated by Chinese herbs

seng [21] reduce the expression of CD40 and the activity of MMP-2. In addition, *Ginkgo biloba* [22], *Curcuma longa* [19,23], *Crataegus pinnatifida [24], Coptis chinensis* [25], and red yeast rice [26] have an inhibitory effect on MMP-2 and/or MMP-9. Table 3 summarizes the target activities of these herbal extracts or compounds in atherosclerosis.

Salvia miltiorrhiza has been widely used in the Chinese population for treating cardiovascular and cerebrovascular diseases. Its specific clinical use is for angina pectoris, hyperlipidemia, and acute ischemic stroke [27], which are all closely associated with atherosclerosis. According to TCM theory, *Salvia miltiorrhiza* promotes blood circulation, removes blood stasis, and relieves pain. Several compounds derived from *Salvia miltiorrhiza* have been well studied in the treatment of atherosclerosis. Protocatechuic aldehyde derived from *Salvia miltiorrhiza* inhibits lipopolysaccharide-induced human umbilical vein EC apoptosis via the regulation of

Herbs	Compound/extract	Target	Reference
Salvia miltiorrhiza	Protocatechuic Aldehyde	Reduce caspase-3, and VSMC migration and proliferation	[28,29]
	Cryptotanshinone	Increase NO; reduce ox-LDL, ICAM-1, VCAM-1, and monocyte adhesion	[30]
	Tanshinone IIA	Reduce ROS, Bax/Bcl-2, caspase-3, LOX-1, NF-κB, ox-LDL, monocyte adhesion, VSMC migration and proliferation, macrophage, cholesterol accumulation, CD 40, TNF-α MMP-2, MMP-9, and platelet aggregation	[34,35,36,43,49]
	Salvianolic acid B	Reduce ICAM-1, E-selectin, NF-κB, ox-LDL, MMP-2, and MMP-9	[31-33]
Panax notoginseng	*Panax notoginseng Saponins*	Reduce ICAM-1, VCAM-1, ox-LDL, IL-1β, MMP-9, MMP-2, NF-κB, CD40, and MCP-1	[4,21,38]
Ginkgo biloba	*Ginkgo biloba* Extract	Increase eNOS/NO; Reduce LDL, VCAM-1, ICAM-1, E-selectin, MMP-2, and NF-κB	[5,14,22,39,40]
Curcuma longa	Curcumin	Reduce LDL, VCAM-1, ICAM-1, MMP-2, MMP-9, TNF-α, and NF-κB	[6,19,23,41]
Crataegus pinnatifida	*Crataegus pinnatifida* extract	Reduce LDL, VCAM-1, ICAM-1, and MMP-9	[7,24]
Paeonia lactiflora	Paeonol	Reduce VCAM-1, ICAM-1, and TNF-α	[42,43]
	Total glucosides of peony	Reduce LDL and TNF-α	[8]
Prunella vulgaris	*Prunella vulgaris* extract	Increase eNOS/NO; reduce LDL, VCAM-1, ICAM-1, and NF-κB	[9,38,44]
Polygonum multiflorum	2,3,5,4'-tetrahydroxystilbene-2-O-beta-D-glucoside (TSG)	Increase eNOS/NO; reduce LDL, VCAM-1, and ICAM-1	[10,15,39,45]
Coptis chinensis	Berberine	Reduce LDL, ox-LDL, VCAM-1, ICAM-1, MMP-9, MCP-1, NF-κB, and TNF-α	[11,12,18,25,40, 46]
Red yeast rice	*Monascus purpureus*-fermented rice extract	Increase eNOS/NO; reduce LDL, VCAM-1, ICAM-1, MMP-9, MMP-2, and NF-κB	[13,16,26,41,42, 47,48]

eNOS, endothelial nitric oxide synthase; ICAM-1, intercellular adhesion molecule; IL-1β, interleukin 1β; LDL, low-density lipoprotein; LOX1, lectin-like oxidized low-density lipoprotein receptor-1; MCP-1, macrophage chemoattractant protein; MMP, matrix metalloproteinase; NF-κB, nuclear factor-kappaB; NO, nitric oxide; ox-LDL, oxidized low-density lipoprotein; ROS, reactive oxygen species; TNF-α, tumor necrosis factor alpha; VCAM-1, vascular cell adhesion molecule-1; VSMC, vascular smooth muscle cells.

Table 3. The target activity of herbal extracts or compounds in atherosclerosis

caspase-3, the migration and proliferation of VSMC, and intravascular thrombosis [28,29]. Cryptotanshinone derived from *Salvia miltiorrhiza* suppresses the increase in endothelial permeability, which is likely because of the restoration of NO bioavailability in EC. Cryptotanshinone also can attenuate monocyte adhesion to EC through inhibiting the expression of adhesion molecules. Salvianolic acid B, a water-soluble antioxidant obtained from *Salvia miltiorrhiza,* can reduce oxidative stress, inhibit LDL oxidation, and reduce oxidized LDL-induced cytotoxicity [31]. Salvianolic acid B also inhibits VCAM-1 and ICAM-1 expression in TNF-α-treated human aortic EC, and attenuates MMP-2 and MMP-9 expression in vivo in apolipoprotein E-deficient mouse aorta and in vitro in LPS-treated human aortic smooth muscle cells [32,33].

Tanshinone IIA, another compound derived from *Salvia miltiorrhiza,* markedly inhibits the elevation of ROS evoked by hydrogen peroxide. Tanshinone IIA significantly decreases the hydrogen peroxide-induced expression of proapoptotic proteins Bax and caspase-3 and significantly increases the expression of antiapoptotic protein Bcl-2 in EA.hy926 cells [34]. Tanshinone IIA inhibits oxidized LDL-induced lectin-like oxidized low-density lipoprotein receptor-1 (LOX1) expression in macrophages by reducing intracellular superoxide radical generation and NF-κB activation [35]. Tanshinine IIA also reduces the expression of CD 40, TNF-α, MMP-2, MMP-9, and suppresses VSMC migration and proliferation, macrophage cholesterol accumulation, and platelet aggregation [36].

Hung et al. [37] report that a low dose (0.015 mg/mL) of *Salvia miltiorrhiza* aqueous extract significantly inhibited the growth of a rat smooth muscle cell line (i.e., A10) under Homocysteine(Hcy) stimulation, and *Salvia miltiorrhiza* aqueous extract treatment decreased the intracellular reactive oxygen species (ROS) concentration in terms of reducing p47 (phox) translocation and increasing catalase activity. The signaling profile suggests that *Salvia miltiorrhiza* aqueous extract inhibits Hcy-induced A10 cell growth via the protein kinase C/ mitogen-activated protein kinase (PKC/MAPK)-dependent pathway [37].

8. Acupuncture and atherosclerosis-related diseases

In addition to herbal medicine, acupuncture has been used for a long time in the treatment of cardiovascular disease in Asia. Acupuncture is applied in the treatment of hypertension and hyperlipidemia, which are risk factors leading to atherosclerosis. Kim et al. [50] demonstrated that electroacupuncture on the *Zusanli* (ST36) (Figure 2) point reduces hypertension by activating nitric oxide synthase signaling mechanisms [50]. Tian et al. [51] report that electroacupuncture on the *Fenglong* (ST40) point downregulates the effect of plasma total cholesterol, LDL, MCP-1, and ICAM-1 in hyperlipidemic rats. Another study by Xiao et al. [52] showed that electroacupuncture on the *Fenglong* (ST40) point effectively lowers serum total cholesterol, LDL, and macrophage TNF-α and IL-6 levels in hyperlipemia rats. Li et al. [53] showed that electroacupuncture of the *Neiguan* (PC6) and *Xinshu* (BL15) points can suppress the increased expression of CD 40 L and MMP-9 proteins of coronary artery tissue in rats with coronary atherosclerotic heart disease.

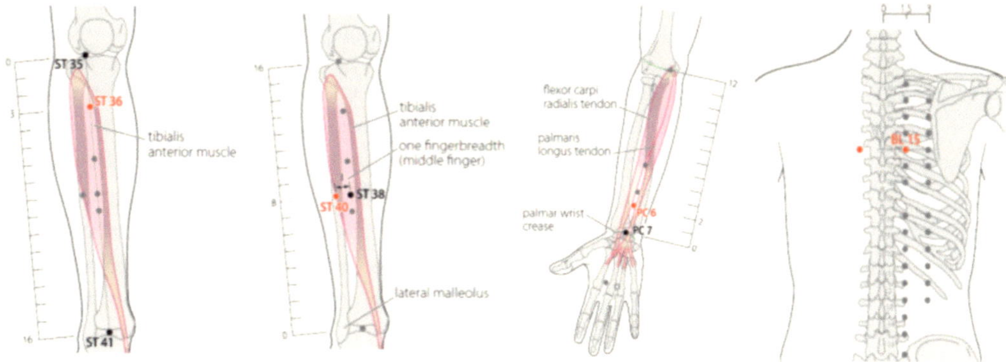

Figure 2. The World Health Organization (WHO) standard acupuncture point locations of ST36, ST40, PC6, and BL15 [54].

9. Mind–body exercise of *tai chi* and yogi

Tai chi chuan (*tai chi*) is a Chinese traditional mind–body exercise with low to moderate exercise intensity. Previous studies have shown that it offers benefits for aerobic capacity, muscular strength, balance, and cardiovascular risk factors such as hypertension, diabetes mellitus, and dyslipidemia. Furthermore, *tai chi* appears to be safe and effective for patients with acute myocardial infarction, coronary artery bypass grafting surgery, congestive heart failure, and stroke [55]. A study conducted in India shows that regular yogic practices can significantly reduce blood pressure, heart rate, body fat, total cholesterol, triglycerides, and LDL.These reactions are beneficial for cardiac and hypertensive patients [56].

10. Meditation, mind, and atherosclerosis

Certain mental disorders and stress are conducive to atherosclerosis. Kroenke et al. [57] revealed that a negative mood is predictive of a greater progression of calcified atherosclerosis, compared to a positive mood. Everson-Rose et al. [58] found that high levels of stress, hostility, and depressive symptoms are associated with a significantly increased risk of incident stroke or transient ischemic attacks in middle-aged and older adults. Stillman et al. [59] and Wang et al. [60] also noted that anxiety can potentially predict a worse outcome through worsening of vascular function in patients with coronary atherosclerotic disease.

Meditation is an alternative medicine practice for mental and physical health. It has salutary effects on patients with anxiety [61, 62], depression [61, 63], and stress [64, 65]. Some articles report that meditation can calm the emotions and produce beneficial effects on the cardiovascular system, particularly with regard to vascular aspects [66-68]. Walton et al. [68] advocate meditation to reduce traditional and novel risk factors for cardiovascular diseases; for example, meditation (1) decreases blood pressure; (2) reduces the use of tobacco and alcohol; (3) lowers the cholesterol level and lipid oxidation; and (4) decreases psychosocial stress.

The mechanism and neurobiological effects of mindfulness meditation involve (1) deactivation of the default mode network, which generates spontaneous thoughts, contributes to the maintenance of the autobiographical self, and is associated with anxiety and depression; (2) the anterior cingulate cortex, which underpins attention functions; (3) the anterior insula, which is associated with the perception of visceral sensation, the detection of the heartbeat and respiratory rate, and the affective response to pain; (4) the posterior cingulate cortex, which helps one to understand the context from which a stimulus emerges; (5) the temporoparietal junction, which assumes a central role in empathy and compassion; and (6) the amygdala, which is implicated in fear responses [69].

11. Further research

There are few studies on formulas or single herbal drugs interaction in the treatment of atherosclerosis. In accordance with evidence-based medicine, well-designed and conducted clinical studies such as randomized control clinical trials will be necessary in the future.

12. Conclusions

Atherosclerosis-related diseases are the primary causes of death. In addition to standard treatment, complementary therapy needs to be face up. Traditional Chinese medicine is a popular complementary and alternative medicine (CAM) in East Asia and throughout the world. There is increasing scientific evidence demonstrating that TCM has potential for treating atherosclerosis and its associated conditions. Acupuncture, *tai chi*, and meditation have beneficial effects for atherosclerosis-related cardiovascular diseases. Extracts or compounds of single herbs of some Chinese herbs such as *Salvia miltiorrhiza, Panax notoginseng, Ginkgo biloba, Curcuma longa, Crataegus pinnatifida, Paeonia lactiflora, Prunella vulgaris, Polygonum multiflorum, Coptis chinensis,* and red yeast rice through their endothelial protective, antioxidative, anti-inflammatory, and lipid-lowering effects may act on multiple mechanisms involved in the pathogenesis of atherosclerosis.

Author details

Yu-Chiang Hung[1,2*], Chun-Ting Liu[1] and Wen-Long Hu[1,3,4]

*Address all correspondence to: hungyuchiang@gmail.com

1 Department of Chinese Medicine, Kaohsiung Chang Gung Memorial Hospital and School of Traditional Chinese Medicine, Chang Gung University College of Medicine, Kaohsiung, Taiwan

2 School of Chinese Medicine for Post Baccalaureate, I-Shou University, Kaohsiung, Taiwan

3 Kaohsiung Medical University College of Medicine, Kaohsiung, Taiwan

4 Fooyin University College of Nursing, Kaohsiung, Taiwan

References

[1] Rafieian-Kopaei M, Setorki M, Doudi M, Baradaran A, Nasri H. Atherosclerosis: process, indicators, risk factors and new hopes. *Int J Prevent Med*. 2014;5:927-946.

[2] Tedgui A, Mallat Z. Cytokines in atherosclerosis: pathogenic and regulatory pathways. *Physiol Rev*. 2006;86:515-581.

[3] Chen Z, Xu H. *Anti-Inflammatory and Immunomodulatory Mechanism of Tanshinone IIA for Atherosclerosis*. Evidence-based complementary and alternative medicine: eCAM. 2014;2014:267976. doi: 10.1155/2014/267976.

[4] Liu Y, Zhang HG, Jia Y, Li XH. Panax notoginseng saponins attenuate atherogenesis accelerated by zymosan in rabbits. *Biol Pharma Bull*. 2010;33:1324-1330.

[5] Zhang Q, Wang GJ, A JY, Wu D, Shu LL, Ma B, Du Y. Application of GC/MS-based metabonomic profiling in studying the lipid-regulating effects of Ginkgo biloba extract on diet-induced hyperlipidemia in rats. *Acta Pharmacol Sin*. 2009;30:1674-1687. doi: 10.1038/aps.2009.173.

[6] Shishodia S. Molecular mechanisms of curcumin action: gene expression. *Biofactors*. 2013;39:37-55. doi: 10.1002/biof.1041.

[7] Zhang J, Liang R, Wang L, Yan R, Hou R, Gao S, Yang B. Effects of an aqueous extract of Crataegus pinnatifida Bge. var. major N.E.Br. fruit on experimental atherosclerosis in rats. *Jf Ethnopharmacol*. 2013;148:563-569. doi: 10.1016/j.jep.2013.04.053.

[8] Li J, Chen CX, Shen YH. Effects of total glucosides from paeony (Paeonia lactiflora Pall) roots on experimental atherosclerosis in rats. *Jf Ethnopharmacol*. 2011;135:469-475. doi: 10.1016/j.jep.2011.03.045.

[9] Hwang SM, Kim JS, Lee YJ, Yoon JJ, Lee SM, Kang DG, Lee HS. Anti-diabetic atherosclerosis effect of Prunella vulgaris in db/db mice with type 2 diabetes. *Am J Chin Med*. 2012;40:937-951. doi: 10.1142/S0192415X12500693.

[10] Gao X, Hu YJ, Fu LC. Blood lipid-regulation of stilbene glycoside from polygonum multiflorum. *Zhongguo Zhong Yao Za Zhi*. 2007;32:323-326.

[11] Kong W, Wei J, Abidi P, Lin M, Inaba S, Li C, Wang Y, Wang Z, Si S, Pan H, Wang S, Wu J, Wang Y, Li Z, Liu J, Jiang JD. Berberine is a novel cholesterol-lowering drug working through a unique mechanism distinct from statins. *Natur Med.* 2004;10:1344-1351.

[12] Hsieh YS, Kuo WH, Lin TW, Chang HR, Lin TH, Chen PN, Chu SC. Protective effects of berberine against low-density lipoprotein (LDL) oxidation and oxidized LDL-induced cytotoxicity on endothelial cells. *J Agri Food Chem.* 2007;55:10437-10445.

[13] Yang CW, Mousa SA. The effect of red yeast rice (Monascus purpureus) in dyslipidemia and other disorders. *Compl Ther Med.* 2012;20:466-474. doi: 10.1016/j.ctim. 2012.07.004.

[14] Ou HC, Lee WJ, Lee IT, Chiu TH, Tsai KL, Lin CY, Sheu WH. Ginkgo biloba extract attenuates oxLDL-induced oxidative functional damages in endothelial cells. *J Appl Physiol.* 2009;106:1674-1685. doi: 10.1152/japplphysiol.91415.2008.

[15] Zhang W, Xu XL, Wang YQ, Wang CH, Zhu WZ. Effects of 2,3,4',5-tetra hydroxystilbene 2-O-beta-D-glucoside on vascular endothelial dysfunction in atherogenic-diet rats. *Plant Med.* 2009;75:1209-1214. doi: 10.1055/s-0029-1185540

[16] Zhu XY, Li P, Yang YB, Liu ML. Xuezhikang, extract of red yeast rice, improved abnormal hemorheology, suppressed caveolin-1 and increased eNOS expression in atherosclerotic rats. *PLoS One.* 2013;8:e62731. doi: 10.1371/journal.pone.0062731.

[17] Zeng Y, Song JX, Shen XC. Herbal remedies supply a novel prospect for the treatment of atherosclerosis: a review of current mechanism studies. *Phytother Res.* 2012;26:159-167. doi: 10.1002/ptr.3587.

[18] Chen FL, Yang ZH, Liu Y, Li LX, Liang WC, Wang XC, Zhou WB, Yang YH, Hu RM. Berberine inhibits the expression of TNFalpha, MCP-1, and IL-6 in AcLDL-stimulated macrophages through PPARgamma pathway. *Endocrine.* 2008;33:331-7. doi: 10.1007/s12020-008-9089-3.

[19] Singh V, Rana M, Jain M, Singh N, Naqvi A, Malasoni R, Dwivedi AK, Dikshit M, Barthwal MK. Curcuma oil attenuates accelerated atherosclerosis and macrophage foam-cell formation by modulating genes involved in plaque stability, lipid homeostasis and inflammation. *Brit J Nutri.* 2014;13:1-14.

[20] Martin-Ventura JL, Blanco-Colio LM, Tunon J, Munoz-Garcia B, Madrigal-Matute J, Moreno JA, Vega de Ceniga M, Egido J. Biomarkers in cardiovascular medicine. *Revista española de cardiología.* 2009;62:677-688.

[21] Liu G, Wang B, Zhang J, Jiang H, Liu F. Total panax notoginsenosides prevent atherosclerosis in apolipoprotein E-knockout mice: Role of downregulation of CD40 and MMP-9 expression. *J Ethnopharmacol.* 2009;126:350-4. doi: 10.1016/j.jep.2009.08.014.

[22] Tsai KL, Chang YL, Huang PH, Cheng YH, Liu DH, Chen HY, Kao CL. Ginkgo biloba extract inhibits oxidized low-density lipoprotein (oxLDL)-induced matrix metallo-

proteinase activation by the modulation of the lectin-like oxLDL receptor 1-regulated signaling pathway in human umbilical vein endothelial cells. *J Vasc Surg*. 2014;S0741-5214:01124. doi: 10.1016/j.jvs.2014.05.098.

[23] Yu YM, Lin HC. Curcumin prevents human aortic smooth muscle cells migration by inhibiting of MMP-9 expression. *Nutri, Metabol Cardio Dis*. 2010;20:125-32. doi: 10.1016/j.numecd.2009.03.001.

[24] Shin IS, Lee MY, Lim HS, Ha H, Seo CS, Kim JC, Shin HK. An extract of Crataegus pinnatifida fruit attenuates airway inflammation by modulation of matrix metalloproteinase-9 in ovalbumin induced asthma. *PLoS One*. 2012;7:e45734. doi: 10.1371/journal.pone.0045734.

[25] Huang Z, Meng S, Wang L, Wang Y, Chen T, Wang C. Suppression of oxLDL-induced MMP-9 and EMMPRIN expression by berberine via inhibition of NF-kappaB activation in human THP-1 macrophages. The anatomical record: *Adv Integ Anat Evol Biol*. 2012;295:78-86. doi: 10.1002/ar.21489.

[26] Lin CP, Huang PH, Tsai HS, Wu TC, Leu HB, Liu PL, Chen YH. Monascus purpureus-fermented rice inhibits tumor necrosis factor-alpha-induced upregulation of matrix metalloproteinase 2 and 9 in human aortic smooth muscle cells. *J pharm pharmacol*. 2011;63:1587-94. doi: 10.1111/j.2042-7158.2011.01364.x.

[27] Zhou L, Zuo Z, Chow MS. Danshen: an overview of its chemistry, pharmacology, pharmacokinetics, and clinical use. *J Clin Pharmacol*. 2005;45:1345-1359.

[28] Xing YL, Zhou Z, Agula, Zhong ZY, Ma YJ, Zhao YL, Xiao XH, Wang SQ. Protocatechuic aldehyde inhibits lipopolysaccharide-induced human umbilical vein endothelial cell apoptosis via regulation of caspase-3. *Phytother Res*. 2012;26:1334-1341. doi: 10.1002/ptr.3720.

[29] Moon CY, Ku CR, Cho YH, Lee EJ. Protocatechuic aldehyde inhibits migration and proliferation of vascular smooth muscle cells and intravascular thrombosis. *Biochem Biophys Res Comm*. 2012;423:116-121. doi: 10.1016/j.bbrc.2012.05.092.

[30] Ang KP, Tan HK, Selvaraja M, Kadir AA, Somchit MN, Akim AM, Zakaria ZA, Ahmad Z. Cryptotanshinone attenuates in vitro oxLDL-induced pre-lesional atherosclerotic events. *Plant Med*. 2011;77:1782-7. doi: 10.1055/s-0030-1271119.

[31] Yang TL, Lin FY, Chen YH, Chiu JJ, Shiao MS, Tsai CS, Lin SJ, Chen YL. Salvianolic acid B inhibits low-density lipoprotein oxidation and neointimal hyperplasia in endothelium-denuded hypercholesterolaemic rabbits. *J Sci Food Agri*. 2011;91:134-141. doi: 10.1002/jsfa.4163.

[32] Chen YH, Lin SJ, Ku HH, Shiao MS, Lin FY, Chen JW, Chen YL. Salvianolic acid B attenuates VCAM-1 and ICAM-1 expression in TNF-alpha-treated human aortic endothelial cells. *J Cell Biochem*. 2001;82:512-521.

[33] Lin SJ, Lee IT, Chen YH, Lin FY, Sheu LM, Ku HH, Shiao MS, Chen JW, Chen YL. Salvianolic acid B attenuates MMP-2 and MMP-9 expression in vivo in apolipopro-

tein-E-deficient mouse aorta and in vitro in LPS-treated human aortic smooth muscle cells. *J Cell Biochem*. 2007;100:372-384.

[34] Jia LQ, Yang GL, Ren L, Chen WN, Feng JY, Cao Y, Zhang L, Li XT, Lei P. Tanshinone IIA reduces apoptosis induced by hydrogen peroxide in the human endothelium-derived EA.hy926 cells. *J Ethnopharmacol*. 2012;143:100-108. doi: 10.1016/j.jep.2012.06.007.

[35] Xu S, Liu Z, Huang Y, Le K, Tang F, Huang H, Ogura S, Little PJ, Shen X, Liu P. Tanshinone II-A inhibits oxidized LDL-induced LOX-1 expression in macrophages by reducing intracellular superoxide radical generation and NF-kappaB activation. Translational research: *J Lab Clin Med*. 2012;160:114-124. doi: 10.1016/j.trsl.2012.01.008.

[36] Gao S, Liu Z, Li H, Little PJ, Liu P, Xu S. Cardiovascular actions and therapeutic potential of tanshinone IIA. *Atherosclerosis*. 2012;220:3-10. doi: 10.1016/j.atherosclerosis.2011.06.041.

[37] Hung YC, Wang PW, Pan TL. Functional proteomics reveal the effect of Salvia miltiorrhiza aqueous extract against vascular atherosclerotic lesions. *Biochim Biophys Acta*. 2010;1804:1310-1321. doi: 10.1016/j.bbapap.2010.02.001.

[38] Wan JB, Lee SM, Wang JD, Wang N, He CW, Wang YT, Kang JX. Panax notoginseng reduces atherosclerotic lesions in ApoE-deficient mice and inhibits TNF-alpha-induced endothelial adhesion molecule expression and monocyte adhesion. *J Agri Food Chem*. 2009;57:6692-7. doi: 10.1021/jf900529w.

[39] Chen YH, Lin SJ, Chen YL, Liu PL, Chen JW. Anti-inflammatory effects of different drugs/agents with antioxidant property on endothelial expression of adhesion molecules. *Cardio Hematol Dis Drug Targ*. 2006;6:279-304.

[40] Zhang S, Chen B, Wu W, Bao L, Qi R. Ginkgolide B reduces inflammatory protein expression in oxidized low-density lipoprotein-stimulated human vascular endothelial cells. *J Cardio Pharmacol*. 2011;57:721-7. doi: 10.1097/FJC.0b013e31821a50a8.

[41] Zhao JF, Ching LC, Huang YC, Chen CY, Chiang AN, Kou YR, Shyue SK, Lee TS. Molecular mechanism of curcumin on the suppression of cholesterol accumulation in macrophage foam cells and atherosclerosis. *Mol Nutri Food Res*. 2012;56:691-701. doi: 10.1002/mnfr.201100735.

[42] Pan LL, Dai M. Paeonol from Paeonia suffruticosa prevents TNF-alpha-induced monocytic cell adhesion to rat aortic endothelial cells by suppression of VCAM-1 expression. *Phytomedicine*. 2009;16:1027-32. doi: 10.1016/j.phymed.2009.04.003.

[43] Nizamutdinova IT, Oh HM, Min YN, Park SH, Lee MJ, Kim JS, Yean MH, Kang SS, Kim YS, Chang KC, Kim HJ. Paeonol suppresses intercellular adhesion molecule-1 expression in tumor necrosis factor-alpha-stimulated human umbilical vein endothelial cells by blocking p38, ERK and nuclear factor-kappaB signaling pathways. *Int Immunopharmacol*. 2007;7:343-350.

[44] Park SH, Koo HJ, Sung YY, Kim HK. The protective effect of Prunella vulgaris ethanol extract against vascular inflammation in TNF-alpha-stimulated human aortic smooth muscle cells. *BMB Rep*. 2013;46:352-357.

[45] Yao W, Huang C, Sun Q, Jing X, Wang H, Zhang W. Tetrahydroxystilbene Glucoside Protects Against Oxidized LDL-Induced Endothelial Dysfunction via Regulating Vimentin Cytoskeleton and its Colocalization with ICAM-1 and VCAM-1. *Cell Physiol Biochem*. 2014;34:1442-1454. doi: 10.1159/000366349.

[46] Huang Z, Cai X, Li S, Zhou H, Chu M, Shan P, Huang W. Berberine attenuated monocyte adhesion to endothelial cells induced by oxidized low density lipoprotein via inhibition of adhesion molecule expression. *Mol Med Rep*. 2013;7:461-465. doi: 10.3892/mmr.2012.1236.

[47] Lin CP, Lin YL, Huang PH, Tsai HS, Chen YH. Inhibition of endothelial adhesion molecule expression by Monascus purpureus-fermented rice metabolites, monacolin K, ankaflavin, and monascin. *J Sci Food Agri*. 2011;91:1751-1758. doi: 10.1002/jsfa.4371.

[48] Xie X, Wang Y, Zhang S, Zhang G, Xu Y, Bi H, Daugherty A, Wang JA. Chinese red yeast rice attenuates the development of angiotensin II-induced abdominal aortic aneurysm and atherosclerosis. *J Nutri Biochem*. 2012;23:549-556. doi: 10.1016/j.jnutbio.2011.02.011.

[49] Li YI, Elmer G, Leboeuf RC. Tanshinone IIA reduces macrophage death induced by hydrogen peroxide by upregulating glutathione peroxidase. *Life Sci*. 2008;83:557-562. doi: 10.1016/j.lfs.2008.08.003.

[50] Kim DD, Pica AM, Duran RG, Duran WN. Acupuncture reduces experimental renovascular hypertension through mechanisms involving nitric oxide synthases. *Microcirculation*. 2006;13:577-585.

[51] Tian JY, Wang Q, Chen YF, Xiao Y, Yue W, Zhang HX. Effect of electroacupuncture stimulation of "Fenglong" (ST 40) on expression of inflammatory cytokines of celiac macrophages in hyperlipidemia rats. *Zhen Ci Yan Jiu*. 2014;39:282-287.

[52] Xiao Y, Le W, Huang H, Zhou L, Tian JY, Chen YF. Effect of electroacupuncture of "Fenglong" (ST 40) on levels of blood lipid and macrophage TNF-alpha and IL-6 in hyperlipidemic rats. *Zhen Ci Yan Jiu*. 2013;38:459-464.

[53] Li M, Cai RL, Sun X, Hu L, Wang KM, He L, Peng CY. Effects of electroacupuncture intervention on blood lipid levels and expression of CD 40 L and MMP-9 in the coronary artery tissue in coronary heart disease rats. *Zhen Ci Yan Jiu*. 2013;38:123-128.

[54] World Health Organization Regional Office for the Western Pacific (WPRO). *WHO Standard Acupuncture Point Locations in the Western Pacific Region*. WPRO: Manila; 2009. p. 64, 66, 107, 154. ISBN 978-92-9061-248-7.

[55] Lan C, Chen SY, Wong MK, Lai JS. Tai chi chuan exercise for patients with cardiovascular disease. Evidence-based complementary and alternative medicine: eCAM. 2013;2013:983208. doi: 10.1155/2013/983208.

[56] Pal A, Srivastava N, Tiwari S, Verma NS, Narain VS, Agrawal GG, Natu SM, Kumar K. Effect of yogic practices on lipid profile and body fat composition in patients of coronary artery disease. *Comp Ther Med.* 2011;19:122-127. doi: 10.1016/j.ctim. 2011.05.001.

[57] Kroenke CH, Seeman T, Matthews K, Adler N, Epel E. Mood patterns based on momentary assessment of positive and negative moods over a day and coronary artery calcification in the CARDIA study. *Psychosom Med.* 2012;74:526-534. doi: 10.1097/PSY. 0b013e3182583e68.

[58] Everson-Rose SA, Roetker NS, Lutsey PL, Kershaw KN, Longstreth WT Jr, Sacco RL, Diez Roux AV, Alonso A. Chronic stress, depressive symptoms, anger, hostility, and risk of stroke and transient ischemic attack in the multi-ethnic study of atherosclerosis. *Stroke.* 2014;45:2318-2323. doi: 10.1161/STROKEAHA.114.004815.

[59] Stillman AN, Moser DJ, Fiedorowicz J, Robinson HM, Haynes WG. Association of anxiety with resistance vessel dysfunction in human atherosclerosis. *Psychosom Med.* 2013;75:537-544. doi: 10.1097/PSY.0b013e31829a0ae3.

[60] Wang G, Cui J, Wang Y, Deng B, Liang X, Bai J, Guo S, Yang Z, Huang L, Li C. Anxiety and adverse coronary artery disease outcomes in Chinese patients. *Psychosom Med.* 2013;75:530-536. doi: 10.1097/PSY. 0b013e3182984317.

[61] Goyal M, Singh S, Sibinga EM, Gould NF, Rowland-Seymour A, Sharma R, Berger Z, Sleicher D, Maron DD, Shihab HM, Ranasinghe PD, Linn S, Saha S, Bass EB, Haythornthwaite JA. Meditation programs for psychological stress and well-being: a systematic review and meta-analysis. *JAMA Internal Med.* 2014;174:357-368. doi: 10.1001/ jamainternmed.2013.13018.

[62] Orme-Johnson DW, Barnes VA. Effects of the transcendental meditation technique on trait anxiety: a meta-analysis of randomized controlled trials. *J Alt Comp Med.* 2014;20:330-341. doi: 10.1089/acm.2013.0204.

[63] Jain FA, Walsh RN, Eisendrath SJ, Christensen S, Rael Cahn B. Critical analysis of the efficacy of meditation therapies for acute and subacute phase treatment of depressive disorders: a systematic review. *Psychosomatics.* 2014; pii: S0033-3182(14)00167-4. doi: 10.1016/j.psym.2014.10.007

[64] Ruotsalainen JH, Verbeek JH, Mariné A, Serra C. Preventing occupational stress in healthcare workers. The Cochrane database of systematic reviews. 2014;12:CD002892. doi: 10.1002/14651858.CD002892.pub4

[65] Hartley L, Mavrodaris A, Flowers N, Ernst E, Rees K. Transcendental meditation for the primary prevention of cardiovascular disease. The Cochrane database of systematic reviews. 2014;12:CD010359. doi: 10.1002/14651858.CD010359.pub2.

[66] Koike MK, Cardoso R. Meditation can produce beneficial effects to prevent cardiovascular disease. *Horm Mol Biol Clin Invest*. 2014;18:137-143. doi: 10.1515/hmbci-2013-0056.

[67] Barnes VA, Orme-Johnson DW. Prevention and treatment of cardiovascular disease in adolescents and adults through the transcendental meditation(®) Program: a research review update. *Curr Hyperten Rev*. 2012;8:227-242.

[68] Walton KG, Schneider RH, Nidich S. Review of controlled research on the transcendental meditation program and cardiovascular disease. Risk factors, morbidity, and mortality. *Cardiol Rev*. 2004;12:262-266.

[69] Ngô TL. Review of the effects of mindfulness meditation on mental and physical health and its mechanisms of action. Santé mentale au Québec. 2013;38:19-34.

Chapter 2

Acupuncture in Treatment of Chronic Functional Constipation

Shuqing Ding, Xun Jin, Yijiang Ding,
Lingling Wang and Huifeng Zhou

Additional information is available at the end of the chapter

http://dx.doi.org/10.5772/60521

Abstract

Constipation is not only a symptom but is a predominant presenting symptom in many diseases. The prevalence is between 3 and 27% worldwide, and is especially prevalent in the elderly population. The aetiology is multifactorial. Laxative abuse or enema use are usually a norm in patients' constipation. Patients tend not to seek further medical aid after several unsuccessful therapies and this can seriously affect their quality of life.

Acupuncture based on Chinese Medicine approaches the patients holistically. While having experience and potential in treating this condition, it does meet Western Medicine's criteria for diagnosis and effectiveness, which are defined by evidence-based medicine. An integrative pelvic floor centre is a platform for offering a comprehensive diagnosis and treatment, and can further research and training. This chapter focuses on a multidisciplinary and integrated background to incorporate acupuncture as a treatment modality in chronic functional constipation with experience from a national colorectal centre in China with more than 20 years research and clinical experience in treating constipation. This includes using patient-reported outcome instruments in the evaluation of the role of acupuncture as a future treatment option.

Keywords: Chronic functional constipation, Acupuncture, Pelvic floor centre, Patient Report Outcome

1. Introduction

Constipation is not only a functional disorder, it is a major symptom in many diseases. The prevalence is between 3 and 27% worldwide, especially in the elderly population. Functional chronic constipation is defined by Rome III criteria, which comprises two or more abnormalities that must be present for at least three months during the previous year. After excluding a mechanical or secondary cause leading to constipation, these include fewer than three bowel movements per week, hard or lumpy stools, and straining at stools.

The aetiology is multifactorial. Patients do not seek medical aid usually because they lose hope, making laxative abuse or use of an enema (usually for refractory constipation) is common. Although not directly life threatening, this psychosomatic disease has four side-effects of discomfort, depression, dollar costs, and drug toxicity (4D, as an abbreviation), and these can seriously affect the patient's quality of life.

Acupuncture, based on Chinese Medicine, approaches the patient as a whole. The first record of constipation was from "Inner Canon of Yellow Emperor (Huangdi Neijing)" around 4700 years ago and other updated literature resources. While Chinese Medicine and practitioners have experience and potential in this condition, they do not exceed Western Medicine in effectiveness of diagnosis and treatment, based upon evidence-based medicine. An integrated pelvic floor centre is a platform offering comprehensive diagnosis and treatment for research and training.

This chapter focuses on a multidisciplinary and integrated background to highlight acupuncture as an adjunctive treatment option in chronic functional constipation, with data from a national colorectal centre in China with more than 20 years research in constipation, including clinical trials and research using patient-reported outcome instruments in the evaluation of acupuncture's future role.

2. Chronic functional constipation in western medicine

It is clear that constipation represents a major public health problem. The prevalence in North America is estimated between 3 and 27% [1], similar to China's 4 to 13% [2, 3], especially in the elderly population [4]. A large proportion of patients with constipation do not have a known cause and suffer from idiopathic constipation. The aetiology and pathophysiology is unclear and multifactorial[5], including diet or environmental issues, psychiatric disorders, metabolic and endocrine disorders such as hypothyroidism and diabetes, connective tissue disorders such as lupus and scleroderma, neurologic illness, and medication side-effects. Before labelling the symptoms as a functional disorder, pathologies that could cause obstruction should be excluded. Additionally, laxative abuse is a key factor associated with refractory constipation.

Two sets of formal criteria have been developed to define chronic functional constipation as a specific concept, as follows. One is the Rome III [6] diagnostic criteria, which comprises two or more of the identified abnormalities, which must be present for at least three months during the previous year — fewer than three bowel movements per week, hard or lumpy stools, and straining more than 25% of the time. Other symptoms include a sensation of incomplete evacuation, or anorectal obstruction or blockage, or manual manoeuvres to facilitate the evacuation etc. Another criterion developed by the American College of Gastroenterology is a simpler and perhaps more clinically relevant definition. This defines unsatisfactory defecation as that characterized by infrequent bowel movements, difficult stool passage, or both. Patients can be further classified as belonging to subsets, such as slow transit constipation (motility disorders), irritable bowel syndrome (IBS), and obstructed defecation syndrome (ODS), or mixed subsets above in this chapter.

Traditional medical therapies for constipation include lifestyle changes, the intake of fibre, over the counter medication (magnesium hydroxide, lactulose, PEG 4000 bisacodyl, and senna), or phosphate enemas, among others. A recent review has shown that 15% of patients were completely satisfied and another 28% of patients were fairly satisfied, while a majority (51%) were "not particularly" or "not at all" satisfied with their medical therapy [7].

2.1. Slow-transit constipation

The main symptoms of slow-transit constipation (STC) are infrequent bowel movements fewer than three times per week, bloating, and abdominal cramping [8]. These symptoms need to be attributed to either the colon or to generalized symptoms affecting the colon as well as the stomach and small bowel. STC accounts for 16% to 40% of chronic constipation. Slow transit constipation may be due to abnormality of the myenteric plexus, associated with alteration of the interstitial cells of Cajal (ICC) and neuronal cells of the enteric nervous system [9,10]. Some research shows that it may derive partly from the anthraquinone laxative abuse [11,12].

2.2. Investigations

A diagnosis of slow transit constipation is usually done by a colonic transit study, described first by Arhan [13]. The methodology is not standardized in radiopaque marker and the abdomen plain X-ray film taken time. A positive result was defined as more than 20% of the radiopaque marker remaining on day five (120 h later), as indicative of slow transit time according to a plain X-ray film of the abdomen [14].

Other options for investigation of constipation include anorectal manometry, colonic scintigraphy, defecography, and use of a wireless motility capsule [15]. Patients are usually treated conservatively with exercise, diet modification, fibre supplementation, and laxatives or enemas. However, the success of controlling symptoms is unsatisfactory. Numerous patients choose cathartic stimulants such as phenolphthalein, rhubarb, senna, and aloe which contain anthraquinones, resulting in melanosis coli and affecting the intestinal nerves. Their side-effects make the symptoms complicated and challenging. When cathartic and other conservative measures fail, invasive treatment options are considered, including antegrade colonic enemas [16], sacral nerve stimulation [17], or subtotal colectomy to relieve the severe symptoms [18], and sometimes a stoma creation. Surgical excision of the colon can be successful in

50–75% of patients, but abdominal pain and constipation can reoccur and patients also run a risk of developing a post-operative small bowel obstruction or faecal urgency/incontinence [19]. Hence, surgery should be accepted in a very select population.

2.3. Constipation-predominant Irritable Bowel Syndrome (IBS-C)

Symptoms of IBS-C are usually associated with abdominal pain or discomfort, bloating, hard stools, fewer than three bowel movements per week, or straining, etc. The main characteristic difference from STC is discomfort that is relieved after defecation and the presence of normal-transit constipation. Some female patients have bowel symptoms that typically worsen immediately before their period and have tendencies to develop anxiety and depression.

Due to the heterogeneity of the symptoms, a single medication or treatment is usually insufficient to achieve symptom control, hence a more comprehensive strategy is required: including diet counselling, medications affecting prokinetic intestinal spasms, and treatment using mental and behavioural therapy, [20] etc. Treatment should be tailored to the patients' needs. The primary treatment of choice is fibre. Other laxatives recommended are lactulose, polyethylene glycol (PEG) 4000, etc. Some patients need a simultaneous supplement of probiotics. If the regimen fails for a time, or if patients develop tolerance to a therapy, a different agent or perhaps an additional treatment will be needed.

2.4. Obstructive Defecation Syndrome (ODS)

Obstructive Defecation Syndrome refers to a series of symptoms such as prolonged and repeated straining at bowel movements, the sensation of incomplete emptying, and the frequent need to support the perineum or the posterior vaginal wall in manual manoeuvres (digital disimpaction) [21]. ODS can have subsets such as dyssynergic defecation, pelvic floor relaxation etc.Dyssynergic defecation is most often associated with an inability to coordinate abdominal, rectoanal, and pelvic floor muscles during defecation. The condition often represents an acquired behavioural disorder. On rectal examination, the patient may have a high resting pressure, and on bearing down, pelvic floor movement may be poor or paradoxical [22]. Pelvic floor relaxation patients may have a normal or lower resting tone, and on bearing down the perineum descends a great deal more and may manifest a rectocele, intussusceptions, or even pelvic organ prolapse of the rectum, uterus, or bladder [23]. Anal physiology testing — including anorectal manometry, cine defecography, anal ultrasound, and EMG findings — may uncover the morphological and functional abnormalities in order to diagnose the symptoms. Overlap between the various sub types of constipation can coexist. Relative subtleties such as rectal compliance, rectoanal inhibitory reflex, and balloon expulsion tests are perhaps less reliable, but abnormalities in these areas no doubt contribute to the overall assessment of the patient's function [24].

The spectrum of therapeutic options in obstructive defecation syndrome has developed in the last decade from nonsurgical to surgical. The first line of treatment is biofeedback therapy. Electromyography biofeedback is more popular but is not superior to pressure biofeedback. The success of biofeedback depends on appropriate patient selection, a well-trained therapist, and treatment compliance. Biofeedback effectively relieves symptoms of defecatory disorders in 69% of affected adults [25]. It is more focused on the modulation of pelvic floor muscles and reflex dysfunction from behavioural or other secondary reasons.

Aetiologies like internal rectal prolapse (or intussusception) and rectocele are the primary or secondary pathologies of ODS, and surgical management provides some options for those patients who do not respond to more conservative treatment. These include stapled transanal rectal resection (STARR) [26,27], Transtar, laparoscopic ventral rectopexy [28], and sacral nerve stimulation [17,29], which have some benefits. However, these approaches are still associated with a significant expense and potential morbidity [30]. Their use must be tempered by the fact that benign conditions are being treated with the aim of improving quality of life. The balance of risk versus benefit must be fully understood by both patients and clinicians.

Patients and physicians have different criteria for defining and describing constipation. Accurate identification of the specific features of chronic constipation reduces the likelihood of unnecessary or inappropriate testing, and improves the chances of treatment success for currently available therapies which are not uniformly effective across all constipation subtypes [31].

Patients suffering from long-term constipation symptoms may have psychological issues. In our experience of 90 cases of chronic functional constipation, 35 (38.9%) cases have this problem, of which 14 cases are mild to moderate, while 21 cases are severe; almost all the patients have a sleeping dysfunction. Additionally we noted fatigue, weakness, and some female patients had menstruation disturbances or weight loss due to endocrine or nutritional dysfunction [32]. Although not directly life threatening, this psychosomatic disease adversely affects a patient's social and personal life as via the 4Ds: discomfort, depression, dollar costs, and drug toxicity.

3. Diagnosis and management of chronic functional constipation in Chinese herb medicine

Traditional Chinese Medicine (TCM) lists constipation as a symptom or syndrome, referring to infrequent bowel movements, a consistency that is too hard, and evacuation that is too difficult, which includes acute and chronic constipation. Chinese Medicine approaches the patient as a whole. Four methods of diagnosis are looking, listening, questioning, and feeling the pulse. Collecting data from asking the patients questions is essential, including: stools issue (sensation, consistence, interval time, colour, odour, and amount); occurrence; onset time, such as after childbirth, postpartum, menopause, or old age; the course of symptoms; how they alleviate the problem; and which accompanying symptoms such as abdominal distension, loss of appetite, fatigue, depression, insomnia, etc.

The basic aetiology and pathology of chronic constipation is abnormal not only in intestinal motility but is closely related to other whole organs and meridians, blood or body fluids, and mental or emotional functions. In diagnosis, the subsets' differentiation of constipation from Western Medicine's definition, combined with the syndrome differentiation (Zheng) from Traditional Chinese Medicine, have a unique advantage in clinical practice communication [33].

Five types of syndromes are identified as excessive heat and body fluid loss, liver and spleen disharmony of Qi stagnation, lung and spleen Qi deficiency, deficiency of liver-yin and kidney-yin, and Yang deficiency of spleen and kidney. The syndromes' processes are mainly deficiency oriented: Qi and Yin deficiency goes through and extends to yang deficiency, with pathogenic damping, heat, phlegm, and blood stasis products.

3.1. Excessive heat and body fluid loss

Patients sometimes have symptoms that are hard stools, scanty dark urine, anal burning, abdominal bloating, thirst and halitosis, red in the face and anxiety, dry and yellow coating tongue, and a fast and slippery pulse. Clear heat through bowel therapeutic principle is used, with the common herbs Gardenia jasminoides, Coptis, Scutellaria baicalensis, Citrus aurantium, and Peach kernel, etc.

3.2. Liver and spleen disharmony of Qi stagnation

Patients sometimes have symptoms that include the urge to defecate but a obstructed sensation, anal fullness, abdominal or chest distension, loss of appetite, frequent belching but incomplete flatus, pink and thin coating tongue and string pulse. Dispel melancholy and strengthen spleen Qi therapeutic principle is used. Common herbs used for treatment are Bupleurum, Radix Paeoniae Alba, Rhizoma Atractylodis Macrocephalae, Poria cocos, Chinese yam, etc.

3.3. Lung and spleen Qi deficiency

The symptoms are mainly an urge to defecate, with soft stools, but being too weak to push them out after exertion; sweating and loss of breath; fatigue; pale in the face and tongue; and a weak pulse. Invigorate Lung and Spleen Qi of the life essence therapeutic principle is used as the common herbs are Astragalus membranaceus, Codonopsis pilosula, Rhizoma alismatis, Fructus aurantii, Magnolia officinalis, Cimicifuga, Ge Gen, among others.

3.4. Liver-yin and kidney-yin deficiency

The symptoms include hard stools like chestnuts, a pale and dull appearance, delayed bowel movements about three days even one week, straining defecation, a reddish and thin coating on the tongue, and a weak pulse. Enriching body essence fluid of Liver and Kidney therapeutic principal is used as the common herbs are Figwort, Radix Rehmanniae Preparata, Ophiopogon japonicus, Cornus officinalis, Chinses Angelica, and Coptis cinnamon etc.

3.5. Yang deficiency of spleen and kidney

Symptoms include no urge to defecate or being too weak to push stools out; with sweating or lack of breath; chills; soreness and weakness of the waist and knees; use of laxatives; a pale, thick, and greasy tongue; and a deep, delayed pulse. Invigorating spleen and kidney warming Yang for relaxing the bowels is used, as the common herbs are Monkshood, Dried ginger, Epimedium, Allium macrostemon, and Pinellia, among others.

4. Perception of chronic functional constipation in acupuncture

Acupuncture based on Chinese Medicine, approaches the patients as a whole. The first record for constipation was from "Inner Canon of Yellow Emperor (Huangdi Neijing)" [34] around 4,700 years ago. He said "In case of abdominal fullness and difficulty in bowel movement, acupoints of the Kidney Meridian of Foot-Shaoyi are punctured" and "In case of occurrence of epigastric pain, abdominal distension and fullness, and constipation, Acupoints of the Spleen Meridian of Foot-Taiyin are punctured". Other works include the Canon of Acumoxibustion (Zhenjiu Jiayijing). Acupuncture has been practiced in China for several millennia, and the technique is now being increasingly accepted by practitioners and patients worldwide, including in the United States [35–37]. Since the side-effects of laxatives used over the long-term are not acceptable, and the outcomes after surgery are frequently unsatisfactory, alternative therapies to treat constipation are attractive to both patients and practitioners.

From Liu's literature research [38], we know that constipation has been relevant to 229 ancient sources, with 148 acupoints involved. The most commonly used acupoints and meridians are listed in Table 1 and Table 2, as are the frequency or times of treatment. Constipation is identified as the first ranked disease spectrum in acupuncture therapy, meaning that only acupuncture can be efficacious in providing a clinical cure [39].

KI6 (Zhaohai)	SJ6 (Zhigou)	ST36 (Zusanli)	SP3 (Taibai)	LR13 (Zhangmen)	RN8 (Shenque)	BL25 (Dachangshu)
34	22	16	15	15	15	14
RN6 (Qihai)	KI3 (Taixi)	KI4 (Dazhong)	BL57 (Chenshan)	SP6 (Sanyinjiao)	BL28 (Pangguangshu)	KI1 (Yongquan)
13	11	10	9	8	8	8

Table 1. Acupoints' frequency, using ancient literature on constipation

BL	KI	RN	SP	ST	LR	TE
93	80	65	54	39	30	25

Table 2. Acupoints' frequency in meridians (times)

Due to its effectiveness and safety, acupuncture treatment in chronic functional constipation has gradually become accepted and is being now investigated. Before the treatment, the patient's history, symptom characteristics, severity, underlying causes, and a physical test should be reviewed by a well-trained multidisciplinary team able to offer a comprehensive protocol of acupuncture and other remedies. Based on our literature and clinical research, we are describing the research and clinical from our practice.

4.1. Acupoints' selection [32]

The acupoints used were divided in two different sets. Group Set 1 included: Bilateral ST25 (Tianshu), SP15 (Daheng), SP14 (Fujie), CV6 (Qihai), CV4 (Guanyuan), ST36 (Zusanli), and ST37 (Shangjuxu). Group Set 2 included: Bilateral BL20 (Pishu), BL23 (Shenshu), BL25 (Dachangshu), BL33 (Zhongliao), BL34 (Xialiao), and GV20 (Baihui).

4.2. Local points and direct stimulation

ST25 (Tianshu) is the Front-mu point of the large intestine and BL25 (Dachangshu) is the Back-shu point of the large intestine. The locations of the points meet the extension of the large intestine on the body's surface. They are close to the Zang-fu organ and are the most directly effective acupoints for the treatment of dysfunction of the large intestine. Concerning the distribution of nerve segments, the nerve segment of BL25 (Dachangshu) is distributed at L3 and that of ST25 (Tianshu) is at T10, which correspond to the distribution of nerve segments from T10 to L3 and the sacral plexus [40]. The pilot research of Ding et al. [15], titled "Effect of acupuncture on neurons in the intestinal nervous system in rats", verified, through the protein gene product 9.5 (PGP 9.5), that acupuncture assisted the improvement of ganglion cell function after the destruction of neurons in the intestinal nervous system.

4.3. Local points and indirect stimulation, BL33 and BL34

Miraculous Pivot: Nine Needles and Twelve Yuan Points (Lingshu: Jiuzhen Shier Yuan) stated that: "Key to needling is qi arrival". By manipulating the piercing direction and distance, the needling sensation is transmitted to the diseases sites, which maintains a satisfactory result. Constipation of dyssynergic defecation and pelvic floor relaxation is partially due to dysfunction of the pelvic floor muscles. After puncturing at BL33 (Zhongliao) and BL34 (Xialiao), the needling sensation may be conducted to the perineum. Patients may usually feel a tightening or lifting sensation in the sacrococcygeal region or around the anus and/or vagina, which becomes much more obvious with electric stimulation. BL33 (Zhongliao) and BL34 (Xialiao) are located in the sacral region, which are the nearest ones to the area (S2–S4) in which the pelvic nerve has an input in the junior defecation control system. The stimulated S4 reaction induces anus contraction and a lifting sensation of the perineum [41]. Hence, acupuncture on BL33 (Zhongliao) and BL34 (Xialiao) modulate the motion and function of pelvic floor muscle, probably by exciting the relevant nerves. Due to the variability of the human sacrum, exact positioning and punching deep in the sacral foramen still requires further research [42].

http://dx.doi.org/10.5772/60521

4.4. Combination of distal points and holistic regulation

From Chinese Medicine theory, constipation pathogens lie in the large intestine, lung, liver, spleen, and kidneys. Combination of distal points has two roles: firstly, indicating the disorders located on the distal of the running course of the affected meridian, like ST36 (Zusanli) and ST37 (Shangjuxu) are applied for disorder of the abdomen. BL57 (Chengshan) is divergent to the anus. Secondly, based on syndrome differentiation and holistic regulation, like KI6 (Zhaohai) communicates with the Yin Heel Vessel that dominates yin in the whole body. KI6 (Zhaohai) can nourish yin and promote bowel movement. In the "two-element holographic unit" theory, the internal malleolus corresponds to the umbilicus, and BL57 (Chengshan) is corresponds to the anus. Hence, the distal point in the lower limb can treat constipation [38]. Cao et al. [43], by applying electric stimulation at ST36 (Zusanli) on rats, discovered that colon substance P (SP) content increased significantly and that gastrointestinal motility was promoted. The effect of the combination of the nearby points and the distal points is better than that achieved by only treating the distal points.

4.5. Communicating with Du Meridian in regulating mental conditions

The incidence of abnormal mental disorders is high in cases of chronic constipation. In addition, patients with chronic functional constipation often also experienced varying degrees of psychological or emotional issues having an effect on sleep; this complicated the situation due to the prolongation of sickness. It was reported by Nehra et al. [44] that 65% of the patients with stool disturbance and constipation suffered from psychological disorders. In research into 90 cases of chronic constipation, 34 cases (38.9%) accounted for 37.8% confirmed diagnoses of depression and anxiety by psychiatric doctors, in which slow transit constipation and dyssynergic defecation patients accounted for 40% and 56.7%, respectively [32]. Slow transit constipation patients lack in confidence in the treatment of the long-term disease and respond poorly to usual medical management. This may the reason of increased psychological issues in these patients. If patients get a good and rapid response from acupuncture, the psychological disorder will accordingly gradually get released. Anxiety or depression is common in dyssynergic defecation patients, which may increase the pelvic floor muscle tension and paradoxical contraction in defecation, boosting a psychological vicious circle. If it is combined with psychological counselling or psychiatric medication in some candidates, then efficiency and patient tolerance will be improved.

Modern research [45] has proved that the intestinal tract is controlled by the central nervous system, with the involvement of the brain-gut axis. Acupuncture was applied to GV20 (Baihui), GV14 (Dazhui), GV10 (Lingtai), and others to modulate Qi of the Du Meridian, to promote Yang in the meridian, nourish the brain, and regulate sleeping and mood. Moreover, the needling technique of qi conduction could enhance the relieving of psychological issue. Zhang et al. [46] found that acupuncture could increase the content of of 5-hydroxytryptamine (5-HT) of model rate, and modulate the norepinephrine (NE) and 5-HT which two substances were related to alleviate depression.

4.6. Technique

A supine posture was required in the treatment using Group Set 1 and a prone position was required in the treatment using Group Set 2. A disposable needle of Hwato brand, 0.32 mm × 75 mm, was selected and prepared. After routine sterilization of local skin, the needles were inserted perpendicularly at ST25 (Tianshu), SP15 (Daheng), SP14 (Fujie), and BL25 (Dachangshu), 40 to 50mm in depth, and the even needling technique was applied after the arrival of Qi. Perpendicular puncturing was applied to CV6 (Qihai), CV4 (Guanyuan), and BL23 (Shenshu), 40 mm in depth, and to BL20 (Pishu), 13 to 25 mm in depth. The reinforcing technique was used after the arrival of Qi. Perpendicular puncturing was applied to ST36 (Zusanli) and ST37 (Shangjuxu), 25 to 40 mm in depth and the even needling technique was used after the arrival of Qi. The lifting, thrusting, and rotating technique was applied to GV20 (Baihui) at a low frequency and small amplitude, operated for two or three minutes. In BL33 (Zhongliao), BL34 (Xialiao), after being inserted into the posterior foramen, oblique puncture was applied, 65 mm in depth with the tip toward the medial aspect and the base of thigh. The angle of 30° was formed between the needle body and the longitudinal axle of the human body, and 60° was formed with the skin. The even needling technique was used after the arrival of Qi to ensure the needling sensation was radiating to the anus or perineum. Deep puncturing of abdominal acupoints is usually used in slow transit constipation patients to improve intestine motility. Obstructive defecation syndrome(ODS) also needs deep puncturing of BL33 (Zhongliao) and BL34 (Xialiao) in the sacral foramen. Irritable bowel syndrome needs shallow puncturing for gut hypersensitivity.

Electroacupuncture was combined on BL33 (Zhongliao), BL34 (Xialiao), ST25 (Tianshu), and ST37 (Shangjuxu). Electroacupuncture apparatus (Han's, LH 202 H) was connected to the needle-handles by disperse-dense wave, 2/15 Hz and at a suitable intensity based on patients' tolerance.

4.7. Course and follow-up

Routinely, the two sets of acupoints were used alternately, one set per day, with 20 sessions being a therapeutic course. Every session lasts for 30 minutes, once daily. Comparing a four-week acupuncture treatment period satisfaction between the dyssynergic defecation patients and pelvic floor relaxation patients, usually the former group responded better, but if the treatment period prolonged to eight weeks, the latter group would be better. It means some patients maybe need a prolonged treatment course if the efficacy displayed slow. Another phenomenon may observed in some patients of the "acupuncture resistance phenomenon", which means that at the beginning of the acupuncture treatment period patients have a good response but when acupuncture continued, symptoms recur despite other new additional treatments added. In these cases, it is beneficial to temporarily stop acupuncture for around one or two weeks interval and then continue the sessions. This results in the return of the previous good effects.

Patients were followed up with telephone calls at one and three months after the conclusion of treatment by a research fellow. The follow-up data included the Wexner Constipation Score [47], stool consistency, awareness of defecatio and PAC-QOL (Patient Assessment of Constipation Quality of Life questionnaire) [48]. Follow-up time is important and prolongs the treatment session intervals after the regular sessions, since functionality after acupuncture may deteriorate with time. Prolonging the treatment interval to come to a gradual cessation is a way to obtain long-term efficacy. If symptoms recur, acupuncture is still effective.

4.8. Difference of effects

Acupuncture has bidirectional holistic and physiological limit modulation effects in treatment. Bidirectional modulation, namely, an unbalanced (hyperactive or hypoactive) pathophysiological state can be normalized by acupuncture based on the patient's individual physique; it is not a purely excitatory or suppression process [49]. Holistic modulation means acupuncture has multi-target and multi-system effects through meridians by adjusting the Yin and Yang [50]. Acupoints and meridians have specific roles to play in the human body. It is an option in treating complex pathological mechanism diseases such as chronic constipation. For example, the Stomach Meridian of Foot-Yangming and the Bladder Meridian of Foot Taiyang go through the abdomen and back, respectively; the effect will reach the meridian site in which chronic constipation pathological changes are mostly involved. Physiological limit modulation means regulation depends on the relevant organ structure's integrity and potential functional reserve. Symptoms are the patient's clinical manifestations of the disease, which generally has similar symptoms and pathology, but the same disease at different stages, or patients in different functional states, will exhibit the differences individually. Acupuncture protocol design should consider the difference may affect the treatment results, such as needle instruments; acupoints combination; treatment timing and course; reinforcement and reduction needling technique; electroacupuncture parameters; and patients' physiological, pathological, or psychological states, etc. Another concerning is how to design the control group. For acupuncture, the control method could be pseudo-acupuncture or no treatment. However, because of the nature of acupuncture, such methods are difficult to operate.

Acupuncture treatment for chronic constipation is explained by two theories, the traditional meridian theory and the modern nerve-electrophysiology theory. From the neuroanatomy point of view, human colonic function is dominated by the central nervous system (CNS), autonomic nervous system (ANS), and enteric nervous system (ENS). ANS innervation comes from C6 to T2 and S2 to S4 segments of the spinal cord and controls the gastrointestinal function. It has been suggested that acupuncture could influence the visceral sensory system by stimulating the somatic sensory system. A series of investigations undertaken on somatoautonomic reflexes have provided good evidence of the importance of cutaneous input in autonomic control of GI motility [34]. The ENS takes its input from the intestine's myenteric plexus and Cajal cells, while CNS involves the brain-gut axis. Stimulation of the corresponding points on the head (GV20 or EX-PN1) and back (BL23, BL25, and BL31–34, from the first to the fourth sacral foramen, respectively) and abdomen (ST25, SP14, SP15, CV4, and CV6) will modulate the intestinal function. It has been proven that stimulation of the sacral nerve can promote colonic motility, and improve pelvic floor sensation [17,51]. Brain imaging studies have demonstrated two potential routes of pain modulation by acupuncture via deactivation of descending nociceptive pathways and by decreased limbic activity during acupoint stimulation [52]. These neurophysiological findings [53,54] influenced our selection of acupoints for clinical study. In our research on 90 cases of chronic functional constipation, over 90% of patients have dysfunctional sleep. We found that the acupoint GV20 or EX-PN can improve insomnia quickly, and has an effect on bowel movement (unpublished data).

STC and IBS-C are subsets of constipation, the symptoms mainly localized in the colon. The former is due to colon motility weakness whereas the latter is due to gut hypersensitivity and spasms. Dyssynergic defecation and pelvic floor relaxation symptoms are localized in the rectum and pelvic floor. The pelvic floor is composed of muscles and ligaments that connect with three different compartments, including the bladder and urethra, vagina and uterus, and rectum and anus. All of these organs are controlled in the same central nervous system. Etiology of constipation from pelvic floor dysfunction is quite complicated, such as from behavioral or reflex loss etc. If it is not optimized by acupuncture, combination with other methods, such as moxibustion [55] and cupping [56], is recommended. Concerning the different dynamic mechanisms of constipation, the electroacupuncture parameters (frequency, waveform, and stimulation intensity) should be optioned rationally [57].

"Acupuncture resistance phenomenon" may be solved by postponing treatment sessions for one or two weeks if it occurs [58]. Related health education should be emphasized and offered as part of the treatment. When a patient has finished treatment in hospital, home training, acupoint pressure, and other remedies may prolong the short-term results. Jin's research [32] showed short-term efficacy rank in constipation subsets was: STC, IBS-C, and either dysynergic defecation or pelvic floor relaxation by acupuncture.

Chronic constipation is challenging in clinical practice. Patients may abuse laxatives, have insomnia, anorexia, and psychological issues, among other problems, and have a poorer quality of life than healthy people [32]. Acupuncture is a potential resource and form of treatment, when integrated into Western Medicine in diagnosis, and evidence-based medical treatment and research. It is appealing for research, and can be included into standard protocols to be carried out in multidisciplinary pelvic floor centers.

5. Multidisciplinary model implement

For patients' overlapping symptoms, as mentioned above, an effective pelvic floor multidisciplinary team (MDT) needs to be introduced for a comprehensive and efficient treatment. Our clinical experience has demonstrated the advantages of promoting acupuncture research in this context.

5.1. Organization

In a leading pelvic floor centre, a leader's interest and training in managing this group of patients who are challenging and demanding is the first step. Besides a pelvic floor physiologist, gastroenterologist, and a specialist nurse who undertakes diagnostic evaluation of pelvic floor abnormalities and optimizes conservative management, surgical input from the colorectal, urological, and gynaecological teams is essential. Psychologists, biofeedback rehabilitation experts, and a dedicated dietician are needed to give accurate advice to some long-term intractable patients. It is clear that those with complex issues often need a novel approach to managing the physical and psychological symptoms with appropriate experts. A well-trained acupuncturist is the key for successful treatment. The importance of the MDT cannot be overstated and it is the basis for a rigorous case presentation and discussion, consensus decision making, and mutual education. Multidisciplinary environments are places where individuals can be counselled and advised on diagnosis, treatment options, and realistic outcomes. For accurate assessment of ODS, a specialist in radiology of defecography, dynamic pelvic magnetic resonance imaging (MRI), or dynamic ultrasound for routine reporting of these studies, are also required.

Initially, the study can begin at a constipation specialist clinic, which reviews patients and refers some to the MDT, to discuss interesting or challenging cases and make decisions at a monthly meeting. Furthermore, many trainees are searching for comprehensive experience and this is rewarded by the presence of interested juniors and visitors, and is also essential for the research fellow's efforts in data collecting.

5.2. Questionnaires and database

The ability, and indeed the desire, to unearth underlying constipation pathology is dependent on carefully gathering a history, and putting simple and pertinent questions to the patient. For example, one must look deeper into why a 70-year-old woman presents with a sudden onset of constipation and haemorrhoidal symptoms. After ruling out cancer, questionnaires will unearth longstanding issues relating to bowel function that can be attributed to pelvic floor dysfunction. A systematic approach to history taking, particularly with the routine incorporation of a quality of life instrument, also lays the foundation for a system of structured prospective data collection and audit. Examples of a simple structured questionnaire are the Wexner constipation severity score. Clues to this may be found in bowel habits that have become excessive, with repeated visits to the toilet due to incomplete emptying, the requirement of assisting defecation by supporting the perineum or posterior vaginal wall, or the presence of post-defecatory soiling in the absence of significant urge incontinence. These are some key factors that suggest existing pelvic floor problems, frequently resulting from rectal intussusception or pelvic floor relaxation syndrome. Thus, a real potential cause of constipation can be found in these conditions. This relies on the standard history questionnaires being logically extended to standardized means of follow-up assessment, using quality of life instruments.

If, in the research stage, all data is collected by research fellows who do not participate in any aspect of patient care but are only responsible for data collection, then the result can be the collection of unbiased data. The data are then imported into a customized database which includes items about the patient's history, symptoms, investigations, treatment protocol, bowel diary, and follow-up data monitored by therapist and nurses. The doctor in charge is responsible for treatment protocols and management.

5.3. Efficacy evaluation methodology

There is little clinical consensus about the appropriateness of acupuncture in treating constipation. Many outcome measures were used to assess its effectiveness and there is as yet a lack of evidence as to which outcome measures are the most appropriate. Heterogeneous datapoints in research are: varying signs and symptoms; lack of use of a standardized constipation severity instrument (Wexner Constipation Scoring System [47]: with this system the increasing severity of constipation correlates to increased scores); lack of accordingly technique or protocol of different constipation subsets; treatment sessions and other interventions combined; research designs; and the efficacy perceptions of the patients and doctors.

Patient requested	STC		IBS-C		Dyssynergic Defecation		Pelvic Floor Relaxation	
	Pre-	Post-	Pre-	Post-	Pre-	Post-	Pre-	Post-
Days with spontaneous bowel movements	√√√	*****	√√	NS	√√√	**	-	-
Straining severity	-	-	√√√	****	√√	NS	√√√	**
Minutes per bowel movement	√√	NS	-	-	√√	NS	√√	NS
Incomplete evacuation sensation	√√	NS	√√	***	√√√	**	√√√	*
Stool consistency	√√	*****	√√√	****	√√	NS	√√	NS
Awareness of defecation	√√	NS	-	-	-	-	-	-
Bloating score	√√	***	√√	**	√√	NS	√√	NS

*Data from Nanjing Pelvic Floor Center: a 90 cases questionnaire research in 2007. Patients received the same acupuncture protocol and the endpoint was after 20 completed sessions.

STC: Slow transit constipation. IBS-C: Constipation-predominant Irritable Bowel Syndrome.

Pre-acupuncture treatment: √√√: means patient request most to release symptom rank over 50%. √√: means patient request most to release symptom rank over 30% and less than 50%. - : means not mentioned or less than 30% patients' choice..

Post-acupuncture treatment: *****,****,***,**,*: means rating the improved symptoms in the four subsets and itself before treatment respectively (*P<0.001*). NS:means no significance.

Table 3. Patients' chief complaint ranking of chronic functional constipation subsets (pre- and post-acupuncture treatment)

Besides those listed above, different efficacy evaluation objectives lead to inconsistencies in various research reporting. For example, to evaluate STARR in obstructed defecation syndrome, the primary responder endpoint collection is the obstructed defecation score (ODS) reduction ≥ 50% at one year, the secondary endpoint is PAC-QOL (Patient Assessment of Constipation Quality of Life questionnaire) and a continence grading scale. (The operation may result in faecal incontinence and this needs to be demonstrated [59]. The same efficacy evaluation parameters, however, are not suitable for acupuncture treatment.)

Thirdly, the Wexner Constipation Scoring System offers the total score of the main symptoms. Patients' chief complaints, however, frequently lie in the subsets, as our research has shown in Table 3. Thus different primary and secondary endpoint parameter weights vary if the Wexner CSS is used, resulting in some bias. Physiology and morphology test findings have a poor relation to the treatment results. Therefore, it is necessary to establish a symptom domain and score weight instrument for constipation subsets evaluation. This will facilitate assessing the results of the same regimen in different subsets, as well as different regimens in the same subset.

6. General effect criteria

Most of the trials reported an effective rate on a four-point scale [33], namely:

Clinical recovery, that is complete disappearance of the symptoms that the patients were most keen to resolve.

Marked improvement, where the symptoms that patients required most to be dealt with were alleviated by over two thirds as compared with the period before treatment.

General improvement, where the symptoms that patients required most to be dealt with were alleviated by one third, but less than two thirds as compared with pre-treatment.

No improvement, meaning the symptoms that patients required most to be dealt with were alleviated by less than one third as compared with pre-treatment.

Jin's clinical efficacy data on acupuncture in chronic functional constipation (n=90) showed [32], total efficacy was achieved in 61 cases (67.7%), of which three cases were a clinical recovery (3.3%), 10 cases showed marked improvement (11.1%), 48 cases showed general improvement (53.3%), and 29 cases showed no change (32.3%).

7. Patient-reported outcomes

For acupuncture, the merits are multiple factor modulations according to the patient's individual bodily constitution as defined by Chinese Medicine Theory. Evidence-based medicine requires blind, randomized controlled research data collecting, but this is controversial and inconsistent with methods in acupuncture. While patient-reported outcomes are measurements of any aspect of a patient's health status coming directly from the patient [60], such measurements may encourage clinicians to focus more on the patient as an entity rather than as an organ system [61]. For constipation patients, information collected using standardized questionnaires may facilitate detection of physical or psychological problems that might otherwise be overlooked. PRO measurement in clinical care may also be used to monitor outcomes as a strategy for quality improvement, or to reward presumed superior care [62]. Disease-specific Patient-Reported Outcomes questionnaire can be adopted for the efficacious assessment for the symptoms that patients required most to improve.

7.1. Seven specific symptoms score on constipation

Days with a spontaneous bowel movement: once every one or two days: Score = 0; once every three or four days: Score = 1; once every five or six days: Score = 2 ; once in a period longer than six days: Score = 3; inability of natural defecation without the aid of a drug, manipulation, or an enema: Score = 4. Patients recorded the bowel movements (yes/no) during the treatment period. The responses were divided into three time periods, to reflect the progress of treatment, and the days with bowel movements were calculated for each week of treatment.

Straining severity: without strain: Score = 0; defecation with a little effort: Score = 1; defecation with great effort: Score = 2; difficult defecation and need of assistance: Score = 3.

Minutes per bowel movement: 1–10 min: Score = 0; 11–20 min: Score = 1; over 20 min: Score = 2.

Incomplete evacuation sensation: no sense: Score = 0; mild sense: Score = 1; obvious sense: Score = 2; intolerable sense: Score = 3.

Stool consistency: like a sausage, smooth and soft: Score = 0; like a sausage, with cracks or soft: Score = 1; hard piece: Score = 2; separate hard lumps: Score = 3.

Symptoms	Pre-treatment	Post-treatment
Days with spontaneous bowel movement	2.19±1.76	0.87±1.43*
Straining severity	2.39±0.83	1.30±1.04*
Minutes per bowel movement	1.41±0.82	0.69±0.78*
Incomplete evacuation sensation	1.62±0.76	0.92±0.76*
Stool consistency	1.84±1.04	0.54±0.74*
Awareness of defecation	0.34±0.48	0.02±0.15*
Bloating score	2.15±0.39	0.87±0.32*

* Symptoms' score reduced after acupuncture treatment (All P value <0.01).

Table 4. Seven specific symptoms' scores on constipation in acupuncture (Score)

Awareness of defecation:: Patients recorded an urge to defecate as either "yes" or "no" each day during the treatment period. Having the sense: Score = 0; no sense: Score = 1.

Bloating score: Patients were asked to assess the subjective degree of bloating according to the following scale: no bloating: Score = 0; mild bloating: Score = 1; moderate bloating: Score = 2; severe bloating: Score = 3. The responses were divided into three time periods, to reflect the progress of the treatment's effect, and the mean bloating score was calculated for each week of treatment.

In a 90 case study [32] of the Nanjing Pelvic Floor Center, seven symptoms' scores reduced after acupuncture, as shown in Table 4.

7.2. Patient Assessment of Constipation Quality of Life Questionnaire (PAC-QOL)

The PAC-QOL is a brief but comprehensive assessment of the burden of constipation on patients' everyday functioning and well-being. Multinational studies have demonstrated that the PAC-QOL is internally consistent, reproducible, valid, and responsive to improvements over time [63]. Its assessment includes four subcategories: worries/concerns, physical discomfort, psychosocial discomfort, and satisfaction. There are 28 items, which are classified into five grades from a mild degree to a severe one, corresponding to scores of 1–5 point, respectively. The total score is 117, and the higher the score the worse the quality of life [48]. It has also been translated into Chinese and validated by the author [64]. The questionnaires were administered before and after treatment follow-up. All of the questionnaires were completed by patients during the study period.

It is preferred at our centre, that a specific symptom questionnaire on constipation subsets efficacy assessment — which usually includes symptoms such as frequency of spontaneous bowel movements, straining severity, minutes per bowel movement, incomplete evacuation sensation, stool consistency, awareness of defecation, and quality of life — is conducted using a PAC-QOL, both before and after treatment.

Groups		Physical	Psychosocial	Worries	Satisfaction	Total
Control (n=90)		5.92±2.41	13.04±5.84	15.86±1.03	8.10±0.57	42.92±17.72
STC(n=20)	Pre-	14.36±3.0#	20.93±8.27*	39.07±3.12#	16.50±1.77#	90.86±6.70#
	Post-	9.00±3.46*	13.43±3.31	24.00±8.41*	11.29±2.36	57.71±15.00*
IBS-C(n=16)	Pre-	11.88±2.90#	17.63±6.99#	28.75±3.48#	16.38±1.36#	74.63±6.61#
	Post-	7.67±2.42*	12.50±4.32	18.00±4.05*	11.17±5.27	49.33±8.71*
Dyssynergic Defecation (n=30)	Pre-	11.96±3.01#	18.54±5.70#	34.54±1.73#	17.13±0.95#	82.17±3.57#
	Post-	10.64±3.25	16.29±5.06*	29.21±10.42*	12.79±4.25*	68.93±16.96*
Pelvic Floor Relaxation (n=24)	Pre-	12.44±3.11#	15.94±2.12	32.33±3.72#	16.59±1.07#	73.53±5.50#
	Post-	9.20±3.67*	13.07±5.161	23.47±8.07*	12.87±3.72*	58.60±4.25*

#: Constipation four subsets PAC-QOL pre-acupuncture treatment vs. normal control (90 healthy adults matched the year and gender of the constipation subsets group), P<0.01

*: Constipation four subsets PAC-QOL pre- and post-acupuncture treatment, P<0.05.

Table 5. Chronic functional constipation PAC-QOL Score (pre- and post-treatment vs. normal control)

Although the total score showed improvement, compared with the normal control group, it was still high and it was difficult to return patients to normal functioning. Glia use PGWB (the Psychological General Well-Being) and GSRS (the Gastrointestinal Symptom Rating Scale) to evaluate the QOL of 102 constipation patients (mean score: 85.5 vs. 102.9), the result of which is similar to our research [65].

7.3. Chronic Constipation PRO Rating Scale (CC-PRO)

Although PAC-QOL is a well-used patient reported outcome questionnaire in constipation efficacy evaluation, it is still insufficient in revealing the advantages and quality of life of acupuncture treatment as the Chinese cultural background difference.

Chronic Constipation PRO Rating Scale (CC-PRO) was designed by our centre's research team [66], following the PRO guideline frame from FDA [60], in order to establish a comprehensive index system combining symptoms and syndromes from Chinese Medicine theory. The implementation process included establishing a theoretical model of the questionnaire from four domains: physiological aspects (specific symptoms of chronic constipation and effectiveness index of syndrome), psychological aspects, social function aspects, and patients' satisfaction. We collected popular expressions on chronic constipation from searching the Chinese language literature; interviewing patients with different educational levels, genders, and ages; and establishing a 96 items pool of the draft questionnaire. After two rounds of screening the items from physicians and patients, the questionnaire reduced to 45 items in four domains, which included physiological aspects was 29 items, psychological aspects was 9 items, social function aspects was 3 items and patient's satisfaction aspect was 4 items accordingly. After a multicentral trial enrolling 521 chronic constipation patients and 76 healthy adults as a control, and completion of the questionnaire, its reliability, validity and responsibility were tested, and the four-level rating scale was determined as: slightly poor (88<total score≤121), poor (121<total score≤160), very poor (160<total score≤199), and quite poor (total score>199), which compared to the normal (total score≤88), For now, only the Chinese version is updated, and further application of acupuncture before and after treatment is on the way [67].

8. Conclusion

Laxative abuse can cause damage to the intestinal structure, damage function, and aggravate constipation, whereas acupuncture is a safe and a non-toxic choice with no side-effects. Biofeedback therapy is a form of behavioural management and is the first line of therapy for obstructive defecation syndrome patients. Candidates need much cognition and compliance to participate in a relatively long-term training programme to reset physical reflexes. Acupuncture demands little from the patients but can achieve a fairly quick response if applied appropriately. Compared to herbal medicine, acupuncture is not only a physical stimulation for the body but a face-to-face doctor-patient communication process, which involves the role of psychological counselling in daily treatment. Acupuncture itself can also improve mental and sleeping disorders through neural regulation.

Acupuncture should not be perceived as just a needling technique depending on the individual's needs; other therapies integrated in a timely fashion can also improve efficacy because the capacity of a human body to self-adjust and repair has certain limits. For those long-term and complicated patients facing a plateau in their condition, when only acupuncture has limitation in modulation, other remedies can compensate and fully arouse the body's potential regulation system.

Optimized protocols with different acupuncture techniques, integrated to accommodate different subsets of chronic constipation, to meet the patients' characters and best indications is the best practice we need. From our clinical experience, if the patient does not respond to acupuncture, then with biofeedback, electrical stimulation, herb medicine, or moxibustion maybe still have desired effects. However, if one of the therapies is partially successful in integrating, others may shorten the working threshold time and enhance efficacy. Whether or not to integrate acupuncture for long-term efficacy is still pending further study.

Optimizing the best indication, choosing the acupoints, manipulating (needling technique, depth of insertion, electroacupuncture etc), and investigating the mechanism of action are required works later. Enthusiasm for research is growing, and collaboration in a multidisciplinary group will speed up this development. In the near future, the efficacy of modern acupuncture treatment protocols based on Patient-Reported Outcomes can treat not only chronic constipation but be extended to other functional gastrointestinal disorders, such as faecal incontinence, functional pelvic pain, and others.

Acknowledgements

I extend my sincere gratitude to Dr. Zutshi Massarat from Cleveland Clinic Ohio of United States for reviewing this article.

Supported by China Jiangsu Province Chinese Medicines Bureau Research Funding, from project " Standardization acupuncture protocol of slow transit constipation: a multi-center prospective study",NO.LZ13104

Author details

Shuqing Ding[1*], Xun Jin[2], Yijiang Ding[2], Lingling Wang[1] and Huifeng Zhou[1]

*Address all correspondence to: njgczx@gmail.com

1 3rd Affiliated Hospital of Nanjing University of Chinese Medicine, Pelvic Floor Center, Nanjing, China

2 Nanjing University of Chinese Medicine, Acupuncture and Moxibustion School, Nanjing, China

References

[1] Higgins PD, Johanson JF. Epidemiology of constipation in North America: a systematic review. Am J Gastroenterol 2004; 99(4) 750–759.

[2] Guo XF, Ke MY, Pan GZ, et al. Beijing area adults chronic constipation whole group, stratified, random epidemiological investigations and related factors. Chinese Journal of Digestion 2002; 22 (10) 637–638.

[3] Yu PL, Li ZJ, Zheng H, et al. Preliminary analysis of epidemiological characteristics of elderly constipation patients. Chinese Journal of Geriatrics 2001; 20 (2) 132–134.

[4] Cai YQ, Wang HJ, Zhang X, et al. Prevalence of constipation in the elderly and its relationship with the sub-health symptoms investigation in Nanjing of China (Chin). Chinese Journal of Geriatrics 2004; 4 (23) 267–269.

[5] Hagiwara, N, Tomita R. Pathophysiology of chronic constipation of the slow transit type from the aspect of the type of rectal movements. Hepatogastroenterology 2008; 55 (85) 1298–1303.

[6] Drossman, DA. The functional gastrointestinal disorders and the Rome III process. Gastroenterology 2006; 130 (5) 1377–1390.

[7] Schiller LR, Dennis E, Toth G. An internet-based survey of the prevalence and symptom spectrum of chronic constipation. Am J Gastroenterol 2004; 99(10) S234.

[8] Nam YS, Pikarsky AJ, Wexner SD, et al. Reproducibility of colonic transit study in patients with chronic constipation. Dis Colon Rectum 2001; 44 (1) 86–92.

[9] Wattchow D, Brookes S, Murphy E, et al. Regional variation in the neurochemical coding of the myenteric plexus of the human colon and changes in patients with slow transit constipation. Neurogastroenterol Motil 2008; 20 (12) 1298–1305.

[10] Bassotti G, Villanacci V. Slow transit constipation: a functional disorder becomes an enteric neuropathy. World J Gastroenterol 2006; 12 (29) 4609–4613.

[11] Ding YJ, Ha NL, Ding SQ, et al. Synapse substance P and vasoactive intestinal peptide findings in slow transit constipation (Chin). Chinese Journal of Gastrointestinal Surgery 2005; 7 (6) 485–487.

[12] Ding SQ, Ding YJ, Ji XT, et al. Effect of acupuncture on PGP9.5 expression in rat model of constipation (Chin). World Journal of Gastroenterology 2009; 17 (21) 2184–2187.

[13] Arhan P, Devroede G, Jehannin B, et al. Segmental colonic transit time. Dis Colon Rectum 1981; 24 (8) 625–629.

[14] Bouchoucha M, Devroede G, Arhan P, et al. What is the meaning of colorectal transit time measurement?. Diseases of the Colon and Rectum 1992, 35(8): 773–782.

[15] Rao SSC, Camilleri M, Hasler WL, et al. Evaluation of gastrointestinal transit in clinical practice: position paper of the American and European Neurogastroenterology and Motility Societies. Neurogastroenterology and Motility 2011, 23 (1): 8–23.

[16] King SK, Sutcliffe JR, Southwell BR, et al. The antegrade continence enema successfully treats idiopathic slow-transit constipation. J Pediatr Surg 2005; 40 (12) 1935–1940.

[17] Dinning PG, Fuentealba SE, Kennedy ML, et al. Sacral nerve stimulation induces pan-colonic propagating pressure waves and increases defecation frequency in patients with slow-transit constipation. Colorectal Dis 2007; 9 (2) 123–132.

[18] Zutshi M, Hull TL, Trzcinski R, et al. Surgery for slow transit constipation: are we helping patients? Int J Colorectal Dis 2007; 22 (3) 265–269.

[19] FitzHarris GP, Garcia-Aguilar J, Parker SC, et al. Quality of life after subtotal colectomy for slow-transit constipation: both quality and quantity count. Dis Colon Rectum 2003; 46 (4) 433–440.

[20] Tuteja AK, Talley NJ, Joos SK, et al. Is constipation associated with decreased physical activity in normally active subjects? Am J Gastroenterol 2005; 100 (1) 124–129.

[21] Gorissen KJ, Gosselink MP. Obstructed Defecation Syndrome: Pelvic Floor Disorders: Surgical Approach. Springer Milan, 2014; 95–102.

[22] Rao SSC, Tuteja AK, Vellema T, et al. Dyssynergic defecation: demographics, symptoms, stool patterns, and quality of life. J Clin Gastroenterol 2004; 38 (8) 680–685.

[23] Law YM, Fielding JR. MRI of pelvic floor dysfunction: review. American Journal of Roentgenology 2008, 191(6_supplement): S45–S53.

[24] Andromanakos N, Skandalakis P, Troupis T, et al. Constipation of anorectal outlet obstruction: pathophysiology, evaluation and management. J Gastroenterol Hepatol 2006; 21 (4) 638–646.

[25] Heymen S, Jones KR, Scarlett Y, et al. Biofeedback treatment of constipation. Dis Colon Rectum 2003; 46 (9) 1208–1217.

[26] Schwandner O, Stuto A, Jayne D, et al. Decision-making algorithm for the STARR procedure in obstructed defecation syndrome: position statement of the group of STARR Pioneers. Surg Innov 2008; 15 (2) 105–109.

[27] Corman ML, Carriero A, Hager T, et al. Consensus conference on the stapled transanal rectal resection (STARR) for disordered defaecation. Colorectal Disease 2006; 8 (2) 98–101.

[28] Collinson R, Wijffels N, Cunningham C, et al. Laparoscopic ventral rectopexy for internal rectal prolapse: short-term functional results. Colorectal Dis 2010; 12 (2) 97–104.

[29] Ortiz H, de Miguel M, Rinaldi M, et al. Functional outcome of sacral nerve stimulation in patients with severe constipation. Dis Colon Rectum 2012; 55 (8) 876–880.

[30] Pescatori M, Boffi F, Russo A, et al. Complications and recurrence after excision of rectal internal mucosal prolapse for obstructed defaecation. Int J Colorectal Dis 2006; 21 (2) 160–165.

[31] Wald A. Constipation in the primary care setting: current concepts and misconceptions. Am J Med 2006; 119 (9) 736–739.

[32] Jin X, Ding YJ, Wang LL, et al. Efficacy of acupuncture in chronic functional constipation. World Journal of Acupuncture-Moxibustion. 2011; 21 (1) 18–24.

[33] Lin L W, Fu YT, Dunning T, et al. Efficacy of traditional Chinese medicine for the management of constipation: a systematic review. J Altern Complement Med 2009; 15 (12) 1335–1346.

[34] Takahashi T. Acupuncture for functional gastrointestinal disorders. J Gastroenterol 2006; 41(5) 408–417.

[35] Kaptchuk TJ. Acupuncture: theory, efficacy, and practice. Ann Intern Med 2002; 136 (5) 374–383.

[36] Eskinazi DP, Jobst KA National Institutes of Health Office of Alternative Medicine-Food and Drug Administration Workshop on Acupuncture. J Altern Complement Med 1996; 2 (1) 3–6.

[37] Lao L, Schyner RN. Society for Acupuncture Research 2007 Conference "The Status and Future of Acupuncture Research: 10 Years Post-NIH Consensus Conference", Baltimore, MD. J Altern Complement Med 2008; 4 (7) 857.

[38] Liu LG. Browse of Acupuncture-Moxibustion Books on Intractable Disease (Chin). Shanghai: Shanghai Scientific and Technical Publishers; 2007: 95–110.

[39] Du YH, Li GP, Lin X, Li J. Research on disease menu of acupuncture and moxibustion therapy in digestive-system. J Clin Acup-Mox (Chin) 2006; 22 (3): 1–3.

[40] Li ZR. Experimental Acupuncture and Moxibustion (Chin). Beijing: China Press of Traditional Chinese Medicine; 2003: 117.

[41] Wexner SD, Duthie GS. Constipation. Second edition, Oxford: Butterworth-Heinemann; 2006:16–22.

[42] Zhou HF, Ding SQ, Ding YJ et al. Eight liao acupoints (sacral foramen) positioning, measurement and point selection methodology research. Chin Acup-Mox (Chin) 2013; 33 (8) 703–707.

[43] Cao DY, Niu HZ, Zhao Y, Du JQ. Stimulation of acupoint induces release of substance P through primary afferent reflex. Chin Acup-Mox (Chin) 2001; 21 (10): 623–625.

[44] Nehra V, Bruce BK, Rath-Harvey DM, Pemberton JH, Camilleri M. Psychological disorders in patients with evacuation disorders and constipation in a tertiary practice. Am J Gastroenterol, 2000; 95 (7) 1755–1758.

[45] Zhang YL. Interactions between enteric nervous system and immune system. Foreign Med: Scisurgery (Chin) 2004; 31(4):196–198.

[46] Zhang JB, Wang LL, Lü M, Liu LY, Li D. Effects of acupuncture on serotonin and norepinephrine in hippocampus of depressed model rats. J Chin Med Res (Chin) 2006; 6 (8): 844–846.

[47] Agachan F, Chen T, Pfeifer J, et al. A constipation scoring system to simplify evaluation and management of constipated patients. Dis Colon Rectum 1996; 39 (6) 681–685.

[48] Marquis P, De La Loge C, Dubois D, et al. Development and validation of the Patient Assessment of Constipation Quality of Life questionnaire. Scand J Gastroenterol. 2005; 40 (5) 540–551.

[49] Cho ZH, Hwang SC, Wong EK, et al. Neural substrates, experimental evidences and functional hypothesis of acupuncture mechanisms. Acta Neurologica Scandinavica, 2006; 113 (6) 370–377.

[50] Han JS. Opioid and antiopioid peptides: a model of Yin-Yang balance in acupuncture mechanisms of pain modulation [M]. Clinical Acupuncture. Springer Berlin Heidelberg, 2001: 51–68.

[51] Yuan R, Lin Y. Traditional Chinese medicine: an approach to scientific proof and clinical validation. Pharmacol Ther 2000; 86 (2) 191–198.

[52] Wu MT, Hsieh JC, Xiong J, et al. Central Nervous Pathway for Acupuncture Stimulation: Localization of Processing with Functional MR Imaging of the Brain — Preliminary Experience 1. Radiology 1999; 212 (1) 133–141.

[53] Shen EY, Chen FJ, Chen YY, et al. Locating the acupoint Baihui (GV20) beneath the cerebral cortex with MRI reconstructed 3D neuroimages. Evid Based Complement Alternat Med, 2011.

[54] Kalavapalli R, Singareddy R. Role of acupuncture in the treatment of insomnia: a comprehensive review. Complement Ther Clin Pract, 2007; 13 (3) 184–193.

[55] Wang LJ, Wang LL. Randomized controlled study on chronic functional constipation treated with grain-shaped moxibustion and acupuncture. Zhongguo zhen jiu. Chinese acupuncture and moxibustion (Chin) 2011; 31 (4) 320–324.

[56] Jiang ZY, Li CD, Li JC, et al. Clinical observation on moving cupping therapy combined with moxibustion for treatment of senile habitual constipation. Zhongguo zhen jiu. Chinese acupuncture and moxibustion (Chin), 2005, 25 (12): 853–854.

[57] Zhou HF, Ding SQ, Ding YJ, et al. Observation on effect characteristics of electroacupuncture for different types of functional constipation. Zhongguo zhen jiu. Chinese acupuncture and moxibustion (Chin), 2014; 34 (5) 435–438.

[58] Jin GY. Clinical Acupuncture Reflexology (Chin). Beijing: Beijing Science and Technology Press; 2004: 124.

[59] Schwandner O, Fürst A, German STARR Registry Study Group. Assessing the safety, effectiveness, and quality of life after the STARR procedure for obstructed defeca-

tion: results of the German STARR registry. Langenbecks Arch Surg, 2010; 395 (5) 505–513.

[60] U.S. Department of Health and Human Services FDA Center for Drug Evaluation and Research. Guidance for industry: patient-reported outcome measures: use in medical product development to support labeling claims: draft guidance. Health Qual Life Outcomes 2006; 4: 79.

[61] Fung CH, Hays RD. Prospects and challenges in using patient-reported outcomes in clinical practice. Qual Life Res 2008; 17 (10) 1297–1302.

[62] Valderas JM, Kotzeva A, Espallargues M, et al. The impact of measuring patient-reported outcomes in clinical practice: a systematic review of the literature. Qual Life Res 2008; 17 (2) 179–193.

[63] Wald A, Burgio K, Holeva K, et al. Psychological evaluation of patients with severe idiopathic constipation: which instrument to use. Am J Gastroenterol, 1992; 87 (8) 977–980.

[64] Jin X, Ding YJ, Ding SQ, et al. Patient Assessment of Constipation Quality of Life questionnaire (PAC-QOL): Chinese version of the reliability validity and reactivity. World Journal of Gastroenterology (Chin), 2011; 19 (2) 209–213.

[65] Glia A, Lindberg G. Quality of life in patients with different types of functional constipation. Scand J Gastroenterol 1997; 32 (11) 1083–1089.

[66] Jin X, Ding YJ, Ding SQ, et al. Construction and screening of the item pool for the Patient-Reported Outcome of Chronic Constipation rating scale. World Journal of Gastroenterology (Chin) 2012; 20 (29) 2855–2859.

[67] Jin X, Ding SQ, Ding YJ, et al. Validation and score meaning of the Patient-Reported Outcome of Chronic Constipation rating scale. World Journal of Gastroenterology (Chin) 2013; 14 1360–1365.

Chapter 3

Patients Suffering from Intractable Diseases Treated Effectively with Medicines of Kampo and TCM

Yasuyo Hijikata

Additional information is available at the end of the chapter

http://dx.doi.org/10.5772/60573

Abstract

There are diseases that cannot be cured by conventional therapies.

In Japan, more than 90% of medical practitioners treat patients with alternative medicines such as Kampo medicine (herbal medicine based on Japanese Kampo theory) or traditional Chinese medicine (TCM) that do not respond to conventional treatments.

The author also treated these patients suffering from cardiovascular diseases, vasculitis diseases, nephrosis, hyperlipidemia, and female disorders including menstruation disorders, incurable pain diseases such as glossodynia and herpes zoster or herpes virus infectious diseases, and other diseases such as female-related ones and diseases that need five-face theory to cure and the administration of gui-zhi-fu-ling-wan (桂枝茯苓丸) before aspiration biopsy, in breast cancer patient, to raise the detection rate of cancer cells.

Interestingly, diseases specified as "intractable diseases" by the Japanese Ministry of Health, Labor, and Welfare sometimes respond to TCM treatment quite successfully, probably because TCM and Kampo medicine systems have their own theories and their own medicines quite different from that of conventional therapies.

Finally, I often experienced plural number of prescriptions for the problematic organs (based on five element theory) administered simultaneously often lead to dramatical improvement. This will mean problematic organs treated simultaneously will lead to quick recovery through synergistic actions among organs. The successfully treated clinical courses after the administration of TCM or Kampo medicines are described here.

Keywords: Alternative medicines, Kampo medicine, Traditional Chinese medicine (TCM), Intractable diseases, Synergistic action

1. Introduction

There exist diseases that cannot be cured by conventional therapies.

In Japan, more than 90% of medical practitioners treat patients with Kampo medicine (herbal medicine based on Japanese Kampo theory) or traditional Chinese medicine (TCM) that do not respond to conventional treatments.

Furthermore, about 80% of universities with medical departments have sections that deal specifically with Kampo medicine.

Many Japanese doctors use Kampo medicines, because of the existence of patients who are not successfully cured after trying all possible conventional therapies

I have been engaged in TCM treatment for more than 35 years, and I have used Kampo medicines or herbs selected based on TCM principles in patients who do not respond to conventional therapies including those who suffer terrible side effects with conventional medicines or cannot take them, for other reasons.

Interestingly, diseases specified as "incurable" by the Japanese Ministry of Health, Labor and Welfare, often respond to TCM treatment quite successfully.

TCM and Kampo medicine are treatment systems that have their own theories and their own medicines which consist of natural remedies.

These systems can be used as complementary or alternative therapy for conventional therapies.

In this chapter, I will introduce clinical courses after the administration of TCM or Kampo medicines, in cases of cardiovascular diseases, vasculitis diseases, nephrosis, hyperlipidemia and female disorders including menstruation disorders, incurable pain diseases such as glossodynia (burning mouth syndrome) and herpes zoster or herpes virus infectious diseases and other female-related diseases, and diseases that need five-face theory to cure.

Finally, by the administration of gui-zhi-fu-ling-wan (桂枝茯苓丸) before aspiration biopsy, in breast cancer patient, the detection rate of cancer cells was found to increase. Hereafter, the name of organ starting with capital letter means organ in TCM. The terminology of TCM is mainly based on WHO International Standard Terminologies on Traditional Medicine in the western Pacific region.

2. Cardiovascular disease

Case 1: 72-year-old Japanese female diagnosed with hypertrophic cardiomyopathy.

Main Complaint: Difficulty in breathing when walking

Past History: Tuberculous hilar lymphadenitis during childhood caused the patient one year off school. At age 39, her right ovary cystoma was resected.

Present Illness: Since the patient turned 40-years-old, she had suffered sudden difficulty in breathing and beating. Since she was 52-years-old, she easily got edema on the frontal part of her lower limbs and was diagnosed with hypertrophic cardiomyopathy. She had been taking drugs for hypertension. Menopause started at 45-years-old. She has been taking sleeping drug because of insomnia and excessive dreaming during sleep.

Her feet got chilly and cramped easily and often had to urinate in the night. She felt dizzy on standing up and easily got purple spots. The sole of her feet felt hot.

Present States: The patient was 161cm tall and weighed 51kg. Her pulse was 72 beats/min and was strong, slippery, string-like, both left and right chi-mai (尺脈) were somewhat weak, the tongue body was red, without fur, but with somewhat swollen sublingual collateral vessels, and her blood pressure (BP) was 150/76 mmHg.

Identification: Deficiency of Heart and Kidney·Blood stagnation with water flood·Heart deficiency with Lung collapse [1].

Treatment: Tonify Heart and Kidney and warm Lung. Activate blood to remove stasis. Promote diuresis, promote Yang circulation.

Prescription: Decoction of modified combinations of Zhi-gan-cao-tang (炙甘草湯), Guan-Xin-er-hao-fang (冠心二号方) and Ba-wei-di-huang-wan (八味地黄丸): Zhi-gan-cao-tang (30g) added with chuan-xiong (川芎)2, jiang-xian (降香)2, dan-shen (丹参)3, hong-hua (紅花)1.5, dang-gui (当帰)3, chai-hu (柴胡)2, pao-fu-zi (炮附子)1, fu-ling (茯苓)3, shan-zhu-yu (山茱萸)3, mu-dan-pi (牡丹皮)3, huang-qi (黄耆)3, chen-pi (陳皮)2 (numerals mean g/day).

Assessment: I created a scale to difficulty in breathing. 0: not effective; 1: slightly effective, 2: effective, 3: quite effective, 4: very effective.

The patient began treatment at level 0.

Clinical course: The patient first visited me on January 29, X year. She started to take the full dose of the above medicines each day.

X year, February 24: She had improved to breathing score 0 to 1 when walking. From this day, her intake was decreased to 0.5 of the initial volume. On April 2, her score was 2. From this day on, she took 0.4 of the initial volume. By June 17, her breathing had improved to score 3. And her dosage changed to 0.3 of the initial volume.

This improved situation (Score 3) had continued for more than 4 years at the time of writing except when patient worked too hard, or does not get enough sleep.

Discussion: The patient's difficulty in breathing and palpitation when walking due to the Heart yang deficiency improved significantly by taking the prescription mentioned earlier.

Under the TCM theory, Zhi-gan-cao-tang (炙甘草湯) would not only tonify Heart yin and yang but also tonify the Lung qi and yin. Ba-wei-di-huang- wan (八味地黄丸) tonifies Kidney yin and yang and also supports the Lung through engendering route between Kidney and Lung. Additionally, Guan-xin-er-hao-fang (冠心二号方) removes blood stagnation and restores blood circulation. These formulas work synergistically to produce good overall condition. Guan-xin-er-hao-fang is composed of chi-shao-yao (赤芍薬)5, chuan-xion (川芎)5, hong-hua (紅花)4, dan-shen (丹参)5, and Jiang-xian (降香) 4g/day. This formula was first reported at zhon-guo-yi-xue-ke-xue-yuan.

Conclusion: For 72-year-old Japanese female with hypertrophic cardio- myopathy, modified combinations of Zhi-gan-cao-tang (炙甘草湯), Guan-xin- er-hao fang (冠心二号方), and Ba-wei-di-huang-wan (八味地黄丸) have been very effective.

Case 2: A 53-year-old Japanese male. 167cm tall, weighing 54kg

Main Complaint: Dyspnea and palpitations

Past History: The patient suffered from a stomach ulcer at age 43. At this point he gave up cigarette and alcohol. He also suffered from irregular pulse and tachycardia.

Present Illness: The patient's first visit to our clinic was on June 4, 1986. Beginning in the middle of the preceding April, he often suffered dyspnea to the extent that he was unable to breathe for 8 seconds at a time; he also experienced tachycardia (160/min). Although he underwent a heart examination at the Red Cross Hospital including angiography, all results proved to be within normal limits. Because he suffered nettle rash as a side effect of certain injections, the medical doctor in charge denied him any prescription.

Due to the condition of his health, he was unable to play his favorite game, golf, and therefore wished to try herbal therapy.

The patient had little energy and his limbs felt cold. He liked to take hot things, and hated cold things.

Present States: The patient has a fair complexion. His pulse (72/min) is sunken and weak. BP was 120/76 mmHg.

Identification: Deficiency of Heart qi.

Treatment: Tonify Heart qi and yin.

Prescription: Zhi-gan-cao-tang (炙甘草湯): Zhi-gan-cao (炙甘草)3, dried sheng-jiang (乾生姜)1, Gui-zhi (桂枝)3, Ma-zi-ren (麻子仁)3, Da-zao (大棗)3, Ren-shen (人参)3, Di-huang (地黄)6, Mai-men-dong (麦門冬)6, E-jiao (阿膠) 2 numerals g/day.

Clinical Course: By June 17, 1986, the patient's dyspnea had improved and palpitations had decreased remarkably. By July 16, 1986, his dyspnea and palpitation disappeared. He continued taking this precription to prevent recurrence.

But gradually he decreased his intake to half of the initial volume in August, 2006. He wrote a letter of thanks to me saying that he was able to lead a happy life and play golf three times/month without any trouble and that he would take this medicine throughout his life. His last request for this prescription was on September 8, 2006 (73-year-old).

Conclusion: For one 53-year-old Japanese male with incurable dyspnea and palpitation, Zhi-gan-cao-tang (炙甘草湯) worked remarkably.

3. Immune system, connective tissue and joint-related diseases including Churg–Strauss syndrome and Henoch–Shönlein-purpura

3.1. Introduction

Kampo medicines improved blood test results and the quality of life (QOL) in two cases of vasculitis cases. One with Churg–Strauss-syndrome (CSS) and with Henoch–Shönlein-purpura (HSP), after inadequate treatment with conventional therapies

3.2. Summary

Objective: Two vasculitis syndrome patients, one with CSS (Case 1) and one with HSP (Case 2) exhibited persistent symptoms and abnormal blood tests after treatment with conventional therapies.

To improve their situation, based on the tenets of traditional Chinese medicine (TCM) theory, herbal medicines were applied.

Methods: Both cases were diagnosed with "blood stagnation" [1] and "dampness and heat" [2, 5, 6] and Case 1 had a "yang deficiency" [3]. Following TCM theory, we applied selected Kampo medicines.

Results: In Case 1, the patient presented with hypereosinophilia, venous thrombosis, pulmonary infarction, a decreased platelet count, ulnar nerve palsy and Raynaud's phenomenon, which led to a diminished QOL. After starting the Kampo medicines, the patient improved quickly and recovered within 11 months. In Case 2, persistent purpura, abdominal pain, and bloody feces quickly improved and disappeared after Kampo medicine treatment. Prednisolone was stopped at 21 days after starting the Kampo medicines and there has been no sign of relapse to date.

Conclusion: Kampo medicines helped clear the persistent abnormal symptoms and improve laboratory findings of two vasculitis syndromes, Churg–Strauss syndrome (CSS) and Henoch–Shonlein purpura (HSP), which had responded inadequately to the conventional therapies administered.

3.3. Introduction

Churg–Strauss Syndrome (CSS) and Henoch–Sholein purpura (HSP) are classified as vasculitis syndromes, in which inflammation and blood vessel damage are common and may lead to various pathologies. CSS is rare, and necrotizing vasculitis involves small-and medium-sized arteries, capillaries, veins, and venules. The histopathological features of CSS are granulomatous reactions in the various tissues of any organ in the body, but lung involvement is predominant, with manifestations in the skin, cardiovascular system, kidney and peripheral nervous system, and also occasionally the gastro- intestinal tract. Although its pathogenesis is uncertain, it has a strong association with asthma, eosinophilia, granuloma and vasculitis.

HSP is usually seen in children, and is characterized by palpable purpura, arthralgia, gastro-intestinal signs and glomerulonephritis. It is a small-vessel vasculitis. The pathogenic mechanism is presumed to be immune-complex deposition. A skin biopsy specimen is useful to confirm leuko-cytoclastic vasculitis with IgA and C3 deposition by immune-fluorescence.

These diseases usually exhibit a good response to corticosteroid hormones. However, some patients do not completely recover and suffer from an incomplete remission state with degraded QOL.

The present CSS case improved to some degree with conventional therapies in a university hospital at the acute stage, but at the chronic stage he continued to exhibit hypereosinophilia, venous thrombosis, pulmonary infarction, decreased platelet count and Raynaud's phenomenon. The patient with HSP showed improvement primarily with steroidal hormones. However, his condition worsened soon after a tapering down of the prednisolone.

From the standpoint of TCM theory, we diagnosed the pathogenesis of these diseases as being related to "static blood" [1] and in vasculitis, as related to "dampness-heat" [2, 5, 6], primarily in the morbid vessels, and also, in Case 1, a yang deficiency (coldness of the fingers and limbs and/or sensitive to coldness) [3].

Case 1: A 13-year-old-boy with CSS

Main Complaints: Hypereosinophilia, left femoral venous thrombosis, pulmonary infarction, decreased platelet count, Raynaud's phenomenon, ulnar nerve palsy

Past History: For three years prior to his admission to the university hospital, the patient suffered from malaise, petechiae, purpura and allergic rhinitis. Hay fever also began from last year.

Present Illness: For 3 years prior to admission, main complaint started and also experienced pain with edema of the legs after extended walking, despite conventional therapies. He was diagnosed with CSS with hypereosinophilia, vasculitis with extravascular eosinophil accumulation, diffuse pulmonary infiltrate, and ulnar nerve palsy.

He also had left femoral deep venous thrombosis and pulmonary infarction. On the 5th day after hospitalization for suspected pneumonia with septic shock, he received pulse doses of methyl-prednisolone and gabexate mesilate. Following this treatment, his fever, chest pain, and diffuse pulmonary infiltrate disappeared and his eosinophile count normalized (Figure1). For the persistent left femoral deep venous thrombosis and pulmonary infarction, he was given heparin and warfarin with prednisolone which are continued to be administered even after his discharge from the hospital (Figure 2). The pulmonary segmental shadow caused by the pulmonary infarction disappeared after 6 months. The left femoral deep venous thrombosis and ulnar nerve palsy disappeared after 9 months (Figures1, 2, 3).

At 81 days after the patient's discharge from the hospital, the Kampo medicine "Chi-ling-tang (柴苓湯)" (TJ 114) [4] was started (2packs/day: for adult 3 packs is required; 3 pack includes 9 g of herbal mixtures consisting of 3g of excipient and 6g of dried herbal extracts. Dried herbal extracts/day is derived from chai-fu (.柴胡)7 g, zhu-ling (猪苓)3g, ze-xie (沢瀉)5 g, ren-shen (人

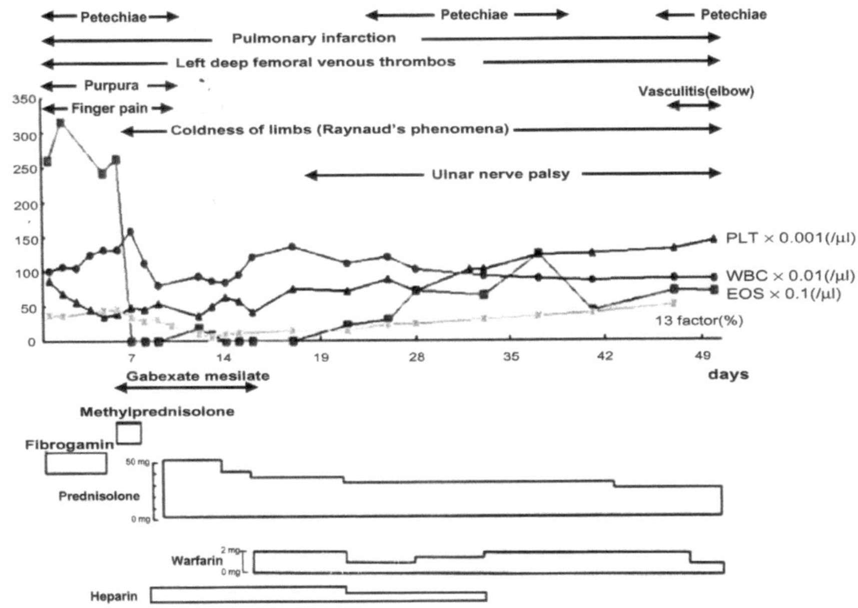

Figure 1. Clinical course during hospitalization of case 1.

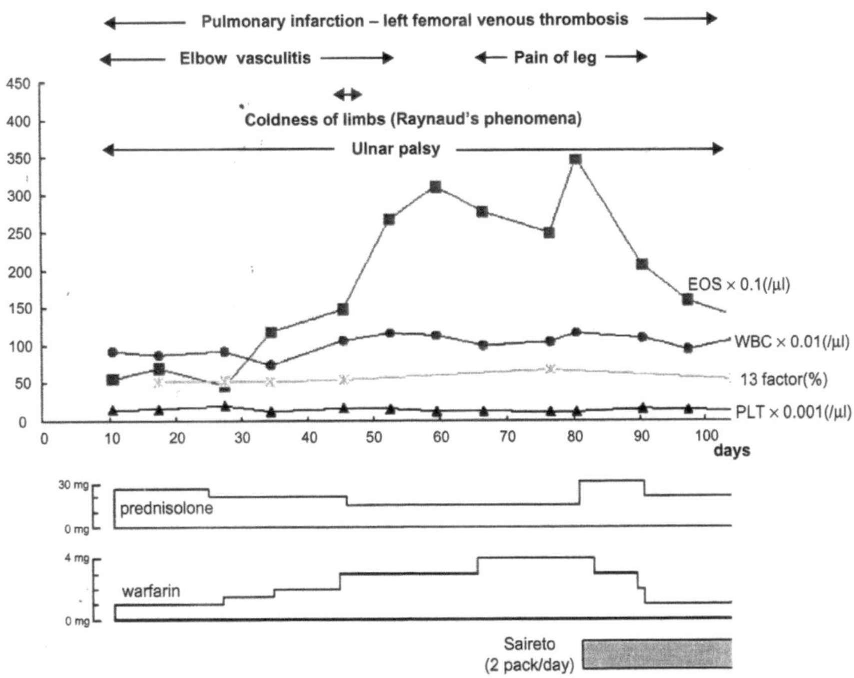

Figure 2. Clinical course after discharge from the hospital of Case 1.

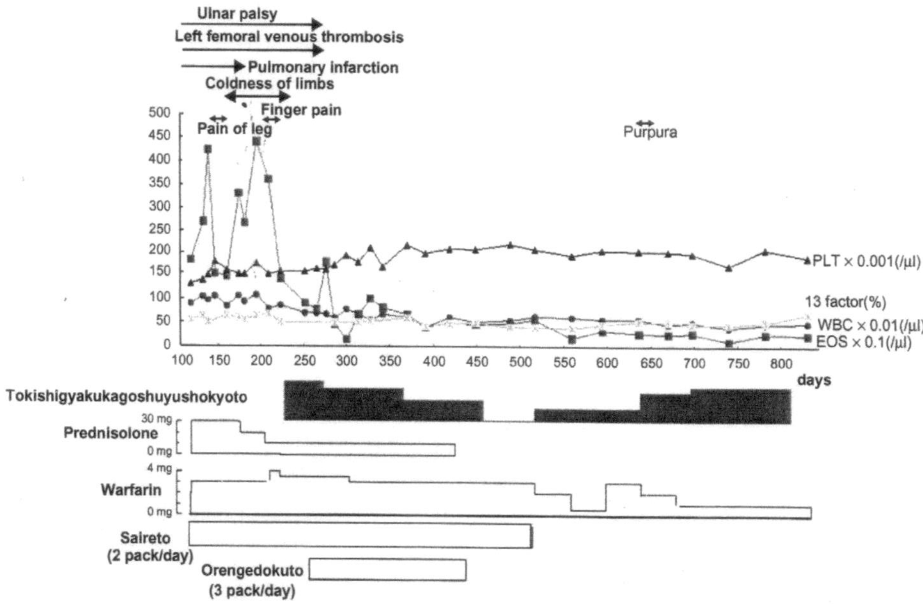

Figure 3. Clinical course after discharge of case 1

参)3g, ban-xia (半夏)5g, fu-ling (茯苓)3g, huang-qin (黄芩)3g, gan-cao (甘草)2g, to prevent the side effects of prednisolone. TJ indicates that this is a product of Tsumura Co (Akasaka, Minatoku, Tokyo, 107-8521 Japan).

The doctor in chief decided to apply Kampo medicine, because even at 7 months after discharge there were no signs of improvement and the patient's QOL was suffering. The patient visited the author's clinic on the 224th day after discharge from the hospital.

Present States: The patient's height was 166cm and weight was 65kg. He had a floating, fine, and weak chi mai (尺脈) (indicating Kidney yang deficiency). His tongue body was pale red and showed thin tongue fur. Sublingual collateral dark vessels were swollen.

Identification: Following TCM theory, the patient was diagnosed as having "static blood" [1] based on thrombosis and infarction of the blood vessels and dark vena sublingualis, as well as "dampness-heat" [2, 5] in the affected vessels, based on vasculitis, and as having "yang deficiency" [3] based on his cold limbs, sensitivity to coldness, and Raynaud's phenomenon.

Treatment: Activate blood to remove stasis. Add and promote yang circulation.

Prescription: Dan-gui-si-ni-jia-wu-zhu-yu-sheng-jiang-tang (当帰四逆加呉茱萸生姜) (Table 1) [7] for Yang deficiency to warm the channels, disperse cold, nourish the blood and unblock the blood vessels. For "blood stasis", mu-tan-pi (牡丹皮) [8], tau-gen (桃仁) (Table 1) [9], zhe-chong (虫) [10], and shui-zhi (水蛭) [11] were added and to remove dampness-heat, huang-lian-jie-du-tang (黄連解毒湯) (TJ-15) (Table 2) [12–14] was prescribed.

Name of the herb	Main function
Radix Angelicae Sinensis(当帰:dang gui)3	Tonify and invigorates the blood
Radix Paeoniae Lactiflorae (芍薬:bai shao)3	Strengthen the tonifying action of 当帰
Ramulus Cinnamomi Cassiae(Keishi:gui zhi)3	Warm the meridian and disperses cold
Herba cum Radice Asari(細辛:xi xin)2	Disperses both internal and external cold
Radix Glycyrrhizae Uralensis (甘草: gan cao)1	Augument the Qi and strengthen the Spleen
Fructus Zizyphi Jujubae(大棗:da cao)5	Augument the Qi and strengthen the Spleen
Caulis Mutong(木通:mu tong)3	Facilitate the flow in the channels and vessels
Fructus Evodiae Rutaecarpae (呉茱萸:Wu zhu yu) 2	Warm the middle, disperse cold, promotes the movement of Qi
Zingiberis Officinalis Recens(dried) (生姜: heng jiang)1	Release the exterior and disperses cold

*1 Tangkuei Decoction for Frigid Extremities plus Evodia and Fresh Ginger (Name in USA) Ref 13. numerals mean weight of dried herbs(g/day). For case 1, 2g of Mutanpi(牡丹皮) & Tao-ren(桃仁) and 0.5g of Zhe-chong(蟅虫) & shui-zhi(水蛭) were added to the above Prescriptions to decoct with water.

Table 1. Composing herbs of : Dan-gui-si-ni-jia-wu-zhu-yu-sheng-jiang-tang (当帰四逆加呉茱萸生姜湯)*1 and main function of respective herbs in Human.(Decoction)

Name of the herb (Japanese:Chinese),N(g/day)	Main function
Rhizoma Coptidis (黄連:huang lian),2	Clear heat and dry dampness
Radix Scutellariae (黄芩:huang qin),3	Clear heat and dry dampness
Cortex Phellodendri (黄柏:huang bai),1.5	Clear heat and dry dampness
Fructus Gardeniae (Jasminoidis) (梔子:zhi zi),2	Clear heat and eliminates irritability

*2 Coptis Decoction to Relieve Toxicity(Name in USA) :Ref 18
Huang lian jie du tang(Name in china)

Table 2. Composition of herbs in Orengedokuto (黄連解毒湯) and main function of respective herbs

Clinical Course: After Kampo medicines were initiated, the patient's Raynaud's phenomenon, cold and painful limbs, and abnormal platelet count quickly normalized, and his hypereosinophilia gradually improved to a normal level, with transient deterioration, over a period of 10 months. The left femoral venous thrombosis and ulnar nerve palsy had disappeared by 9 months of treatment (Figure 2, 3).

Discussion: The Kampo medicines selected in this case were chosen for the particular activities of the herbs. They work synergistically to produce improvement.

Case 2 A 2-year-old boy

Main Complaint: Purpura, abdominal pain, bloody feces

Past History: In the middle of April 2000, the patient caught a common cold. On April 25, petechiae appeared on his right leg and then spread to his left leg and both forearms. Abdominal pain with watery diarrhea, bloody stool, and knee joint pain were also noted, with the latter appearing and recovering spontaneously.

Present Illness: As the purpura became aggravated, the patient was hospitalized and diagnosed with HSP. He was treated with prednisolone successfully for the abdominal pain and bloody stool, but the symptoms reappeared with the tapering of the drug (Figure 4). The family of the patient requested treatment with Kampo medicine.

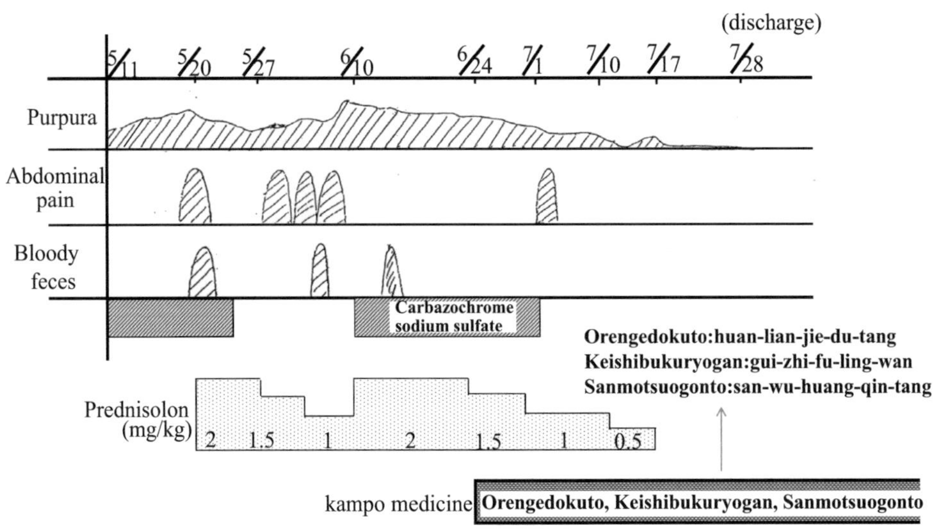

Figure 4. Clinical course of case 2 during hospitalization

Present States: The boy was very nervous and crying, and the doctor in chief was unable to examine him.

Identification: Following TCM theory, he was diagnosed with "blood stagnation" for his purpura. Yin deficiency with yang hyperactivity [15] for his rapid pulse (90/min) and excita-

Name of herbs	Main function
Ramulus Cinnamomi Cassiae (桂枝:gui zhi)	unblock the blood vessels and promote blood circulation
Sclerotium Poriae Cocos (茯苓:fu ling)	transform phlegm and promote urination nourishes the qi and calm the spirit
Radix Paeoniae(芍薬:shao yao)	relax spasm and alleviate abdominal pain
Cortex Moutan Radicis(牡丹皮:mu dan pi)	cool and invigorates the blood and dispel blood stasis
Semen Persicae(桃仁:tao ren)	invigorates the blood and dispel blood stasis

*3 Cinnamon Twig and Poria Pill(Name in USA). Gui zhi fu ling wan(Name in China).
:Ref 22

Table 3. Composing herbs of Keshibukuryogan (桂枝茯苓丸)*3 and main functions of respective herbs in human

bility, and with "dampness-heat" [2, 5] based on the existence of vasculitis and his preference for cold rather than hot food. We prescribed Keishi-bukuryogan: Gui-zhi-fu-ling-wan (桂枝茯苓丸) (Table 3) (TJ 25) for "blood stagnation" [1]. San-wu-huang-qin-tang (三物黄芩湯) (TJ 121: One day's dose include di-fang 6g, ku-shen 3g, and huang-qin 3g) [13, 16–18] for Yin deficiency with yang hyperactivity and Huan-lien-jie- du-tang (黄連解毒湯) (TJ 15) for "clearing dampness-heat" [2, 12–14].

As shown in Figure 4, in spite of the tapering down of the prednisolone, soon after the administration of the Kampo medicines, the purpura and abdominal pain drastically decreased and the bloody stool subsided. Despite the fact that the patient stopped the prednisolone 3 weeks after starting the Kampo medicines, his improved condition continued, leading to his discharge from the hospital [19].

Discussion: In Case 1, the platelet decrease might have been the result of a pulmonary infarction. The prednisolone pulse therapy may have aggravated the infarction despite the patient's good QOL. In CSS with eosinophilia and systemic vasculitis, "blood stagnation" is present due to the pulmonary infiltrate of eosinophils caused by the vasculitis. As mentioned earlier, mu-tan-pi (牡丹皮) [8], tau-ren (桃仁) [9], zhe-chong (虫) [10], and sui-zhi (水蛭) [11] resolved the blood stagnation and accelerated blood flow.

In the United States, Tokisigyakukagosyuyusyokyoto (Japanese pronun- ciation), Dan-gui-si-ni-jia-wu-zhu-yu-sheng-jiang-tang (当帰四逆加呉茱萸生姜) named as "The Decoction For Frigid Extremities plus Evodia and Fresh Ginger" [7], which means warm the channels, disperse cold and unblock blood vessels in TCM.

Inflammation implies "dampness-heat" in TCM, Huan-ren-jie-du-teng (黄連解毒湯) which traditionally relieves heat and dampness was applied. These formulas and remedies are considered to work synergistically to prompt recovery.

In Case 2, as in Case 1, vasculitis has the characteristic of "heat and dampness", for which Huan-lien-jie-du-tang was applied. Deposits of immune complex in the blood vessels or purpura mean blood stagnation in TCM, for which Gui-zi-fu-ling-wang (桂枝茯苓丸) was applied. The fact that the patient preferred cold drink, and was feverish with a rapid pulse rate suggested Yin deficiency with internal heat [15], for which San-wu-huang- qin-tang was prescribed (TJ-121). These prescriptions are also believed to work synergistically to effect a quick recovery.

These cases of systemic vasculitis had "blood stagnation" and "dampness-heat" in TCM terminology. Properly selected remedies for "blood stagnation" and "heat and dampness" seemed to help to achieve patient improvement.

4. Kidney diseases

4.1. Alternative treatment for nephrotic syndrome with Kampo medicines including Ba-Wei-Di-Huang-Wan [20]

4.1.1. Abstract

The dose of steroid hormone was decreased or eliminated by the addition of Kampo medicines to cure patients suffering from nephrotic syndrome.

In two cases refractory to steroid hormone, the combination of ba-wei-di- huang-wan (八味地黄丸), gui-zhi-fu-ling-wan (桂枝茯苓丸), and dang-gui- shao-yao-san (当帰芍薬散) or ba-wei-di-huang-wan, chai-ling-tang (柴苓湯), and the addition of various herbs (*Captis chinensis* Franch, *Gardenia jasminoides* Ellis, etc.) was very effective.

Based on these formulations, the new combination of Ba-wei-di-huang- wan (八味地黄丸), Xiao-chai-hu-tang (小柴胡湯), Si-wu-tang (四物湯), and huang-lian-jie-du-tang (黄連解毒湯) (hereafter this combination of four prescriptions shortened to BXSH) proved to be effective in eight cases (one case refractory to steroids and therefore without steroid treatment, one case with steroid dependency and six cases with nephrotic syndrome). This combination was effective in five of six patients with proteinuria. In one recurrent case, the combination of Ba-wei-di-huang-wan and Bu-in-tang (補陰湯) led to recovery. These results show that these formulas may exert a synergistic effect responsible for improvement in urinary protein excretion.

4.2. Introduction

Patients with nephrotic syndrome commonly take steroid hormones. However, some patients experience many side effects. To decrease these steroidal side effects, Chai-ling-tang (柴苓湯) was often applied [4].

Because some side effect may persist, we tried to create new herbal combination.

Ba-Wei- Di- Huang-Wan is effective in treating oliguria, edema [21], and proteinuria [22]; xiao-chai-hu-tang (小柴胡湯), as a part of chai-ling-tang (柴苓湯), huan-lien-jie-du-tang (黄連解毒湯) as antiphlogistic and si-wu-tang (四物湯) (di-huang, dang-gui, shao-yao, chuan-xiong) to tonify and accelerate the blood circulation are chosen to treat nephrotic syndrome. We describe our promising results below.

4.3. Material and methods

We studied eight adults and three children who were diagnosed with nephrotic syndrome at other medical facilities that followed our instructions.

A treatment was deemed very effective (+2) when more than 2 years had passed without recurrence even after quitting steroid hormones after a combination therapy consisting of four prescriptions (BXSH) in steroid refractory and dependent cases. Another very effective (+2) case is without relapse for more than 2 years who took only Kampo medicines without steroid hormone. A treatment was deemed effective (+1), only during the intake of Kampo medicines, improvement was observed in the form of a reduction in daily proteinuria of more than 50% compared to patient's condition without Kampo medicines, or when the required steroid volume was reduced. And another effective (+1) case is as follows. The patient took a combination of steroids and Kampo medicine and proteinuria disappeared within 6 months, subjective symptoms improved and no recurrence was observed in more than 2 years after steroid hormones were stopped.

We obtained powdered prescriptions of ba-wei-di-huang-wan (八味地黄丸) (di-huang: 地黄 6,fu-ling: 茯苓 3, shan- zhu-yu: 山茱萸 3, mu-dan-pi: 牡丹皮 2.5, san-yao: 山薬 3, gui-pi: 桂皮 1; ze-xie: 澤瀉 3 and fu-zi: 附子 0.5; numbers indicate g/day), xiao-chai-hu-tang (小柴胡湯) (chai-fu.7g, ban-xia.5g, dried sheng-jiang.1g, huang-qin.3g, da- zao.3g, ren-shen.3g, gan-cao.2g; numbers indicate g/day), huang-lian-jie-du-tang (黄連解毒湯), and Si-wu-tang (四物湯). Hereafter, we refer to the mixture of the above mention- ed four prescriptions as BXHS. For adults, we prescribed full ~ half dose of ba-wei-di-huang-wan depending on weight. Infants were prescribed, 1/2 of the adult volume of ba-wei-di-huang-wan, and 1/3 of xiao-chai-hu- tang, huang-lian-jie-du-tang, and si-wu-tang (BXHS).

(Composition of herbs respective prescriptions are listed in Reference 16.)

Sometimes to other cases ba-wei-di-huang-wan added with bu-zhong-yi- qi-tang (補中益気湯), bu-in-tang (補陰湯), dang-gui-shao-yao-san (当帰芍薬散), and gui-zhi-fu-ling-wan (桂枝茯苓丸) could be prescribed.

We obtained these prescriptions in powder form from Matsuura Yakugyo Co, Ltd (24–21, Enjo-Cho, Showa-Ku, Nagoya 466-0054, Japan) or Tsumura Co. LTD. These powdered prescriptions are made from filtrate of decoctions followed by spray drying.

The components of the decoction were derived from "Keiken Kampo Shoho Bunryo syu" [23]. We obtained appropriate herbs from Tochimoto Tenkaido Co, LTD (3–21 Suehiro_cho, Kita-ku, Osaka 530-0053, Japan).

When several different prescriptions were combined to make a single new prescription for decoction, and when the same herb was used in more than two prescriptions we used the largest volume of herb.

We prepared the decoction using with market boiling instrument. Kampo medicines are usually taken before meal. In cases of digestive system trouble, they are taken after a meal.

4.4. Results

1. Effects to steroid-resistant nephrotic syndrome

Case 1. M.O female. First onset at age 7

Three months' steroid treatment did not work for her. At the first visit to my clinic, her proteinuria score on the paper test was +4. She showed moon face, red striae and polytrichia.

At the insistence of the patient's mother, any conventional therapy including steroid hormone was stopped and 1/2 of the adult volume of ba-wei-di-huang-wan (八味地黄丸), gui-zhi-fu-ling-wan (桂枝茯苓丸) and dang-gui-shao-yao-san (当帰芍薬散) were prescribed which made her proteinuria disappear after 2 weeks.

She continued taking the same prescription for 4.7 months. At the time of the writing, more than 10 years have passed and she has had no recurrence.

Her treatment was estimated very effective (+2).

Case 2.T.K female. First onset at the age 45 (Figure 5)

Nine years of conventional therapy at other hospital brought no improve- ment in this patient's condition. When she first visited my clinic, she was taking 10 mg of prednisolone and 50mg of cyclophosphamide every other day.

Her proteinuria level was 4.7g/day. For 25 weeks, she was treated with a decoction of a mixture of xiao-chai-hu-tang, huang-lian-jie-du-tang, and si-wu-tang (chai-fu.7g, ban-xia.5g, dried sheng-jiang.1g, huang-qin.3g, da- zao.3g, ren-shen.3g, gan-cao.2g, huang-lian.1.5g, huang-bo. 1.5g, zhi-zi 2g, dang-gui.4g, chuan-xiong.4g, di-huang.4g) with ba-wei-di-huang-wan (pill form: 1 day's full dose) which reduced her proteinuria to 1.1g/day. When she overworked herself, her proteinuria increased temporarily to 4.3g/day. We changed to a combination of bu-yin-tang (補陰湯) and ba-wei-di-huang-wan which decreased her proteinuria to ca 2g/day and more recently decreased further to approximately 1g/day (Figure 5).

In Figures 5 and 6, ba-wei-di-huang-wan (八味地黄丸) is expressed as Hj. shao-chai-fu-tang (小柴胡湯) is expressed Ss, si-wu-tang (四物湯) is expressed Sm, huang-lian-jie-du-tang as Og, and bu-yin-tang (補陰湯) as Hi based on Japanese pronunciation.

When she was 59 years old, the doctor in chief stopped all her conventional therapies. We assessed her treatment was effective (+1).

Case 3. T.F. female. First onset at age 21

She relapsed five times whenever her intake of prednisolone reduced to below 20 mg/day. Betamethasone gabexate mesylate(B), and pulse therapy did not work at all. When a hematoma was produced by her kidney biopsy, her proteinuria level increased to 25g/day which then decreased with a dose of 60 mg of prednisolone/day. Cyclophosphamide was restarted at a

http://dx.doi.org/10.5772/60573

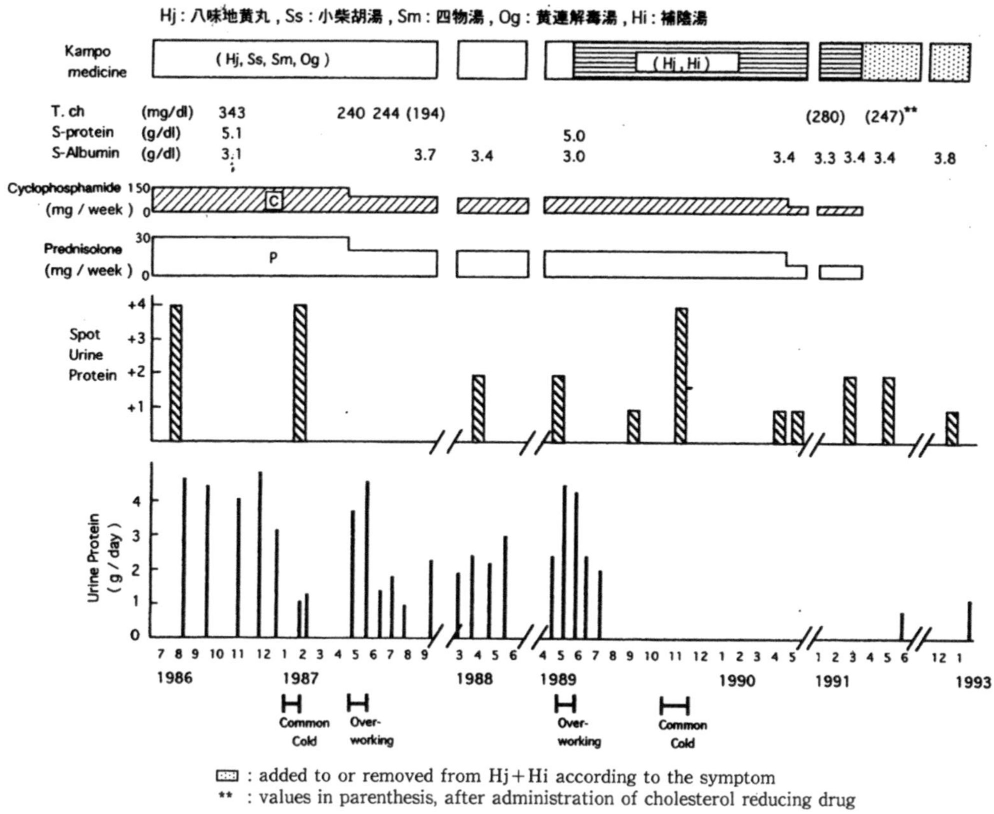

Figure 5. T.K. 6ly. f. (corresponds to table 1).

dose of 50mg/day, and 2 months later when the patient's intake of prednisolone was reduced to 17.5g/day, no relapse occurred. And when her prednisolone was decreased to 15mg/day, she started taking BXHS mix prescriptions. After 13 months, she had no proteinuria and her intake of prednisolone was further reduced to 5mg/day. She had been taking 2.5mg of prednisolone to prevent relapse. But now more than 20 years had passed without any recurrence. We estimate her treatment effective (+1) (Figure 6).

2. Effects on steroid-dependent nephrotic syndrome

Case 4. H.S. female. First onset at age 60.

This patient's initial proteinuria level was 10g/day with membranous nephropathy. When her intake of prednisolone decreased from 40mg/day to 5 mg/day, her nephropathy relapsed. At her first visit to my clinic, she was taking prednisolone at a dose of 15mg/day, and her proteinuria level was 2.2 g/day. After 26 weeks of intake of BXHS mix prescriptions, her proteinuria level had fallen to 0.7g/day which meant that the treatment was judged to be effective (+1). The patient was later able to reduce her intake of prednisolone to 2.5mg/day. At 3 years after discontinuing BXHS mix prescriptions, the patient recurred with a proteinuria level 3g/day despite intake of prednisolone. She was assessed to be effective (+1).

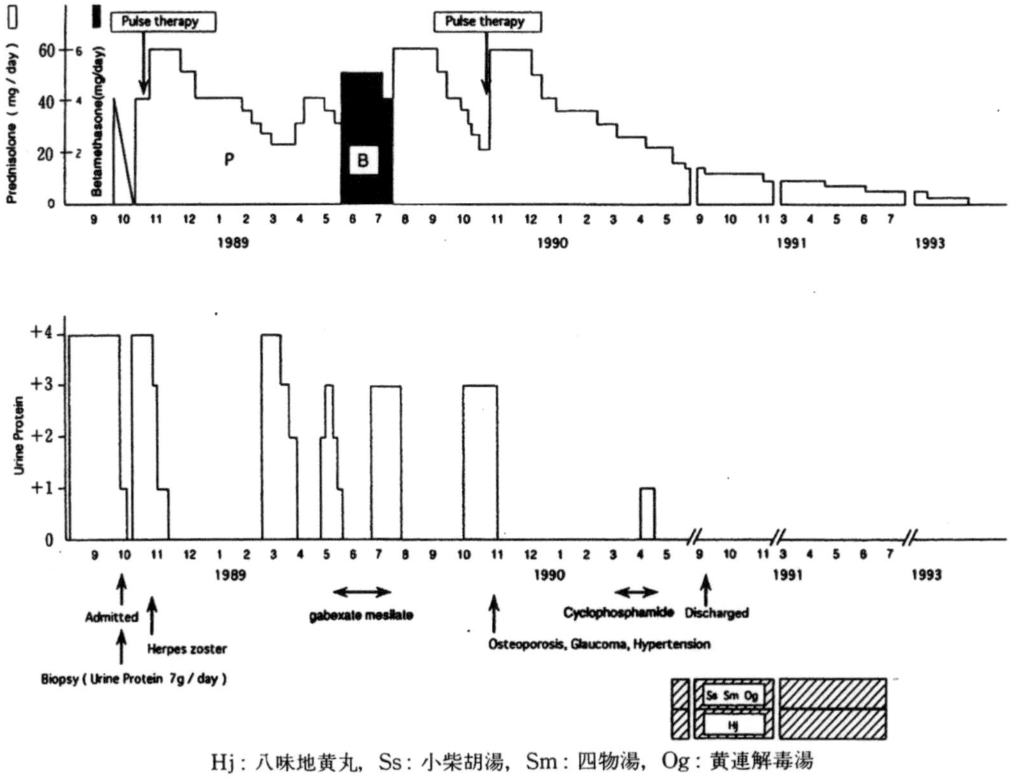

Figure 6. f. (corresponds to table 1)

Case 5. Y.M male. First onset at age 7.

This patient suffered from proteinuria (+4 with test paper) after being vaccinated for influenza. With the full-dose administration of betamethasone, his proteinuria disappeared. But a reduction in the intake (administration on a schedule of 3-days on, 4-days off), caused his proteinuria to reappear at a level of +1 with test paper. In order to break away from the betamethasone, he began taking BXHS mix prescriptions and 2 months later his proteinuria disappeared. Twenty months after starting BXHS together with betamethasone, he stopped taking betamethasone but continued BXHS for an additional 7 months. He has had no relapse for more than 20 years.

He will be evaluated very effective (+2).

Other cases: One male patient. First onset at age 36.

After spontaneous recovery from proteinuria, suffered a relapse (+4 with test paper) due to the aggravation of chronic prostatitis. His proteinuria level was 10 g/day and he was hospitalized. He was treated with steroid therapy which worked. To achieve steroid withdrawal, BXHS was prescribed with the goal of being protein-free. And he succeeded at 8 weeks. Three years after starting BXHS the patient's steroid was reduced to 7.5mg/day and further reduced to 5mg and finally stopped after 22 months. Since the start of BXSH, there has been no relapse for 9.2 years. Recently, although the patient's chronic prostatitis was again aggravated, there was no relapse indicating complete recovery. He was deemed very effective (+2).

2. Quick start of BXHS together with steroid therapy

One of two cases, was effective. We present the effective case.

Case 6. H.H female. First onset at age 44.

Since 1 year ago, this patient was made aware of her proteinuria.

(+1~+2 with test paper) with membranous nephropathy. She was hospitalized with proteinuria (5 g/day). But it reduced to 2 g/day with 60mg/day of prednisolone. When steroidal intake decreased to 50mg, she started BXHS. After approximately 3 months' intake of BXHS, her urinary protein disappeared and she was discharged from the hospital. After taking steroid for 18 months, she stopped and remained protein-free for more than 4 years. She had been taking 1/4 of initial volume of BXHS without relapse more than 10 years. She was assessed very effective (+2).

2. To nephrotic syndrome cured by only Kampo medicines

Case 7. Y.O female. First onset at 50.

Proteinuria (2.7g/day) disappeared approximately 15months later after BXHS was started with a gradual decrease and then stopped after 4 years and 2 months. The patient took this medicine for more than 7 years to prevent relapse. She was deemed very effective (+2).

4.5. Appendix: Efficacy for proteinuria

We applied Kampo medicines to eight patients without postural proteinuria. BXHS worked in seven of eight patients (data not shown).

4.6. Discussion

Generally speaking, the pathology of nephropathy stems from an over permeability of the glomerular basement membrane to serum protein.

Furthermore, blood coagulation can be accelerated. Histologically, thrombosis with fibrin may be observed. The side effects of the administration of steroids for a long time include an increase in blood viscosity and platelet hyperfunction. It is quite natural for antiplatelet drugs to decrease the diapedesis of protein from the kidneys.

We applied ba-wei-di-huang-wan, xiao-chai-hu-tang, huang-lian-jie- du-tang, and Si-wu-tang. Results were described below.

As mentioned above, ba-wei-di-huang-wan warms the Kidney and improve the kidney function. Huang-lian-jie-du-tang worked to remove dampness and heat and also used si-wu-tang to accelerate blood circulation and improving anemic tendency. I also used xiao-chai-fu-tang because it is the component of chai-ling tang which is used to eliminate steroid side effects and for nephrotic syndrome in Japan. Additionally, it was used effectively by Otsuka and Yakazu for proteinuria and nephrotic syndrome [21, 22]. I selected these prescriptions for these reasons. I will propose instead of combination of huang-lian-jie-du-tang and si-wu-tang, wen-qing-tang (温清飲) will be successfully replaced. Because, wen-qing-tang (温清飲) equals combination of huang-lian-jie-du-tang and si-wu-tang.

4.7. Conclusion

The combination of ba-wei-di-huang-wan (八味地黄丸), shao-chai-hu-tang (小柴胡湯), huang-lian-jie-du-tang (黄連解毒湯) and Si-wu-tang (四物湯) works to decrease the intake of steroids or helps the patients to stop taking steroids in steroid-refractory and dependent cases and for general nephrotic syndrome.

5. Leukemia-related diseases

5.1. Abstract

A 41-year-old female was diagnosed with acute lymphocytic leukemia (ALL) at a university hospital. She could not tolerate chemotherapy and started alternative Chinese herbal medicine including zi-xue-tan (紫雪丹) (Table 6) at the time of her fourth recurrence. This provided transient improvement followed by aggravation after her intake was decreased. A blood test suggested complete recovery. Although cyclophosphamide had previously been ineffective, this time together with Chinese medicine, it led to a dramatic improvement.

5.2. Introduction

Conventional therapies for leukemia have developed dramatically and now include such treatments as bone marrow transplantation (BMT). However, there remain the problems of side effects of chemotherapy, age limits for certain treatments, and a shortage of donors for BMT. Based on the clinical course of the case presented here, TCM should be considered as a potential alternative medicine treatment in some cases [24].

5.3. Case report

A 41-year-old female developed bone pain in November, 1989. She had also been suffering from constipation and cold intolerance. She reported in her family history that her mother had been suffering from rheumatism and brain embolism. After a thorough examination, the patient was diagnosed with L2 (by the French–American–British, FAB, classification) acute lymphocytic lymphoma. Chemotherapy with vincristine, prednisolone, daunorubicin, mercaptopurine, methotrexate, L-asparaginase, vindesine, and adriamycin was instituted. Complete remission was achieved and the patient left the hospital in March, 1990.

However, she subsequently suffered relapse three times. After she left the hospital in complete remission in August, 1993, 54.2% peripheral blood blasts appeared simultaneously with hair loss, nausea, diarrhea, candida stomatitis, mycotic pneumonia, and sepsis. As these side effects of chemotherapy were overwhelming, she refused all treatment at the hospital. Her family was told by the doctor that she had only 3 months to live. In April, 1994, she suffered from terrible weariness, insomnia, vertigo, and palpitations. She also suffered from inflammation of the mandibular joint (3–4 times/month) followed by difficulty in chewing food.

Lu Xi of the Lu family, noted for their treatment of acute febrile diseases (Wen bin), diagnosed her with acute febrile disease with stagnation of pathogenic heat, shortage of Qi (vital energy) and Yin including blood (xue) with blood stasis [24]. Her tongue body was pale and her lips were dark, indicating anemia and blood stagnation. Her pulse was thready and barely palpable. The patient elected to start TCM therapy on April 25, 1994.

At the beginning of the therapy, the patient showed the following values: white blood cells (WBC), 68000/μl; red blood cells (RBC), 231×10^4/μl; hemo- globin (Hb), 8.2 g/dl; blasts (sum of blast cells and atypical cells), 61%; lactic dehydrogenase (LDH), 730 (Figure 7).

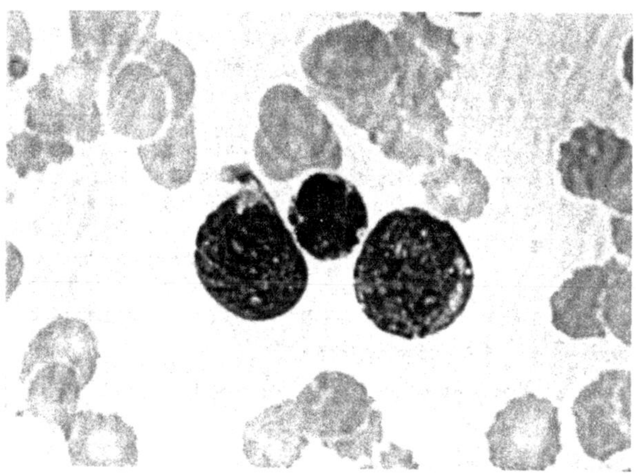

Figure 7. Findings of peripheral blood of patient 2 on May 17, 1994

Treatment was carried out to detoxify by supporting with Qi-tonic and Blood-tonic. The patient took prescriptions I-1, I-2, and I-3 as shown in Table 4 from April 25 to May 6, which increased her WBC to 69800/μl and decreased RBC to 204×10^4/μl, Hb to 7.0 g/dl, and changed blasts from 41480/μl to 66799/μl.

We considered this aggravation to be due to the intake of I-1, I-2, and I-3, that is, Qi-tonic Huang-qi (黄耆. *Astragali radix*), Da-cao (大棗. *Zizyphi fructus*), and Blood-tonic Shu-di-huang (生地黄 *Rehmanniae radix*), Bai-shao-yao (白芍薬 *Paeoniae radix*), Long-yan-rou (竜眼肉 *Longanae arillus*), and Dang-gui (当帰. *Angelicae radix*), which may stimulate a presumably predominant multiplication of blasts with normal WBC. The coexistence of Qi-tonic and Blood-tonic in an environment with malignant cells may lead to a predominant uptake of both tonics preferentially by fast-growing malignant cells, followed by a recurrence of leukemia. Thus the patient started to take Prescription II (Table 5) and modified Zi-xue-dan (紫雪丹) (Table 6), as listed in He-ji-jyu-fang (和剤局方).

Main functions	1-1 (Decoction)	1-2 Extracts of guipiteng (帰脾湯)	1-3 Extracts of baweidihuangwan (八味地黄丸)
・Clearing heat ・Removing pathogenic heat from blood ・Yin-tonic (清熱. 涼血. 補陰)	・REHMANNIAE RADIX (shangdihuang 生地黄 5.0) ・SCROPHULARIAE RADIX (xuanshen 玄参 5.0)		・REHMANNIAE RADIX (shengdihuang 生地黄 3.0)
・learing heal ・Removing pathogenic heat from blood ・Resolving blood stagnation (清熱. 涼血. 活血)	・MOUTAN RADICIS CORTEX (mudanpi 牡丹皮 5.0) ・PAEONIAE RUBRA RADIX (chishaoyac 赤芍薬 3.0)		・MOUTAN RADICIS CORTEX (mudanpi 牡丹皮 2.5)
・Activating blood circuration ・Resciving blood siagnation (活血)	・NOTOGINSENG RADIX (tiangi 田七 2.0) ・SALVIAE MIL TIORRHIZAE RADIX (danshen 丹参 5.0)		
・Detoxification ・Dissipating heat ・Repercussion (清熱. 解毒)	・VESPAE NICUS (ioufengfang 露蜂房 5.0)		
・Promoting the flow of channeis and collaterals ・Clearing heat (通絡.清熱)	・LUMBRICUS (dilong 地竜 3.0)		
・Regulating Ci (理気)	・CITRILEIOCARPAE EXOCARPIUM (qingpi 青皮 3.0)	・AUCKLANDIAE RADIX (muxiang 木香 1.0)	
・Ci-tonic (補気)	・ASTRAGALI RADIX (huangqi 黄耆 8.0) ・ZIZYPHI FRUCTUS (dacao 大棗3.0) ・GLYCYRRHIZAE RADIX (zhigancao 炙甘草 2.0)	・ASTRAGALI RADIX ・ZIZYPHI FAUCTUS (dacao 大棗 2.0) ・GINSENG RADIX (renshen 人参 3.0) ・ATRACTYLODIS PHIZOMA (baizhu 白朮 3.0)	・BATATATIS RHIZOMA (shanyao 山薬3.0)
・Yang-tonic (補陽)			・ACONTI TUBER (fuzi 附子 0.5) ・CINNAMOMI CORTEX (quipi 桂皮 1.0)
・Blood-tonic ・Yin-tonic (補血. 補陰)	・PAEONIAE RADIX (baishaoyao 白芍薬 3.0) ・REHMANNIAE RADIX (shucihuang 熟地黄 5.0)	・LONGANAE ARILLUS (longyanrou 龍眼肉 3.0) ・ANGELICAE RADIX (danggui 当帰 2.0)	・REHMANNIAE RADIX (shucihuang 熟地黄 5.0)
・Promoting digestion (消滞)	・CRATAEGI FAUCTUS (shanzhazi 山楂子 3.0)		
・Stomachic (健胃)		・ZINGIBERIS SICCATUM PHIZOMA (shengliang 生姜 1.0)	
・Diuresis (利尿)		・PORIA (fuling 茯苓 3.0)	・PORIA (fuling 茯苓 3.0) ・ALISMATIS RHIZOMA (zexie 沢瀉 3.0)
・Moderating (調和)		・GLYCYRRHIZAE RADIX (gancao 甘草 1.0) *1	
・Tranquilizing the mind (安神)		・ZIZYPHI SPINOSI SEMEN (suanzaoran 酸棗仁 3.0) *2 ・POLYGALAE RADIX (yuanzhi 遠志 3.0) *2	
・Astringent (収斂)			・CORNI FRUCTUS (shanzhuyu 山茱萸 3.0)

Pulverlzed extracts of I-2 and I-3 were obtained from Tsumura Co., Ltd., Tokyo, Japan.
The lower right number indicates intake (g/day) of respective herbs.
*1: This has the function of Qi-tonic as well.
*2: This has the function of blood-tonic as well.

Table 4. Composition of the formulas applied (I -1, I -2, I -3).

http://dx.doi.org/10.5772/60573

Main functions	II	III
· Clearing heat · Removing pathogenic heat from blood ·Yin-tonic (清熱. 涼血. 補陰)	·REHMANNIAE RADIX (shangdihuang 生地黄 5.0) ·SCROPHULARIAE RADIX (xuanshen 玄参 5.0)	·REHMANNIAE RADIX (shengdihuang 生地黄 5.0) ·SCROPHULARIAE RADIX (xuanshen 玄参 7.0)
· Clearing heat · Removing pathogenic heat from blood ·Resolving blood stagnation (清熱. 涼血. 活血)	·MOUTAN RADICIS CORTEX (mudanpi 牡丹皮 5.0)	·MOUTAN RADICIS CORTEX (mudanpi 牡丹皮 5.0) ·PAEONIAE RUBRA RADIX (chishaoyac 赤芍薬 3.0)
· Activating blood circulation · Resolving blood stagnation (活血. 袪瘀)	·EUPOLYPHAGA SINENSIS (chechong 庶虫 6.0) ·HIRUDO (shuizhi 水蛭 3.0) ·ZEDOARIAE RHIZOMA (ezhu 莪朮 3.0) ·SALVIAE MIL TIORRHIZAE RADIX (danshen 丹参 5.0)	·EUPOLYPHAGA SINENSIS (chechong 庶虫 6.0) ·TABANUS (mengchong 虻虫 2.0) ·MYRRHA (moyao 没薬 3.0)
· Detoxification · Dissipating heat (清熱. 解毒)		·VESPAE NICUS (ioufengfang 露蜂房 7.0)
·Regulating Ci (理気)	·AURANTII NOBILIS PERICAROIUM (chanpi 陳皮 3.0)	·CITRI LEIOCARPAE EXOCARPIUM (qingpi 青皮 3.0)
·Ci-tonic (補気)	·ASTRAGALI RADIX (huangqi 黄耆 5.0) ·GINSENG RADIX (renshen 人参 3.0)	·GINSENG RADIX (renshen 人参 2,5)
·Blood-tonic (補血)	· SPATHOLOBI CAULIS*(a) (jixueteng 鶏血藤 5.0) ·PAEONIAE RADIX (baishaoyao 白芍薬 3.0) ·LONGANAE ARILLUS (longyanrou 龍眼肉 3.0) ·REHMANNIAE RADIX (shucihuang 熟地黄 3.0)	·REHMANNIAE RADIX (shucihuang 熟地黄 5.0)
·Yang-tonic (補遠)		·EPIMEDII HERBA (yinyanghuo 淫羊霍 3.0) ·PSORALEAE SEMEN (ponuzhi 補骨脂 7.0)
·Purging ·Dissipating heat (瀉下.解毒)	·RHEUM PALMATUM RHIZOMA (dahuang 大黄 1.0)	

*(a): This has the function of activating blood circulation as well.

(4 Leukemia-related disease)

Table 5. Composition of prescription II and III

From May 16 to May 19, she was hospitalized for examination and her results were found to have improved remarkably. Her WBC count had fallen from 41900/μl to 28400/μl, with blasts decreasing from 96% to 69%. For anemia, the patient underwent blood transfusion (Figure 8). Her bone marrow, evaluated by tap, showed many malignant cells. Peripheral blood findings are shown in Figure 7.

Main functions	components	(g)
· Clearing heat · Purging fire (清熱、瀉火)	· GYPSUM FIBROSUM (shigao 石膏) · CALCITUM (hanshuishi 寒水石) · KAOLINUM (huashi 滑石) · NATRIUM SULFURICUM (mangxiao 芒硝)	50 50 50 100
· Dissipating excessive heat stagnation (火郁発之)	· POTASSIUM NITRATE (xiaoshi 硝石)	100
· Clearing heat · Removing pathogenic heat from blood · Yin-tonic (清熱、涼血、補陰)	· SCROPHULARIAE RADIX (xuanshen 玄参)	50
· Dissipating heat and detoxifying · Checking the liver and calming the wind (清熱、解毒、鎮肝、熄風)	· ANTELOPIS CORNU (lingyangjiao 羚羊角)	15
· Dissipating heat and detoxifying · Removing pathogenic heat from blood (清熱、解毒、涼血)	· BOS CORNU (niujiao 牛角)	150
· Tranquilization with heavy materials (重鎮、安神)	· MAGNETITE (cishi 磁石)	100
· Warming Zhongjiao* activating Qi (温中行氣)	· AQUILARIAE LIGNUM (chenxiang 沈香) · EUGENIA CARYOPHYLLATA (dingxiang 丁香)	15 15
· Regulating Qi (理氣)	· SAUSSUREAE RADIX (muxiang 木香)	15
· Detoxyfying (解毒)	· CIMICIFUGAE RHIZOMA (shengma 升麻) · GLYCYRRHIZAE RADIX (gancao 甘草)	50 25

***: The middle part of the body from the diaphragm to the umbillcus which contain viscera such as spleen and stomach. Every component was broken to be powderlike by using grinder. 1.5 g of this powder was taken at a time. Modified zixuedan: add nlujiao to and subtract xijiao, zhusha and shexiang from zixuedan (Hejijufang).**

Table 6. Composition of modified Zi-xue-dan written in He-ji-ju-fang, (4 Leukemia-related disease)

Seven days after the patient's discharge from the hospital on May 26, her WBC and blast cells again increased to 52200/μl and 89%, respectively, implying worsening of the disease. This may have been caused by excessive Blood-tonic herbs. We accordingly increased her dose of modified Zi-xue-dan (Table 6) and started Ling-yang-jiao (羚羊角) on May 29. In Prescription III, Qi-tonic and Blood-tonic herbs were decreased. Kidney-tonic Yin-yang-huo (淫羊藿) and Bohuzhi (破胡紙) were added, and an-gong-niu-huang-wan (Table 7) was added to dissipate heat and detoxify. Nevertheless, the patient's high fever continued. Her WBC count increased to 99800/μl on June 6 and retinal bleeding occurred with bone pain unresponsive to indomethacin for which narcotics were required.

Calculus bovis	20%	0.60 g
Radix curcumde	15%	0.45 g
Margarita	10%	0.30 g
Moschus	5%	0.15 g
Asiatici	20%	0.6g
Rhizoma coptidis	15%	0.45 g
Honey	15%	0.45 g
	100%	3.00 g

Table 7. Contents of An-gong-nju-huang-wan (Beijing)

The increase in blastic cells suggests an autocrine phenomenon. Perhaps a different cell line that was suppressed by Zi-xue-dan and Prescription was activated and increased. Based on TCM theory, in prescription III, Yang-tonic yin-yang-huo (淫羊藿) and po-hu-zhi (破胡紙) were included to warm the kidneys and increase kidney function. As in bone marrow, the haemopoietic role will be carried out more with the Yang-tonic herbs.

The patient then took cyclophosphamide at doses of 50mg, 50mg, 50mg, 100mg, 100mg, and 300mg for 7days in this order, even though it had not been effective 6 months earlier. Her WBC count on June 14 had decreased to 17700/μl. During the 7-day treatment with cyclophosphamide, the patient's severe bone pain continued, but disappeared almost completely on the 8th day. She was diagnosed with gout based on clinical symptoms, in spite of normal uric acid levels. Beginning on June 23, she took granulocyte-colony- stimulating factor (G-CSF) for 7 days. Every day, approximately 2 hours after G-CSF intake, she had a fever of 39°C, which was successfully reduced by indomethacin and which resolved when the G-CSF therapy was stopped.

After 750 mg of cyclophosphamide together with TCM for just 1 week, the patient's WBC decreased to near 500/μl, with 4% blasts. This situation continued for approximately 1 month until An-gong-niu-huang-wan was stopped and other Chinese medicines were decreased to 1/4 dosage because her WBC did not increase above 1000/μl. Complete relapse was achieved. The patient's renewed sensitivity to cyclophosphamide may be the result of an interval or partially by the change in her constitution created by taking Chinese medicine.

If we do not stop An-gong-niu-huang-wan and do not decrease Kampo medicine for the time being, the patient might survive longer. Sadly, there remain few treatment options for this patient.

In conclusion, a combination therapy with traditional Chinese herbs and chemotherapeutic agents may make it possible to reduce the total quantity of chemical drugs for some time. This may be particularly useful in cases of refractory leukemia.

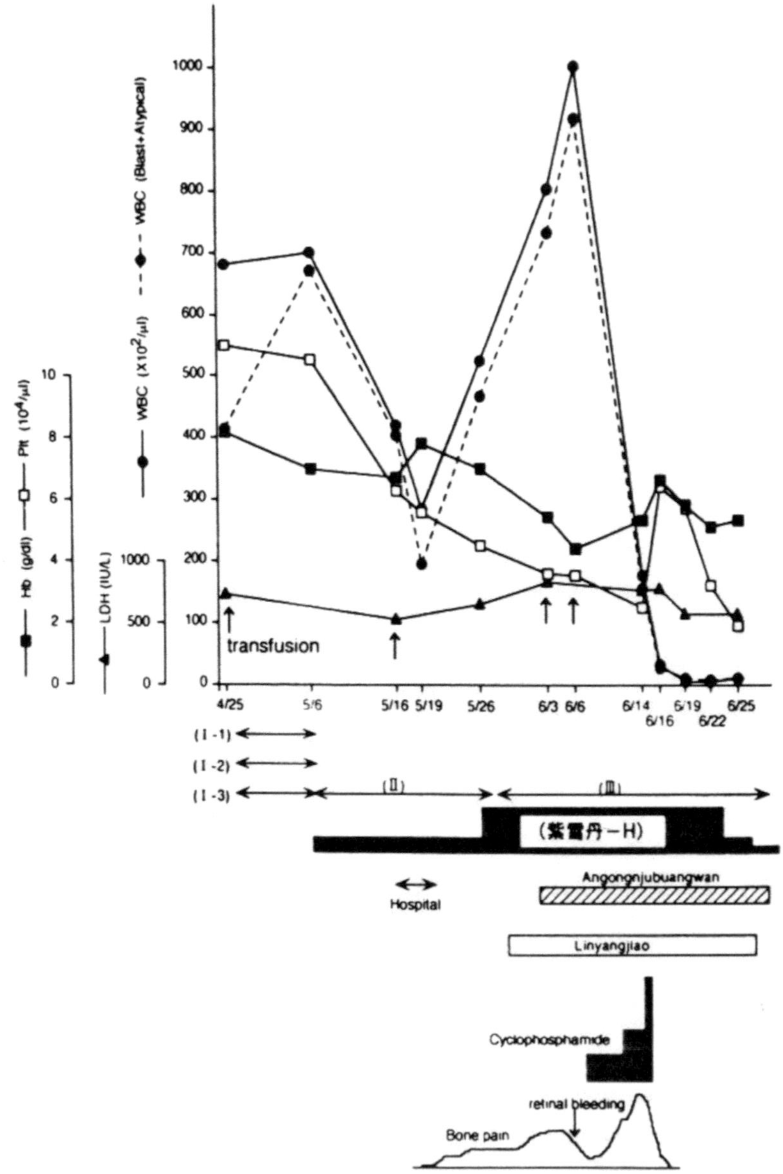

Figure 8. Clinical course of patient 2 since the start of treatment.

We also experienced another case not reported here of leukemia/lympho- blastic lymphoma (LBL) in which the patient was unable to receive chemotherapy due to terrible side effects. Traditional Chinese medical doctor, Lu Gan Fu, applied Zi-xue-dan (紫雪丹) for pathogenic heat and detoxification, which was able to reduce the patient's WBC count including leukemic cells [24]. He could survive 4 years and 10 months, though before starting TCM therapy his physician in charge told his family the patient could live 2 months.

http://dx.doi.org/10.5772/60573

6. Hyperlipidemia-related disease

6.1. Ayurvedic herb, Tinospora cordifolia

Tinospora cordifolia (Tin) is widely used in Southeast Asia as folk medicine for various diseases including diabetes mellitus (DM) [25]. In Japan, mechanism in decreasing blood cholesterol was reported in catabolism to bile acid [26].

We studied the effect of Tin in lowering blood total cholesterol (TC), triglycerides (TGs), very low-density lipoprotein (VLDL) and high-density lipoprotein (HDL) in 4 patients with hyperlipidemia. We prescribed powdered Tin at a dose of 0.75g/day for these four patients for 6 months. We examined blood TC, TGs, VLDL, and HDL before starting, once a month during administration, and at 17 days after stopping this herb.

6.1.1. Abstract

Tinospora cordifolia (Tin) was administered to four patients with hyperlipidemia for approximately 6 months and TC, TGs, VLDL, and HDL were measured once a month.

In three cases, on sampling in December, TGs tended to decrease (Figures 9, 10, and 11, Ayurvedic herb.Tinospora cordiforia) and subsequently kept similar level and increased after discontinuation of Tin. TCs seem to keep similar level during testing period. VLDL tend to decrease during Tin administration in Figures 9, 10, and 11. Tin seems to have some influence on the human lipid metabolism, especially in TG and VLDL. Our subject who had a family history of DM (Figure 12) showed different patterns in TG, VLDL from cases shown in Figures 9, 10, and 11. She may have a different lipid metabolism due to a shortage of insulin action or insulin resistance with her family history of DM, which requires further clarification through continued research in this field.

6.1.2. Materials and methods

The four patients had all been taking their own herbal medicines for their constitutions. We tested the effect of powdered Tin without changing their regularly taken medicines including herbal medicine. For breakfast of test day, they each had a small portion of rice and some pickled vegetables, and tested at my clinic about noon, I drew blood from a vein on the left hand. Their breakfast was small and quite similar every time that blood was drawn.

Case 1: A 78-year-old Japanese female; height: 156cm; weight: 45kg.

She had been suffering from constipation, anal prolapse, and hyperlipidemia, and has adrenal tumor. She had been taking modified bu-zhong-yi-qi-tang (補中益気湯) for 3 years.

Case 2: A 75-year-old Japanese female; height: 154cm; weight: 55kg. She had slight hyperlipidemia and cholelithiasis.

Case 3: A 74-year-old Japanese female; height: 154cm; weight: 45.6kg. She catches cold easily. She has not been strong since childhood and is sensitive to cold. From time to time when she had her blood tested, the doctor informed her that she had hypercholesterolemia. She had been taking modified chai-ling-tang (柴苓湯) with ba-wei-di-huang-wang (half dose/day) for more than 7 months.

Case 4: A 56-year-old Japanese female; height: 155 cm; weight: 56 kg.

Her parents had a family history of DM. She had been taking ba-wei-di- huang-wang (八味地黄丸) and gui-zhi-fuling-wan (桂枝茯苓丸: full dose of 1 day) for more than 1 year.

We prescribed powdered Tin (regular volume, 0.75 g /day) for these four patients for 6 months. I examined blood level of TC, TGs, VLDL, and HDL before starting, once a month during administration, and at 17 days after stopping this herb. LDL was calculated as total-Cho extracted HDL plus 1/5 TGs.

6.1.3. Results and discussion

In Case 1, LDL showed a small increase at the initiation of Tin, but then decreased consistently even after Tin was discontinued and remained low for approximately 1 month. At 2 months after the discontinuation of Tin, however, it started to increase. TG had decreased from 152 to 83 mg/dl at 2 months after initiating Tin, and remained nearly constant until 1 month after stopping Tin. HDL increased from the beginning until 1 month after stopping Tin. In short, in Case 1, LDL and TG kept decreasing and HDL kept increasing. A high level of TC might reflect HDL concentration, which does not necessarily mean bad hyperlipidemia. For her Tin seemed to play a good role to decrease the level of TG, LDL and increase of HDL (Figure 9).

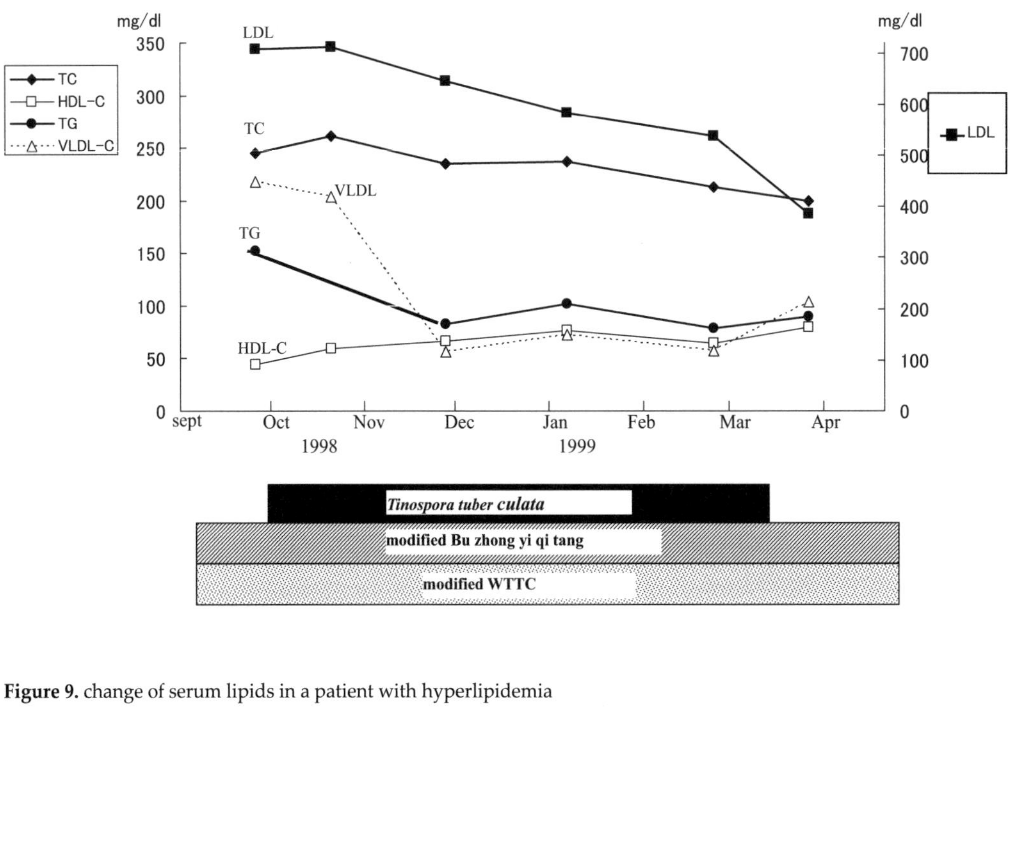

Figure 9. change of serum lipids in a patient with hyperlipidemia

In Case 2, from October 7 till November 28, TC, LDL, and TGs all decreased. However, early in the new year, the patient ate her favorite herring roe every day. At January 7, TC and LDL had increased while TGs kept decreasing. The patient's LDL level at 20 days after stopping herring roe had decreased slightly. The intake of herring roe did no influence to the ability of Tin to decrease TG levels. But after stopping Tin, TG, VLDL, and TC similarly increased which implies that Tin can decrease TG levels. In this case Tin did not influence HDL level (Figure 10).

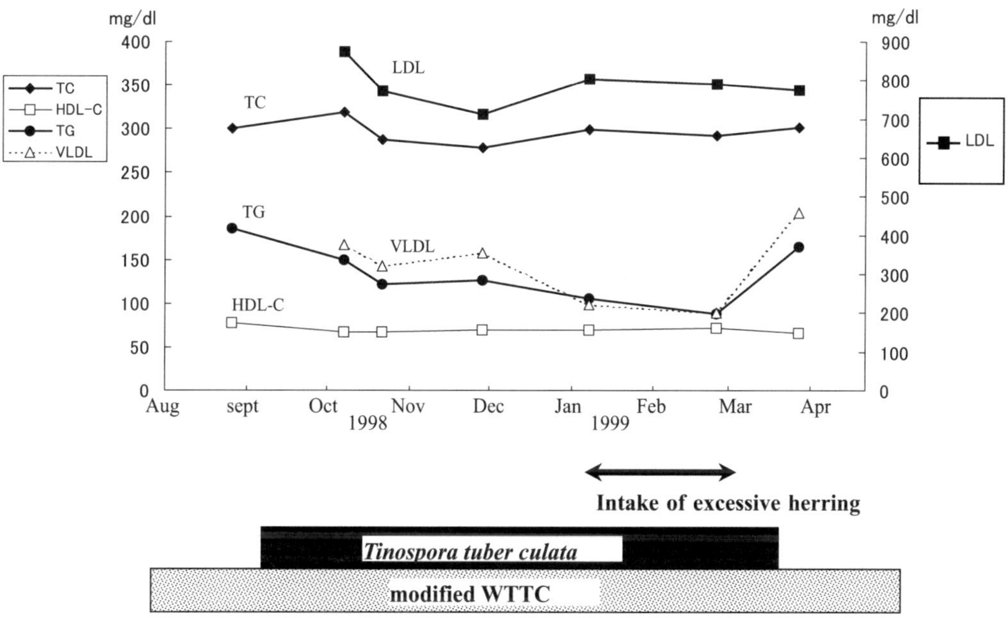

Figure 10. Change of serum lipids in a patient with hyperlipidemia

In Case 3, TC, LDL, and HDL all tend to increase until second sampling, and then increased again after Tin was discontinued.

Until the time of the third sampling, the patient had been taking antibiotics for inflammation associated with otitis externa, which would have influenced her lipid metabolism. After stopping Tin, all levels increased. This may mean that Tin can decrease the blood levels of TC, LDL, VLDL, and TG. But I cannot explain why LDL increased at the beginning of Jan- uary. The patient's TG level tends to remain same normal level (Figure 11).

In Case 4, unfortunately, three spots could not be measured for her private reason, but it is clear that, from January until the time when Tin was continued, all factors increased except HDL and that after Tin was discontinued, they all decreased. This implies that Tin was not effective in decreasing blood levels of TC, LDL, VLDL, or TGs in this case. We therefore recommend that this patient should take conventional medicine for hyperlipidemia (Figure 12). Her family history of DM may play a role in this phenomenon and must be further clarified.

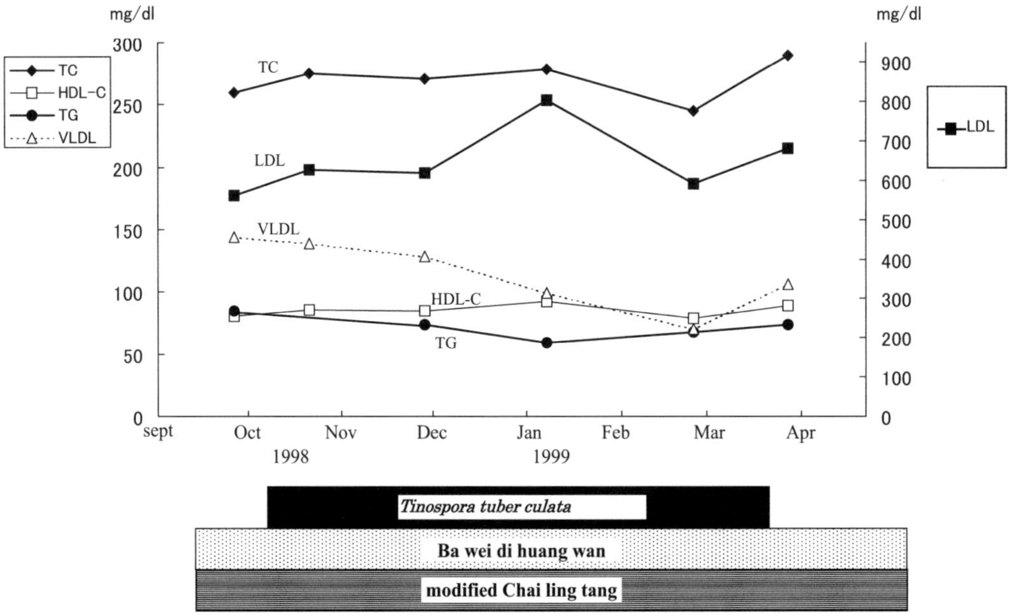

Figure 11. Change of serum lipids in a patient with hyperlipidemia

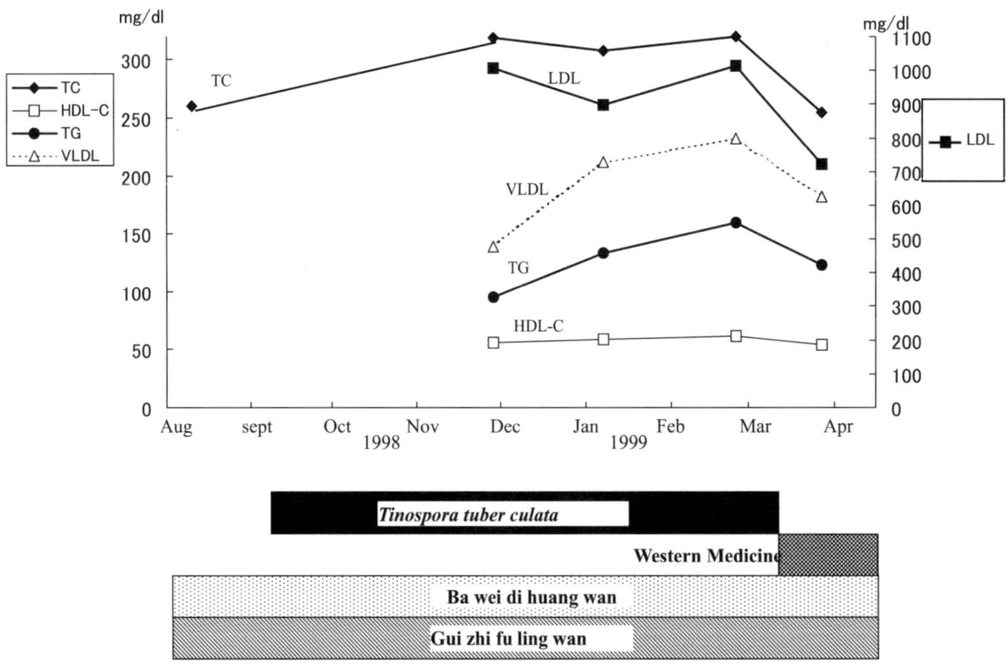

Figure 12. Change of serum lipids in a patient with hyperlipidemia

Finally, except Case 4 with family history of DM, Tin tends to decrease the level of TG and VLDL and tend to increase HDL in Case 1 and 3.

Finally, Tin may play a role to decrease human hyperlipidemia in TG and VLDL level, which must be clarified about the mechanism in future.

6.2. Kampo or TCM (Dandao-paishi-tang)

6.2.1. Abstract

Some patients with hyperlipidemia do not wish to pursue conventional therapies because of their side effects. Two such patients requested that I prescribe herbal medicine to decrease the blood levels of TG and TC. The Chinese herb combination known as modified Dandao-paishi-tang (DDPT; 胆道排石湯) (Table 8) which is generally used to promote the excretion of gallstones, was administered to two patients with high blood TG levels.

Desmodiumstyracifolium.	Jin-qian-cao (金銭草)	6g
ScutellariaeRadix.	huang-qin(黄金)	5g
Poncirustrifoliate	zhi-gu(枳殻)	5g
Rosa banksiae	mu-xiang(木香)	5g
Melia azedarach var.subtrpinnata	chuān-liàn-zǐ(川楝子)	5g
Curcuma aromatic	yu-jin(郁金)	5g
Rheirhizome	da-huang(大黄)	1g
Artemisiaecapillarisspica	yin-chen-hao（茵陳蒿）	2g
Natrii Sulfas	mang-xiao(芒消)	1g

Table 8. Modified Dandaopaishi tang (DDPT:胆道排石湯) (daily dose)

In the first case, a 66-year-old male, TG levels decreased from 634 mg/dl to 273 mg/dl during 4 years' intake (Figure 13). The second case, a 66-year-old Japanese female since 61 year suffering from DM and hyperlipidemia, took DDPT for 4 months. Her TG levels decreased from 815 mg/dl to 442 mg/dl, but then increased again when she decreased the volume of DDPT intake (Fig 14) [27].

Case 1: A 66-year-old Japanese male, 171cm tall and weighing 81kg, first visited our clinic in February 1984, because of hyperlipidemia and cholelithiasis. His blood pressure was 156/100. He had had cholelithiasis previously in 1976 which was left untreated because it improved. Since 1982, when he suffered from acute hepatitis A, he had been diagnosed with hyperlipidemia at every medical checkup. As he suffered occasional bouts of cholelithiasis that had a thick gall bladder wall, I diagnosed him with liver–gallbladder dampness-heat syndrome (Figure 13).

We started modified da-chai-hu-tang (大柴胡湯) consisting of chai-fu (柴胡) 6, ban-xia (半夏)4, gan-sheng-jian (乾生姜)1.5, huang-qin (黄芩)3, da-zao (大棗) 3, zhi-shi (枳実)2, da-huang (大黄)1, huang-lian (黄連)1, gua-lou-ren (栝楼仁)3, and mu-dan-pi (牡丹皮)2g/day in February 1984, and continued treatment until October of 1987 but without success. In October 1987, we changed to modified dan-dao-paishi-tang (DDPT). With this change, the patient's TG levels decreased from approximately 600 mg/dl to 400 mg/dl before cholecystectomy, and further decreased to 203 mg/dl after surgery in April 1991, at which point he stopped taking herbal medicines.

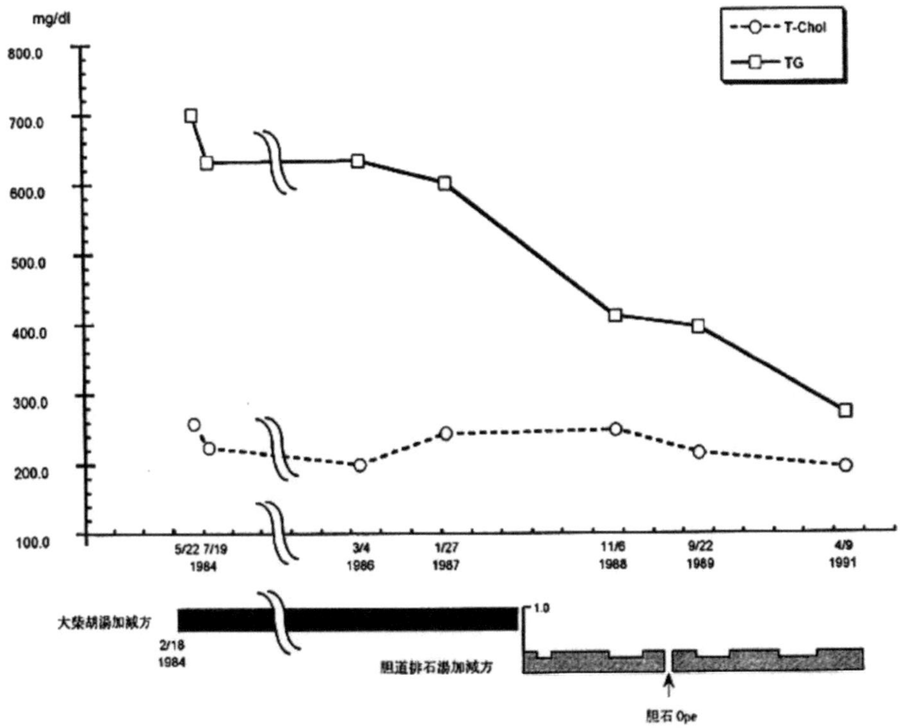

Figure 13. The change of levels of TC, TG in case 1

Case 2: A 60-year-old Japanese female, 152 cm tall and weighing 54 kg, who refused conventional therapy had been taking ba-wei-di-huang-wan (八味地黄丸: full dose/day) with powdered type of extract of zhi-gan-cao-tan (炙甘草湯) and xiao-chai-hu-tang (小柴胡湯) together with gui-zhi-fu-ling-wan (桂枝茯苓丸) because unless she take these prescriptions her fasting glucose level increase above 150 mg/dl. When her TG level surpassed 800 mg/dl in December, 1987, we prescribed modified dan-dao-paishi-tang (DDPT) without changing the medicines described earlier, and her TG level had decreased to 450 mg/dl by April 1988. As she suffered from appetite loss, stomach fullness and loose stool, her intake was reduced to 1/6, which led to 735 mg/dl in May 1989. She repeated the pattern of a high dosage of DDPT followed by a low blood TG level, then digestive system symptoms, then a lower DDPT intake followed by high blood TG. Finally, she persisted in taking only a small amount of DDPT, which led to an increase in TG. TC showed a similar tendency to TG, but was not so conspicuous as TG in this

http://dx.doi.org/10.5772/60573

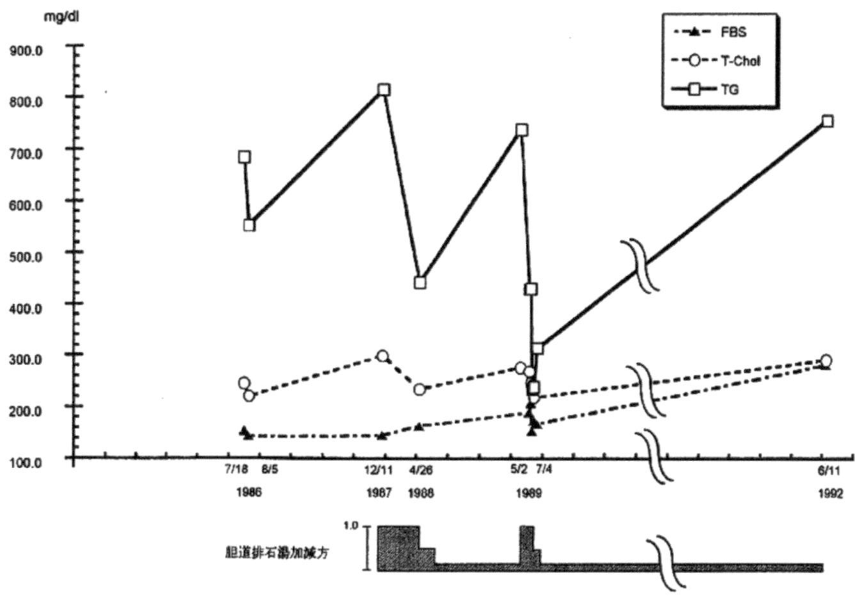

Figure 14. The change of levels of TC, TG in case 2

patient. These results may be related to the patient's DM condition and/or to the fact that she did not excise regularly and was on no specific diet (Figure 13).

6.2.2. Discussion

In Case 1 and 2 and two other cases (data not shown), DDPT was able to decrease TG levels. In Case 2, DDPT seem to work dose-dependently. Unless the digestive system is weak, DDPT can be used without complications. Of course, exercise is required with herbal medicine. It has been suggested that DDPT may promote the secretion of bile acid, which promotes lipid absorption. If this were the case, blood TG levels should be elevated; but in fact the opposite occurs. Further study is required to clarify the actions of DDPT.

7. Pain-related diseases

7.1. Sprains, bruises, and arthritis

7.1.1. Abstract

It takes a long time to recover from sprains, bruises, and arthritis, which often involve both pain and a decline in QOL. We applied two Kampo medicines, zhi-da-pu-yi-fang (治打撲一方: remedy for contusion) (Tsumura & Co. 7.5 g/day) to resolve inflammation and restore injured parts ("dampness- heat" in TCM), and Ba-wei-di-huang-wan (八味地黄丸) to restore presumed minute bone injury and to regulate metabolism (kidney tonic in TCM). We treated sprains, bruises, and arthritis in 10 patients (40–85 years of age; 1 male, 9 female) using the visual analog scale (VAS) to assess pain in the affected body parts before and after the administration of Kampo medicines. In almost all cases, recovery began promptly and pain disappeared within approximately 2 weeks. Large doses for a short time seemed to achieve quicker recovery [28].

7.1.2. Bruises

Case 1: A 67-year-old Japanese female was involved in a traffic accident and suffered bruising of the left hip without bone fracture. The two prescriptions were started immediately. At seven days, her VAS score had improved to 2 from 10. She was completely pain-free 28 days after the accident (Figure 15).

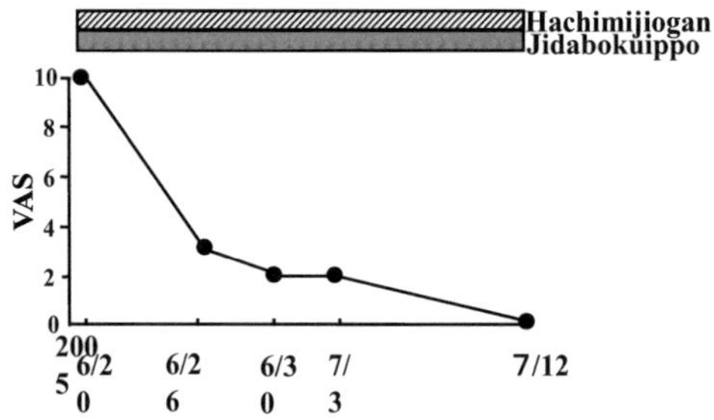

Figure 15. Change in pain (bruises after a traffic accident) after administration of Kampo medicines of a 67-year –old Japanese female

7.1.3. Sprain

Case 2: A 72-year-old Japanese female with osteoporosis and rheumatoid arthritis sprained her right ankle and was treated with the conventional therapies for 1 month without any improvement to her VAS score of 9. After initiating Kampo medicine, her pain disappeared completely after 14 days (Figure 16).

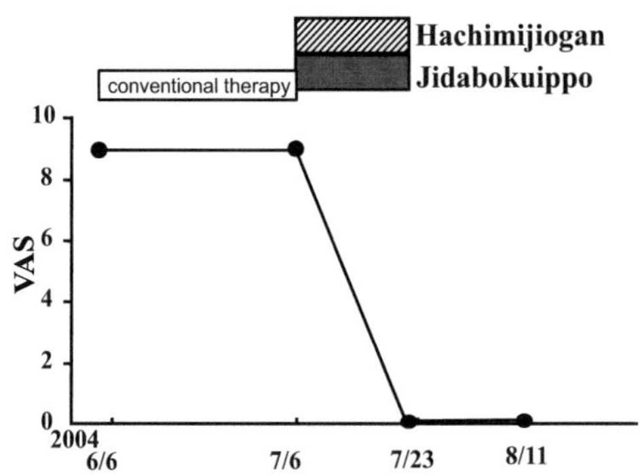

Figure 16. Change of pain (right ankle sprain) after administration of Kampo medicine (72 years female)

http://dx.doi.org/10.5772/60573

7.1.4. Arthritis

A 72-year-old Japanese female had been treated with conventional therapies for more than 6 years without stable recovery. After taking Kampo medicines for 14 days, she reported no pain (Figure 17).

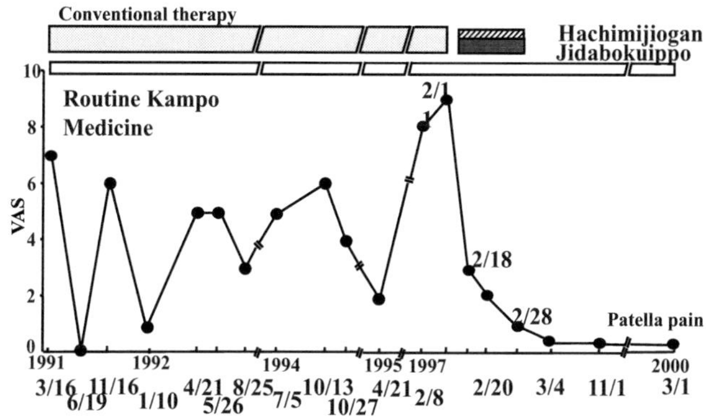

Figure 17. Change of pain of arthritis (patella) after administration of Kampo medicin (72- year-old female)

7.1.5. Discussion

Among components of 治打撲一方, gui-zhi (桂枝: *Chinamomi Cassesiae*) and ding-zi (丁子: *Caryophylli Flos*) promote blood circulation, and chuan-xiong (川芎: *Ligustici Chuanxiong* Rhizoma) accelerates blood circulation and blood stasis. In a Japanese clinical study, chuan-gu (川骨: *Nupharis* Rhizoma) was found to stop bleeding and accelerate the reabsorption of bleeding in the body. Da-huang (大黄: *Rhei* Rhizoma) removes substances produced by a resolving hematoma and other affected parts, which accelerates hematoma resolution. Po-su (樸樕: *Quercus* Cortex) is thought to have detoxifying, antiphlogistic, and astringent properties. Gan-cao (甘草: *Glycyrrhizae Uralensis* Radix) regulates and harmonizes other herbs. With Ba-wei-di-huang-wan (八味地黄丸), it serves as a kidney tonic and accelerates the bone metabolism, which supports the recovery of injured parts with two prescriptions (Tsumura & Co 7.5 g/day).

7.2. Acute herpes zoster [29]

7.2.1. Abstract

The intake of hot water extracts including Ganoderma lucidum or WTMCGEPP (Wisteria floribunda 0.38, Trapa natans 0.38, Miristica agrans 0.38, Coix lachryma-jobi 0.75, cultivated Ganoderma lucidum 0.75, Elfuinga applanata 0.38, tissue cultured Panax ginseng 0.3, and Punica granatum 0.38; numbers designate dry weight g/dose) decreased the pain of acute shingles in five Japanese patients, two with herpes zoster with trigeminal ophthalmia (74 years), one with lower body zoster (70 years), one with herpes zoster oticus (17 years), and one with leg herpes (28 years) without conventional therapies including antiviral drugs. In all patients, pain began to decrease within a few days of the initiation of intake and completely

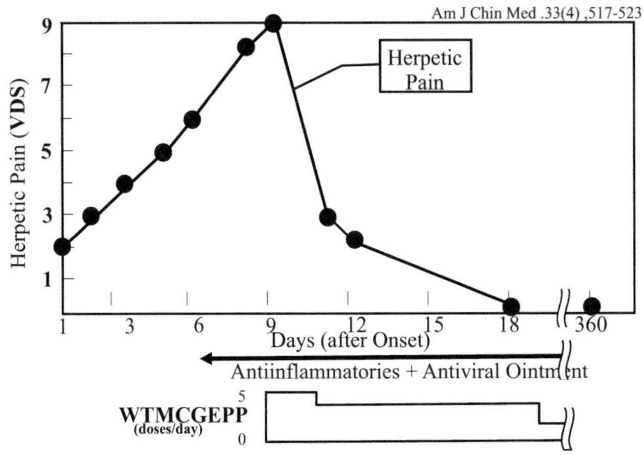

Figure 18. Acute Herpes Zoster with Opthalmia (73 yr male.)

disappeared within 10 days. There were no instances of postherpetic neuralgia (PHN) within a follow-up period of more than 1 year.

Additionally WTMCGEPP increased NK cell activity during intake of for 3 months in 4 females (mean: 51years) and in 9 weak infants who are outpatients of university hospital (data not shown).

Case 1: This patient was 158 cm tall and weighed 65 kg. Several days prior to his consultation, he had been on a bus tour and suffered lack of sleep and fatigue. On day 1, he felt pain on the left sinciput of his face. Vesicles appeared and the left half of his face was swollen with pain at a verbal descriptor scale (VDS) level of 1. His pain increased day by day and reached VDS 5 on the 6th day. He was diagnosed with shingles at a local hospital. Neither antiviral ointment nor anti-inflammatory medicine worked, and his pain increased to VDS 6. By day 8, the pain was intense and the patient's left eye was swollen shut with mucus and deteriorating skin lesions. When he visited us with VDS 9, we prescribed 5 doses per day of WTMCGEPP. After 2 days of administration, his pain started to decrease and his swollen face and eye improved enough that he was able to see clearly (Figure 18). Even though his doses were reduced, his pain continued to decrease, soon reaching VDS 2. By day 12, the patient's rhinorrhea had decreased significantly. On day 18, he achieved complete recovery with a VDS score of 0. At the time of writing, he has been pain-free for more than 10 years. Herbs composing WTMCGEPP was obtained from Tochimoto Tenkaido Co, Ltd.

Case 2: The patient was a 17-year-old Japanese female (165 cm, 54 kg) with acute herpes zoster otitis. She had become very tired due to lack of sleep while studying very hard for exams for 5 days before the onset of this pain. As she felt severe right ear pain, she visited an otolaryngologist, who diagnosed her with acute herpes zoster otitis and recommend starting conventional therapy immediately. However, she refused this treatment because her grandmother insisted on taking herbal medicines and requested WTMCGEPP therapy, which she started (6 doses per day) on the 3rd day from the onset of pain (Figure 19). The pain gradually decreased and, even though she then decreased her intake, her QOL remained satisfactory and her pain continued to decrease. On the 15th day, she was completely free of pain.

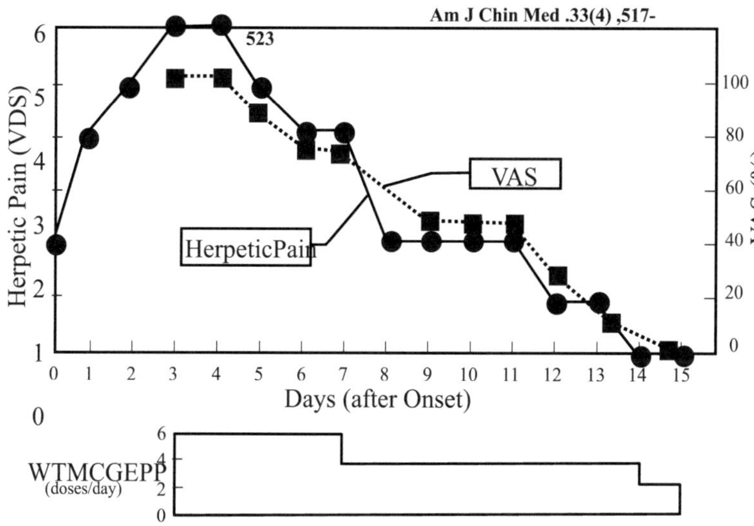

Figure 19. Acute Herpes Zoster Oticus (17 yr female)

Discussion: Only a combination of herbs is able to replace antiviral drugs for shingles. WTMCGEPP therapy can be begun at any time after the onset of shingles, while antiviral drugs must be started before 3 days after onset. This difference may be due to differences in the pain-killing mechanism. Further research is necessary to clarify this issue.

Addendum: WTMCGEPP was presented at the International Congress on Complementary & Alternative Medicines (ICCAM) in 2005, when many acupuncturists wanted to buy. But unfortunately it proved that selling them from Japan to another country was forbidden.

WTMCGEPP may be taken in many different types of cases to reduce pain and improve QOL. Evidences from my own experience include the following cases:

1. In advanced lung cancer who had brain metasis, WTMCGEPP worked to improve various aspects of the patient's degraded QOL, such as general fatigue, cough frequency, and bone pain in the metastatic lesions. The patient's family was told she had 2 months to live, but by taking this remedy, her symptoms almost disappeared and she survived with improved QOL for 2 years.

2. A patient who suffered cough and bone pain due to the metastasis of breast cancer to the lungs took this prescription. Her cough and bone pain gradually decreased and finally disappeared. Tumor marker decreased as well while she was taking this remedy. However, when she stopped taking it, thinking she had achieved complete recovery without consulting with me, she suffered recurrence.

3. WTMCGEPP worked in a weak infant suffering from infections related to Epstein-Barr virus (EBV), cytomegalovirus (CMV), and/or herpes simplex virus that required repeat admissions to the hospital [30, 31].

i. A 5-year-old boy with EBV and CMV infection suffering from frequent bronchial asthma and chronic bronchitis with fever was not cured by conventional therapy, but was cured by WTMCGEPP.

ii. A 6-year-old Japanese girl with herpes labialis suffered pain during eating which disappeared after 3 days of WTMCGEPP treatment.

iii. A 60-year-old man with herpes genitalis felt an unpleasant sensation with genital pain when he was tired. After intake of WTMCGEPP for several days, the pain disappeared. WTMCGEPP is a good choice for this patient because he seemed to develop tolerance for antiviral drugs.

iv. WTMCGEPP works herpes labialis and herpes genitalis very well. But patients with leukemia or lymphoma do not want to take it. Because of a feeling of wrongness. Of course, I never prescribe WTMCGEPP to them. I wish to study to find the reason.

4. In Japan, for patients suffering from hepatitis C, many Kampo medicines are applied. I often added WTMCGEPP not to progress to liver cancer, which seems relatively effective [32].

7.3. Menorrhagia-related pain

In Japan, gui-zhi-fuling-wan (桂枝茯苓丸) to remove blood stasis and accelerate blood circulation is most commonly used for menorrhagia-related pain. If this does not work, the dose is increased or a prescription to warm the Kidney yang, like Ba-wei-di-huang-wan, may be added. In more severe case of blood stasis, she-chong-yin (折衝飲) (tao-ren: 桃仁, 5; hong-hua: 紅花, 2; niu-xi: 牛膝, 3; mu-dan-pi: 牡丹皮, 3; chi-shao: 赤芍, 3; dang-gui: 当帰, 5; chuan- xiong: 川芎, 3; Yan-huo-suo: 延胡索, 3; gui-zhi: 桂枝, 3g/day) will work dramatically. Of course, dan-gui-shao-yao-san (当帰芍薬散) may be used in patients with a weak constitution. Patients with Qi stagnation and a disorder of the menstrual cycle may benefit from xion-gui-tiao-xue-yin (芎帰調血飲).

7.4. Glossodynia-related pain

Glossodynia is often difficult to cure with conventional therapies, but some Kampo medicines have been reported to be effective. I present one case here [33].

Case 1: A 74-year-old Japanese female (height, 150 cm; weight, 35 kg) suffered from sore tongue and appetite loss with atrophic gastritis since 1 year ago. She had had alopecia 5 years previously. On September 20 (X year), both sides of her tongue were reddish and rough. By October, her tongue was sore all over without fur (mirror tongue).

All treatment at a national hospital failed to improve her condition. One dentist recommended that she receive Kampo treatment. At her first visit to my clinic, she was diagnosed with Yin deficiency of the Heart and Spleen, Kidney Yang deficiency, Liver Qi depression tending to transform into fire based on oral dryness and heat, constipation, aversion to the cold, dry skin, depression and insomnia, a reddish tongue body without fur, dark sublingual vessels and string-like, slippery and sunken pulse.

Prescriptions: One-third of 1 day's intake of powder type of extracts of liu-jin-zi-tang (六君子湯) (can- shu: 蒼朮 4; da-cao: 大棗 3; ren-shen: 人参 4; chen-pi: 陳皮 2; ban-xia: 半夏 4; gan- cao: 甘草 1; fu-ling: 茯苓 4; sheng-jiang;生姜 0.5: numbers indicate g/day), and long-dan-xie- gan-tang (竜胆瀉肝湯) (dang-gui: 当帰 1.5, syao-yao: 芍薬 1.5, chuan-xiong: 川芎 1.5, di- huang: 地黄 1.5, huang-lian 黄連 1.5, huang-qin: 黄岑 1.5, huang-bo: 黄柏 1.5, shan-zhi-zi: 山梔子 1.5, lian-qiao: 連翹 1.5, bao- he: 薄荷 1.5, mu-tong: 木通 1.5, ban-fang-feng: 浜防風 1.5, che-qian- zi: 車前子 1.5, gan-cao: 甘草 1.5, and 2 g/day of long-dan: 竜胆; and ze-xie: 澤瀉) and 2/3 of 1 day's intake of ba-wei-di- huang- wan (八味地黄丸) (di-huang: 地黄 6, fu-ling: 茯苓 3, shan- zhu-yu: 山茱萸 3, mu-dan-pi: 牡丹皮 2.5, san-yao: 山薬 3, gui-pi: 桂皮 1; ze-xie: 澤瀉 3 and fu-zi: 附子 0.5; numbers indicate g/day) were administered until Xyear November 26th, when her tongue body was reddish and without fur, indicating a severe Yin deficiency. I added One day's intake of zi-yin-jiang- huo-tan (滋陰降火湯)/day (can-shu: 蒼朮 3, dang-gui: 当帰 2.5, di-huang: 地黄 2.5, mai-men-dong: 麦門冬 2.5; syao- yao: 芍薬 2.5, huang-bo: 黄柏 1.5, chen-pi: 陳皮 2.5, gan-cao: 甘草 1.5, tian-men-dong: 天門冬 2.5, and zhi-mu: 知母 1.5).

Three days later, she telephoned to tell me that her tongue pain had decreased dramatically, and on December 10 her tongue and stomach were pain-free, suggesting that her tongue pain stems from Yin deficiency (Fig.20).

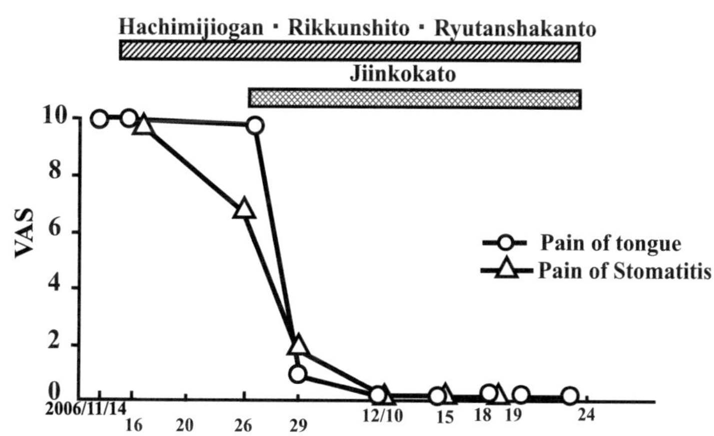

Figure 20. Change of tongue pain of case 1

Discussion: For intractable diseases, I experienced plural number of necessary prescriptions suitable for the organ with diseases (five element theory) are required to improve. As mentioned above, liu-jin-zi-tang (六君子湯) is for Spleen and long-dan-xie-gan-tang (竜胆瀉肝湯) is for Liver and ba-wei-di-huang-wan (八味地黄丸) was for Kidney and for total deficiency of yin, zi-yin-jiang- huo-tan (滋陰降火湯) was prescribed to get quick recovery. This means we finally treat five organs (five element theory) at a time which means the treatment with synergy with pleural prescriptions will be most important for intractable diseases (Fig.20).

8. Other diseases

8.1. Obstetrics- and gynecology-related diseases

1. The Japanese Kampo diagnosis method known as "Zheng" (証) helps to identify the problem in infertile women and, with the proper Kampo medicine treatment chosen based on "Zheng" (証) they may succeed in having a baby [34].

2. Amenorrhea sometimes is difficult to cure. A 23-year-old female (154cm; 50kg) had been taking female hormones for amenorrhea for 4 years. Soon after stopping the hormones, amenorrhea recurred. Intake of Ba-wei-di- huang-wan (八味地黄丸) with wen-jing-tang (温経湯) for 4 months did not work. Based on my diagnosis of Yang deficiency of the kidney and spleen, and dysfunction of the thoroughfare and conception vessels (衝任失調), I prescribed dang-gui-si-ni-jia-wu-zhu-yu-sheng-jiang-tang (当帰四逆加呉茱萸生姜湯) with pig placenta (胎盤) and xiong-gui-tiao-xue-yin (芎帰調血飲). Within 2 months, menstruation started again. Probably, the first two prescriptions cannot improve dysfunction of the thoroughfare and conception vessels and Kidney yang deficiency. But dang-gui-si-ni-jia-wu-zhu-yu-sheng- jiang-tang with Pig placenta tonify and warm Liver meridian, Kidney, and Spleen. Xiong-gui-tiao-xue-yin additionally supported to regulate qi and accelerate blood stasis which succeeded in curing her amenorrhea.

3. Premenstrual syndrome (PMS): Some females suffer from various type of PMS [35].

Case 1. One 46-year-old female who suffer from irritability was successfully treated with xiong-gui-tiao-xue-yin (芎帰調血飲 6 g/day) added with jia-wei-gui-pi-tang (加味帰脾湯 7.5 g/day) (full dose is 7.5 g/day) symptoms disappeared after 8 weeks.

Case 2. One 47-year-old female suffer depression spiritless and headache. She was treated with xiong-gui-tiao-xue-yin and gui-zhi-fu-ling-wan. Four weeks later all symptoms disappeared.

Case 3. One 34-year-old female suffer headache and hypogastrium pain and sensitiveness to cold who was successfully treated with dang-gui-si- ni-jia-wu-zhu-yu-sheng-jiang-tang and xiong-gui-tiao-xue-yin after 4 months' intake [35].

8.2. Epilepsy

To three adult patients with epilepsy refractory to standard antiepileptic medications, bu-yang-huan-wu-tang (補陽還五湯) were administered. All three patients showed substantial improvement in the frequency and severity of seizures. This treatment will rely on the resolution of blood stagnation in cerebrovascular systems [36].

8.3. "Five Elements Theory" must be applied to get the treatment

When we treat patients with various symptoms, we usually treat for severest symptoms like cough, with mai-men-dong-tang. This is for Lung. But sometimes prescriptions for lung did not cure cough at all. Example is shown below.

When patients suffering from chronic cough and various Kampo medicines for the cough do not work. To this case I apply "Five Elements Theory".

1. One 72-year-old female suffer chronic coughing. Her coughing started when she started to feel cold and get sensitiveness to cold probably because of her aging. I thought her aged Kidney deprive vital energy of lung which will cause her chronic cough. Actually, administration of ba-wei-di-huang- wan (八味地黄丸) stopped coughing after intake of 1 month.

2. Another case of diarrhea (38-year-old) which continued more than 3 weeks which did not response to various Kampo medicines for digestive system. I thought this diarrhea would be the result of Liver overwhelm the Spleen. I prescribed jia-wei-xiao-yao-san (加味逍遥散) to suppress Liver. A week later her diarrhea almost disappeared [37].

8.4. Application of Gui-zhi-fu-ling-wan (桂枝茯苓丸) for the diagnosis of breast cancer in diagnostic hormonal therapy

In spite of improvement in imaging technique for breast cancer, many latent microcarcinomas go undetected. Diagnostic hormonal therapy with antiestrogens may induce terrible side effects in some patients. Thus, excisional biopsy is required for an accurate diagnosis of malignancy.

Gui-zhi-fu-ling-wan (桂枝茯苓丸) has been effective in treating mastopathy and has almost no side effects. Thus, we tested its use as an alternative to antiestrogens. Gui-zhi-fu-ling-wan was administered to 116 patients out of 218 with mastopathy. Four were suspected to have breast cancer and were later definitively diagnosed with breast cancer, two by fine-needle aspiration cytology and two by excisional biopsy. Gui-zhi-fu-ling-wan proved to be useful in the diagnostic hormonal evaluation of mastopathy and in the diagnosis of breast cancer [38].

Author details

Yasuyo Hijikata*

Address all correspondence to: hijikata@hcn.zaq.ne.jp

Toyodo Hijikata Clinic, Ibaraki Osaka, Japan

References

[1] World Health Organization. TERMINOLOGIES/Cause of Disease (1.6.0): static blood (1.6.84). *WHO International Standard Terminologies on Traditional Medicine in the Western Pacific Region.* Geneva, Switzerland: World Health Organization; 2007: 45.

[2] World Health Organization. TERMINOLOGIES/Cause of Disease (1.6.0): dampness (1.6.14). *WHO International Standard Terminologies on Traditional Medicine in the Western Pacific Region.* Geneva, Switzerland: World Health Organization; 2007: 40.

[3] World Health Organization. TERMINOLOGIES/Mechanism of Disease (1.7.0): yang deficiency with yin exuberance (1.7.31). *WHO International Standard Terminologies on Traditional Medicine in the Western Pacific Region.* Geneva, Switzerland: World Health Organization; 2007: 48.

[4] Kamimura K, Nanba S, Tojo A, Matsuoka H, Sugimoto T. Effects of sairei-to on the relapse of steroid-dependent nephrotic syndrome. Am J Chin Med 1990;18 (1–2): 45–50.

[5] World Health Organization. TERMINOLOGIES/Cause of Disease (1.6.0): heat (1.6.17). *WHO International Standard Terminologies on Traditional Medicine in the Western Pacific Region.* Geneva, Switzerland: World Health Organization; 2007 40.

[6] World Health Organization. TERMINOLOGIES/Cause of Disease (1.6.0): heat (1.6.33). *WHO International Standard Terminologies on Traditional Medicine in the Western Pacific Region.* Geneva, Switzerland: World Health Organization; 2007: 41.

[7] Bensky D, Barolet R. Formulas that warm the channels and disperse cold. In: Scheid V, Bensky D, Ellis A, Barolet R, eds. Chinese Herbal Medicine: Formulas and Strategies. Vista, CA: Eastland Press;1990: 216–7.

[8] Herbs that clear heat. In: Scheid V, Bensky D, Ellis A, Barolet R, eds. Chinese Herbal Medicine: Formulas and Strategies. Vista, CA: Eastland Press;2004: pp.126–8.

[9] Herbs that regulate the blood. In: Bensky D, Clavey S, Stoger E, Gamble A, eds. Chinese Herbal Medicine: Materia Medica. 3rd edn. Vista, CA: Eastland Press; 2004: pp. 657–9.

[10] Herbs that regulate the blood. In: Bensky D, Clavey S, Stoger E, Gamble A, eds. Chinese Herbal Medicine: Materia Medica. 3rd edn. Vista, CA: Eastland Press; 2004: pp. 657–9.

[11] Herbs that regulate the blood. In: Bensky D, Clavey S, Stoger E, Gamble A, eds. Chinese Herbal Medicine: Materia Medica. 3rd edn. Vista, CA: Eastland Press; 2004: pp. 656–7.

[12] Bensky D, Barolet R. Formulas that clear heat and relieve toxicity. In: Scheid V, Bensky D, Ellis A, Barolet R, eds. Chinese Herbal Medicine: Formulas and Strategies. Vista, CA: Eastland Press; 1990: pp.78–9.

[13] Herbs that clear heat. In: Bensky D, Clavey S, Stoger E, Gamble A, eds. Chinese Herbal Medicine: Materia Medica. 3rd edn. Vista, CA: Eastland Press; 2004: pp.130–4.

[14] Herbs that clear heat. In: Bensky D, Clavey S, Stoger E, Gamble A, eds. Chinese Herbal Medicine: Materia Medica. 3rd edn. Vista, CA: Eastland Press; 2004: pp.95–8.

[15] World Health Organization. TERMINOLOGIES/Mechanism of Disease (1.7.0): yin deficiency with yang hyperactivity (1.7.24). *WHO International Standard Terminologies on Traditional Medicine in the Western Pacific Region*. Geneva, Switzerland: World Health Organization; 2007: 47.

[16] Yasui H. Appendix. Composition and indications of 148 prescriptions: three herbs baikal skullcap decoction. Kampo Acupuncture and Integrative Medicine. 2005; 1 (Special Edition): p.99.

[17] Herbs that clear heat. In: Bensky D, Clavey S, Stoger E, Gamble A, eds. Chinese Herbal Medicine: Materia Medica. 3rd edn. Vista, CA: Eastland Press; 2004: pp.120–3.

[18] Herbs that clear heat. In: Bensky D, Clavey S, Stoger E, Gamble A, eds. Chinese Herbal Medicine: Materia Medica. 3rd edn. Vista, CA: Eastland Press; 2004: pp.144–6.

[19] Hijikata, Y. Kampo medicines improved blood test and QOL in two vasculitis cases of Churg–Strauss syndrome and Henoch–ShOnlein purpura after inadequate treatment with conventional therapies. Int J Gen Med 2010;3: 93–9.

[20] Hijikata Y, et al. Alternative treatment for nephrotic syndrome using Ba-wei-di–huang-wan. J Tradit Med 1994;11: 29–37.

[21] Otsuka K. Tanpakunyo 3 dai, "Otsuka Keisetsu Chosakusyu 4" Shunyodo, pp.325–6, 1980.

[22] Yakazu D. Hachimi-jio-gan. "Rinsyo-oyo-Kampo-Shoho-Kaisetsu", Sogensya, pp.452–7, 1979.

[23] Keiken Kampo Shoho Bunryo syu, Ido no nihonsya.

[24] Hijikata Y, Kaneko J, Lu X, Nasu, M, Yamashita S. Traditional Chinese medicine improves the course of refractory leukemic lymphoblastic lymphoma and acute lymphocytic leukemia: two case reports. Am J Chinese Med 1995;23: 195– 211.

[25] Modak M, et al. Indian herbs and herbal drugs used for the treatment of diabetes. Int J Ayurveda Res 2010;1 (2): 112–21.

[26] Tensan et al. The effect of Tinospora cordifolia in rats hypercholesterol. J Tradit Med.

[27] Hijikata Y, et al. Treatment of hypertriglyceridemia using herbs. J Kampo Med 1999;50: 235–40.

[28] Hijikata Y, et al. Two kampo medicines, Jidabokuippo and Hachimijiogan alleviate sprains, bruises and arthritis. eCAM 2007;4: 463–7.

[29] HijikataY, Yasuhara A, Sahashi Y. Effect of an herbal formula containing Ganoderma lucidum on reduction of herpes zoster pain: a pilot clinical trial. Am J Chinese Med 2005;33: 517–23.

[30] Hijikata Y, Sentou S, Yasuhara A, Yoshida Y. Effect of herbal therapy for chronic inflammation of Epstein-Barr-virus, Varicella-Zoster-virus. J Kampo Med 2003;50: 97–103.

[31] Hijikata Y, Yamada S, Yasuhara A. Herbal mixtures containing the mushroom Ganoderma lucidum improve recovery time in patients with herpes genitalis and labialis. J Altern Complement Med 2007;13: 985–7.

[32] HijikataY. Treatment of liver diseases with Kampo medicine. Toseikampo- kenkyushitsu. 2010;33 (1, 2): 34–46.

[33] Hijikata Y, Makiura N, Kano T, Higasa K, Shimizu M, Kawata K, Mine T. Kampo medicine, based on traditional medicine theory, in treating uncured glossodynia: efficacy in five clinical cases. Am J Chinese Med 2008;36: 835–47.

[34] Kano Z, et al. Analysis based on Kampo medicine and conventional medicine about success in getting live birth with the treatment based on Japanese Kampo diagnosis. J Kampo Med 2008;59: 35–45.

[35] FjiwaraY, Hijikata Y. Modified xiong-gui-tiao-xue-yin (芎帰調血飲) succeeded in improving premenstrual syndrome (PMS) in four cases. J Kampo Med 2013;60 (3): 433–41.

[36] Hijikata Y, Yasuhara A, Yoshida Y, Sento S. Traditional Chinese medicine treatment of epilepsy. J Altern Complement Med 2006;12: 673–77.

[37] Hijikata Y. Application of "Five Elements Theory" for Treating Diseases, in: Kuang H, ed. Recent Advances in Theories and Practice of Chinese Medicine, 2012. http: // www.intechopen.com/books/recent-advances-in-theories- and- practice-of-chinese-medicine/application-of-five-elements-theory-for-treating-diseases

[38] Kotsuma Y, Hijikata Y. Application of keishi-bukuryo-gan for the diagnosis of breast cancer in diagnostic hormonal therapy. J Kampo Med 2000;51: 35–42.

Chapter 4

Low Back Pain from the Perspective of Traditional Iranian Medicine (TIM)

Mohammad Reza Vaez Mahdavi, Mohsen Naseri, Nafiseh Hoseini Yekta, Younes Roohany, Fatemeh Emadi and Soghrat Faghihzadeh

Additional information is available at the end of the chapter

http://dx.doi.org/10.5772/61170

Abstract

In this chapter the attitudes and opinions of Traditional Iranian medicine (TIM) about "low back pain: (LBP)" are considered. According to TIM, several main mechanisms for this very common disorder are explained. The spine, being far from the body heat source (heart) that sets the spine in coldest position, is considered in terms of temperament. The most common type of low back pain is cold temperament, simple or material. However, movements in the joints would cause heating, but the range of motion of the spine is very limited, so that its temperament remains cold, and the most common type of low back pain is caused by a cold temperament. Pain is the most common symptom whichabates with walking, rubbing, and warming, and usually becomes worse with the cold.

There is some adaptation of risk factors and causes of low back pain in conventional medicine compared to TIM attitudes. Traditional Iranian medicine (TIM) represents very interesting fields for research and therapy which can be considered economically effective and lead to prevention and treatment for LBP. TIM's insight clarify that gastrointestinal disorders are one of the most important causes of low back pain, and dyspepsia is at the top of this context. In this chapter there is analysis of the results obtained during a post-after designed clinical trial on patients who have chronic low back pain. It was treated with *Mentha longifolia,* which is known as an effective herbal medicine for dyspepsia chosen as the medicinal plant used in TIM. The results of this trial indicate that intervention was quite effective on both dyspepsia and low back pain. Our results achieved that the reduction of gastrointestinal symptoms leads to decrease in disability and pain symptoms associated with low back pain.

Keywords: Low back pain, Dyspepsia, Traditional Iranian Medicine (TIM), *Mentha longifolia*

1. Introduction

In this chapter, the attitudes and opinions of traditional Iranian medicine regarding the very common disease of "low back pain" are examined and a clinical trial conducted based on a therapeutic theory in Iranian traditional medicine is discussed.

First, the definition of medicine, its division in Iranian traditional medicine, and a brief introduction of traditional Iranian medicine and its attitude toward humans and diseases is given. Then, with this view in mind, low back pain is discussed.

Medicine is a science that studies changes in the human body, which can lead to the preservation of health or to disease.

In his book" Al-Qanun-Fi-Teb", Abu Ali Sina states: "Medicine is a science by which the human body's conditions is known in terms of what causes health and disease in order to preserve health and, in case of loss of health, returns health to the body."

The important point in this definition is that the medical purpose and the physician's main task is to preserve human health. Treatment is second in priority, and still, it is much higher than what is proposed in conventional medicine today as "preventive medicine."

2. Division of the science of medicine

Medical knowledge is divided into two parts: theoretical medicine and practical medicine.

a. Theoretical medicine:

The knowledge that examines the normal human function of body changes and factors affecting this function which lead to health or disease and which finally helps doctors make a diagnosis is called theoretical medicine. It consists of three parts:

1. Natural matters: Matters that are the base of life, consistency and the preservation of physical perfection of the human body (physiology).

2. Factors and causes: The reasons for changes in the human body and their influencing factors and how to check disease incidence (etiology and pathogenesis).

3. Arguments and symptoms: Symptoms and signs which guide the doctor to diagnose health or disease, such as temperament symptoms and the dominance of humors, pulse, and urine (semiotics).

b. Practical medicine:

Practical medicine includes methods for preserving health (health preservation science) and restoring health (treatment science). It consists of three parts:

1. Measures: food measures (food or regime therapy) and other related directives of principle 6, which will be presented.

2. Drug treatments with plant, animal, and mineral medicaments in oral and topical forms.

3. Manual application: Massage, acupressure, reflexology, etc., phlebotomy, and various surgeries.

Briefly, traditional Iranian medicine can be defined as a complete school and system, including diagnostic procedures, etiology, and treatment, based on intrapersonal differences (temperament) and on health preservation and the treatment of disease. Supported scientifically and empirically by several thousand years of Iranians and other nations, it regards the moral and cultural aspects and the Islamic doctrines that were reviewed and established through efforts by great scientists of the Islamic civilization, and the point of its perfection was reached. The characteristics of this school include holism, spiritual, physical, mental, and social trust for humans, a regard for active and passive qualities and the four humors, emphasis on disease prevention by lifestyle modification, strengthening spiritual views, and providing favorable conditions for internal system activity (called management power or nature). In this school, food and natural therapies take priority over drug treatments, single drug treatments take priority over compound drugs, and finally non-invasive treatments take priority over invasive treatments.[1]Temperament or individual differences, the infrastructure of the traditional Iranian medicine viewpoint:

What is considered the base of intrapersonal differences from the perspective of traditional Iranian medicine and upon which each treatment is based is called temperament. They can also be observed in combinations of hot and dry, hot and moist, cold and dry, or cold and moist. The human body is a composition of four elements: earth, water, air, and fire. It should be considered that they are different from earth, water, air, and fire that exist around us and each of these elements have their own especial properties:

- Earth: cold and dry
- Water: cold and moist
- Air: hot and moist
- Fire: hot and dry

A combination of different amounts of these elements creates numerous temperaments. No two people can have the same temperaments. Accordingly, healthy people in a simple classification temperament are divided into four main qualities: hot, cold, dry, and moist. They can also be observed in combinations of hot and dry, hot and moist, cold and dry, or cold and moist. These qualities can be created with or without material if material existed. Temperament is divided as follows: sanguineous (hot and moist), choleric (hot and dry), phlegmatic (cold and moist), melancholic (cold and dry).

Everything around us has a special temperament because each is a composition of the four elements[1].

Every person is born with a temperament. If one remains in compliance with the instructions necessary to preserve health and prevent disease, one's temperament throughout life will have no adverse changes, except those expected in every season, location, and different age periods.

If one does not comply with the given rules and measures for his temperament, however, one's temperament will be changed and will lean toward an adverse health condition, and those changes cause all or part of the function disorder.

The principles of health preservation and disease prevention that can be defined in terms of lifestyle is placed in the framework of six essential principles in Iranian traditional medicine: air, food, and drink; movement and rest; sleep and wakefulness; emotional states; cleansing the body; and keeping the essential material.

The most important part of the treatment program is also set by considering these six principles. These six principles and how they are applied in preventing and treating low back pain will be explained in the following section[1-2].

Given the different perspective of traditional Iranian medicine on categories of health and disease, searching through traditional Iranian medicine resources can be useful for finding different solutions and alternatives to conventional medicine for the prevention and treatment of diseases and for opening a new window to ways of dealing with these problems. Today, an important issue in society health is chronic diseases[3]. Currently, the prevention and control of chronic diseases is a major health concern [4]. Despite surprising advances in medical knowledge, many diseases, including low back pain, remain a mystery [5]. Low back pain, despite having an ancient history, is still epidemic in modern society [6]. This disease is one of the most common health problems in different world societies, especially in industrialized countries [7].

Low back pain is one of the most common causes of low patient referral to health and treatment professionals. It has been declared the fifth leading cause of reference to a doctor in America [8-9]. Between 1/2 and 3/4 of all adults will experience low back pain. About 40% of adults had a low back pain attack in one year, and at any given moment, 15–20% of the adult population suffers from low back pain [10]. Since all individuals with low back pain will not necessarily go to a health center, exact statistics on the prevalence of this disease are not known. In fact, only about 40% of patients with low back pain refer to health professionals for this problem. Previously the prevalence of this disease was considered 7–8%; it has now been declared as 40–50% [11]. In America, 176 million hours of useful work are lost annually due to this disease, and low back pain in the United Kingdom imposes annually £480 million of direct loss and £5 billion of indirect loss on the country's economy [12]. In recent years, $5–10 billion of rising costs in the United States are related to advanced imaging technologies. Low back pain is much more costly than other diseases such as rheumatoid arthritis, respiratory infectious diseases, Alzheimer's, diabetes, depression, multiple bridge sclerosis, embolism, and stroke [13-14]. These costs are direct costs of the disease; its social and indirect costs such as non-routine treatments and sick leave from work in the United States are estimated to be about $75–100 billion. With the variety of available treatments and advances in imaging techniques, it is expected that better treatment results would be seen compared to the past, but the results of these investigations do not indicate improvement [15].

Treatments include conservative measures and prescriptions for topical and systemic analgesic and anti-inflammatory medications or inhibitor drugs, modulators of the immune system, and surgery [9], each of which has its own side effects. A 2001 study in Sweden showed that 53.1% of men and 57.4% of women have cervical disc hernia disease and are treated with non-steroidal anti-inflammatory drugs [16]. Studies show that 15–20% of patients who chronically use non-steroidal anti-inflammatory drugs have ulcers of the stomach or duodenum [17]. Long-term use of these drugs has many complications for the patient, including physical dependence upon the drug, gastrointestinal disorders such as gastritis, nausea and vomiting, respiratory complications, myocardial infarction, and renal failure. Corticosteroid medications are not recommended for long-term use because of their immunosuppressive effects [18].

The efficacy of intrathecal injection is limited, and using an opioid may conversely cause increased sensitivity to pain. Moreover, surgery is sometimes associated with worse complications [15]. It is now suggested that bed rest, long considered a key part of treatment, be limited and only short term, because its effectiveness has not been proven [19]. The proper treatment of this disease is still unknown [20].

Low back pain is usually seen in the working age population, and therefore it imposes high economic costs on society [21]. Pain affects health, functionality, and the quality of life of patients; chronic pain causes physical and mental health involvement in adults and children [22].

Results of this investigation show that low back pain is a costly problem for present-day societies, and in many cases, classic medicine is an ineffective treatment. Given the global approach to supplemental medicine, searching for treatment strategies in schools of thought of supplementation, including that of Iranian traditional medicine, seems imperative.

This chapter has two parts:

1. The attitudes and opinions of traditional Iranian medicine regarding the very common disease of low back pain are examined.

2. Clinical trial conducted based on a therapeutic theory in traditional Iranian medicine is discussed.

3. Low back pain causes in Iranian traditional medicine

Ibn Sina considered low back pain a muscle and tendon disease (what comes from the muscles to the bones). Basically, what will come in the future from causes mainly affects the members, and what causes the members' disorder will have a serious effect on the performance of the spine. These causes are also expressed in conventional medicine for low back pain. Bone disorders are less considered for low back pain, and low back pain is mostly associated with muscle problems. Pain due to muscle spasm has been mentioned as a mechanism for low back pain, and the major role played by muscles in preserving back health has been emphasized.

Since nervous diseases are discussed, muscular disorders are presented, because, by definition in the rule book, the muscle is a part composed of nerves, and because the nerve does not have the capability of binding to the bone, a rougher part, that is the tendon, connects to it that transfers motion commands to the bone. The existing space between the nerves is filled with flesh and a membrane covers it; that, in fact, is a nerve muscle. Muscle relaxation is caused by diluted moisture that muscle strength is lower than normal and seizure in muscle where muscle length is low and its width is high includes a variety of dry and moist adverse health that moist type is condensed due to moisture and frequent and shows symptoms suddenly. Sometimes seizure is bilateral, where the length is high and width is low and is called "TAM-ADOD" [23]. Each of these disorders can also occur in lumbar muscles and cause pain. In other words, the causes given in the following text in most cases affect muscular structure.

1. **Simple hot temperament**: This type of low back pain is related to body heating causes. If any of the causes of heating becomes imbalanced, it can cause hot temperament. This could be in general or due in part to the effect of the cause.

2. **Simple cold temperament or phlegmatic temperament in the back**: The most common types of low back pain are cold temperament, simple or material. The spine, being far from the body heat source (heart) and lacking a range of movement in the coldest position, is considered in terms of temperament. One may propose that the joints are farther to the back. In response, it should be said that a lot of movements in the joints would cause its heating; however, the range of motion of the spine is very limited. Because of this, its temperament is cold, and the most common type of low back pain is caused by a cold temperament.

3. **Excessive sex and fatigue:** This can cause dryness due to the effect of decreased body moisture, and muscle disorder occurs due to dryness. It can stimulate the loss of raw material and condense moisture or phlegm to the area, in which case symptoms would be different.

4. **Anger**: As previously stated, anger can stimulate material and cause phlegm to reach the back. In fact, some factors such as anger, sex, and excessive fatigue can cause low back pain due to the flux of material to the position. If pain on the back or joints occurs due to flux of material, depending on the material dilution or concentration, symptoms such as inguinal hernia and upper or lower limb swelling, enlarged lymph nodes in the inguinal, axillary, and gluteus can be experienced.

5. **Shape change and curvature of the spine**: Anatomical changes can be caused by a hit or, without it, the direction change can be side or front and rear protrusions. From the perspective of Iranian traditional medicine, each factor consists of swelling in one direction, the presence of diluted moisture that causes loss of muscle strength, and/or condensed moisture that increases muscle strength, and shortening its length can change the direction of vertebra and their protrusion and cause low back pain. The risk of curvature of the spine structural disorder in children whose feeding is begun early is high because of the production of condensed moisture.

6. **With the participation of some viscera**:

    a. GI: The four stages in traditional Iranian medicine are expressed for material entering the body to be digested as a part of the organ. First digestion occurs in the stomach, and its disorder can be directly associated with organ dysfunction, because the

http://dx.doi.org/10.5772/61170

material's conversion process will be disrupted by the non-production of adequate mucus. Disruption in weaker organs is expressed more, and organ weakness occurs more in less heated organs. As the back is one of the coldest organs, it will suffer from dyspepsia. When digestion is impaired, more gas is produced in the GI; the existence of these gases can pass through the membranes of the gastrointestinal tract and reach the back area, thus causing low back pain. In traditional Iranian medicine resources, the stomach temperament in most patients with dyspepsia is cold. Clinical trials mentioned in this section also confirmed the result that patients with dyspepsia suffering low back pain are in fact patients who, in most cases, have cold and moist dyspepsia simultaneously in the back and stomach.

b. Kidney: Stones in the urinary tract and kidney failure may be associated with low back pain.

c. Uterine problems**:** Closer to menstruation, delayed menstruation, lack of proximity, delivery pain.

4. **At the critical stage of the disease**: In Iranian traditional medicine, it is believed that some diseases reach a stage in which one symptom is material excretion in urine or stools; in other words, low back pain, urination, or diarrhea are observed [23-24-25].

4. Low back pain Signs and symptoms in Iranian traditional medicine

The signs and symptoms of each type of low back pain and methods of diagnosis will be discussed separately.

1. Low back pain due to simple hot temperament:

This type of low back pain has inflammation in the area and its pain is not with weight. There is no beat. Common symptoms of hot temperament may be chromatic urine and thirst, which abate with the ingestion of cold temperament foods.

2. Low back pain due to simple cold temperament:

Gradual pain without weight that abates with walking, rubbing, and warming and sometimes becomes worse with the cold. Often, the back is cold to the touch.

3. There is raw moisture and phlegm in the back muscles and spine that are produced in the back area:

Gradual pain with weight abates with warming, walking, and rubbing and sometimes becomes worse with the cold and at night. Sometimes the back is cold to the touch.

4. Extreme sex, fatigue, anger, or whatever causes flux phlegm, moisture, and/or gas in the back:

In patients who have mucus loss in the back, sudden severe with weight in the back and constant intensity. If the pain reaches the position by the preceding factors, the pain is like tension and transmitted with less weight.

Sometimes fatigue, heavy loads, bending, and excess sex without loss of materials cause pain which is felt as soreness in the muscles.

5. Due to deviation of the spine and herniated vertebral:

If this condition is caused by an injury, the individual's history indicates it. If it is due to the presence of moisture in the place, the oil when massaged into the skin will not be absorbed. If the low back pain occurs due to dryness of spine deviation, oil absorption will be observed when the back is massaged with oil. Sometimes gas in the spine will cause this, but in this case the pain will be different and spine protrusions will occur after low back pain.

6. In participation with other organs:

If it is partnered with the **digestive system** by dyspepsia, symptoms such as bloating, dyspepsia, and heaviness after a meal will occur. Sometimes there may be nausea and vomiting, and low back pain or constipation may be observed. If it is partnered with the **urinary system:** the symptoms due to stones in the urinary tract and kidney failure may be exist with low back pain.In partnership with **uterus**: Low back pain is also seen at times of childbirth or menstruation and in individuals with irregular menstrual periods, low bleeding, or undesired sexual relations. Low back pain due to crisis: If fullness is in the intestines, diarrhea occurs, and if it is in the kidneys, it takes the form of increased urine volume and changes in urine color and density [23-24-25].

- As noted, the main cause of low back pain in most cases can be traced to muscular disease which, in most cases, includes structural abnormalities including muscle shortening and thickening, becoming long and thin or loss of muscle strength.

Among causes also expressed in modern medicine for low back pain, bone disorders are less considered. Low back pain is mostly associated with muscular problems. The mentioned mechanisms for pain in the back area and pain due to muscle spasm are accepted, and the important role of muscles in the preservation of back health is emphasized. Given the multifactorial nature of low back pain and the controversy in determining its most common cause, specific views exist regarding its natural treatment, some of which have serious opposition; however, the use of active participation methods is confirmed by all [26]. Various exercises influencing different muscles can improve low back pain [27-28-29]. Interestingly, clinical trials have shown that the only therapeutic method proven to be effective in all trials is sports and physical activities. Each of them reinforces one set of muscles of the abdomen and back, including the paravertebrals [30]. In some studies, the relationship between muscle weakness and pain intensity and also that between the muscle cross-sectional area and inability resulting from low back pain has been proven [27], and body muscle dysfunction is acceptable as a cause of low back pain continuity. Even low back pain resulting from psychological states, such as anxiety or anger, has muscle tension and stress, and by decreasing the psychological pressure, the tension and stress will be reduced [28]. traditional Iranian medicine explains this issue as a sudden loss of material in muscles. It has been seen several times at the bedside of a person with severe anger that this person's low back pain is due to a loss of material in the back muscles and tendons. Even in psychological pressure and sensual complication, the role of muscles and their involvement are emphasized and confirmed, and psychotherapy procedures for low back pain also control the removal of muscle spasms [31]. Therapeutic techniques such as water therapy can reduce pain in such patients by increasing the flexibility of muscles, which subsequently reduces muscle spasms [29].

5. Relationship between low back pain risk factors in conventional medicine and from the traditional medicine perspective

In terms of temperament in Iranian traditional medicine, the back is far from the body's heat source (heart) and, being the body's coldest region, has a limited range of motion. The most common type of low back pain is cold type either with or without a medium of material. The low back pain risk factors in modern medicine confirm the traditional medicine viewpoint in this regard; therefore, low back pain risk factors in modern medicine are the factors that, in traditional medicine, cool the temperament [32-1]. They are given in Table 1.

Risk factor of low back pain in modern medicine	Conformity to traditional medicine view about the prevalence of low back pain with cold temperament
Obesity	Obesity is often caused by a cooling body temperament and waste and moisture accumulation.
Age over 50 years	This age in traditional medicine is the period that the body has a cold temperament.
Female	In comparing the two genders, the female is cooler.
Psychological stress and disorders	Major categories of stress cause an inherent heat decrease and a generally cold temperament, and consequently organ temperament.
Body heavy works	Inherent heat decrease causes cooling of the body.
Sitting works	Accumulation of moisture and moderate heat cause heat decrease and cold temperament.

Table 1. Adaptation of risk factors of low back pain in conventional medicine to traditional medicine view

6. Recommendations in traditional Iranian medicine for preventing low back pain

Recommendations for preventing low back pain with respect to the six principles of traditional Iranian medicine are listed in the following text.

Note: Since the most common type of low back pain is the cold type (simple or material), recommendations are provided based on that type.

6.1. Air

Air is the most important of the six causes, and since each person is permanently associated with it, it has a particular effect on health. In order to prevent a recurrence of low back pain, the following are recommended for everyone.

1. Avoid exposure to cold weather for long periods, such as normal weather turning in winter or synthetic cold from air conditioners.

2. Avoid exposure to hot weather for long periods, such as exposure to extreme hot weather in outdoor jobs, like farming.

3. Avoid contact with surfaces that have low temperatures, such as tile, ceramic, and plaster that transfer cold to the organ.

4. Cover the back with a suitable cover at all times.

5. If attempting to carry out business or exercise activities in a cold environment, using a heated cover in the back area is strongly recommended.

6. Avoid living in moist and humid environments.

6.2. Food and drink

Nutrition is another essential cause that has direct relationship with the back, and the relationship between low back pain and dyspepsia are clear. Three major matters 1) how much to eat; 2) what to eat; and 3) how to eat are discussed as they pertain to the prevention and treatment of low back pain.

6.2.1. How much to eat?

Traditional medicine resources and modern medicine emphasize reducing food consumption for the prevention and treatment of low back pain. In terms of the amount and number of calories, this is applicable in three forms.

1. Consume less food in a diet that consists of low-calorie foods; at the same time the quality of food should cause a positive effect on the quality of the disease (eating cold **temperament** foods is less recommended).

2. Maintain consistency in the amount of food consumed, and the diet should consist of low-calorie foods.

3. Reduce the amount of foods, but the diet should not be low-calorie in terms of energy.

Any one of the three diets is selected based on a patient's strengths and weaknesses.

It is important to note that an extreme reduction in food intake can cause a cold temperament and, consequently, low back pain.

6.2.2. *What to eat?*

From research in modern medicine and traditional medicine resources, the following recommendations are summarized:

1. Avoid eating foods that are hard to digest and are more likely to make mucus. Processed foods and fast food fall into this category.
2. Eat foods that are more quickly digested, that cause a lightheadedness after eating them, and that do not put an additional burden on the digestive system.
3. Eating hot **temperament** foods is recommended for these individuals.
4. Avoid eating fruit, especially peaches and plums. Low back pain patients should not eat dried figs.
5. Avoid beets, carrots, and cucumbers.
6. Avoid alcoholic drinks.
7. Avoid meat, particularly beef and pork.
8. Avoid pickles.

6.2.3. *How to eat?*

The importance of the time of eating and drinking is noted in resources of traditional medicine and is summarized in the following:

1. Consider the principles of drinking water and other liquids, including not drinking water with meals, fasting at midnight, or when the body is warm, like after exercise, intercourse, or in the bathroom.
2. Avoid eating at the same time and eating together in the sense that one type of food is eaten at each meal and food intake is done after gastric emptying the previous meal.

6.3. Sleep and wakefulness

traditional Iranian medicine considers the amount and location of sleeping.

6.3.1. *How much sleep?*

1. Avoid sleeping too much, which causes the accumulation of moisture in the body.
2. Avoid too much wakefulness that prevents a person from revitalizing.
3. Avoid long naps during the day.
4. In the treatment of patients with acute low back pain, modern medicine recommends against bed rest for more than 2–3 days; traditional medicine also recommends against excessive bed rest, because it causes a long break moisture decrease.

6.3.2. Where to sleep?

1. Considering the cold quality of the disease, the temperature and location of sleep is important; it is recommended that sleeping in cold and damp locations be avoided.

- **Movement and rest:**

One of the most important causes associated with low back pain is sports. The only method of prevention and treatment confirmed as effective in numerous articles is physical movement. Although the reviewed articles suggested that there is a need for comprehensive research to compare different sport systems, it is clear that exercise is effective in prevention of first, second, and third levels.

Exercising in moderation strengthens, and it is recommended for all. It is not recommended by the experts but after passing acute phase, exercise is recommended at all times. Because of its beneficial and positive role, balanced exercise is approved. Doing extreme movements in terms of quality or quantity can be harmful. In summary, the following recommendations are given regarding physical movement:

1. Do moderate exercise and physical movements to prevent and treat low back pain.
2. Avoid extreme immobilization and high inertia.
3. Avoid heavy work and excessive fatigue. It is recommended that heavy loads be carried in the correct manner. The prevalence of low back pain in people who have heavy work is equal to people who work in an office, but radiological changes are more in people who do heavy work.
4. According to the traditional medicine view on the common temperament of the disease, it seems that using chairs made of metal that transmit cooling could have a negative effect on prevention or treatment of the disease. There is, however, a need for further research.
5. Traditional medicine also recommends that one wear shoes of a natural type that can be helpful in transmitting heat and protecting feet from cold.
6. Avoid sitting in awkward and fixed positions. This is especially recommended for people who work in an office.

- **Emotional states:**

As in all research, the relationship between low back pain and psychological issues has been proven. In traditional medicine, this issue is also important, and one of the causes of low back pain is anger. The following recommendations are provided in this regard:

1. Avoid continuous stress and anxiety-causing situations that can cause muscle spasms.
2. Avoid computer games that cause stress in children and adolescents.

6.4. Cleansing the body and keeping the essential material

If the means of waste disposal in the body are disrupted, the body's moisture retention capacity causes low back pain, such as in menstrual disorders, being deprived of intercourse in the person who is used to having it, menopause, stopping bleeding from hemorrhoids that for some people is a way of disposal, constipation, urinary retention, impaired perspiration, or perspiration breaker treatments, delayed bathing, and similar cases which all can be effective in the development or recurrence of low back pain.

On the other hand, the loss of many materials needed by the body can make the body more prone to this disease, such as too much intercourse, excessive fatigue, prolonged disease, and prolonged and frequent bathing that removes moisture from the body (one sign of this is shriveling finger skin) [1-23-24-25].

7. Conclusion

In most cases, low back pain is a muscular disease that causes pain, and most of its causes and reasons explained in both traditional and modern medicine confirm the important role of muscles. This very common disease is in most cases of the cold temperament type that can be prevented by complying with simple recommendations of health preservation and life style, many of which are approved by both medical points of view. In Iranian medicine, preventive recommendations are in six categories: air, foods, and drinks; movement and rest; sleep and wakefulness; emotional states; cleansing the body; and keeping the essential material, which are known health as principles. Moreover, many of these recommendations are useful in treatment or in preventing a recurrence of the disease.

8. Analysis on a Clinical trial on patients with chronic low back pain based on traditional Iranian medicine issue about participation back and gastrointestinal system

As was discussed in the section on the causes of low back pain, traditional Iranian medicine views gastrointestinal disorders as causes of low back pain, and at the top of this list is dyspepsia. The elders of traditional Iranian medicine initially advised patients with low back pain to treat their disorders of digestion [23]. In order to examine this idea, a clinical trial was performed in which patients with chronic low back pain who were also diagnosed with functional dyspepsia were treated with an effective drug for dyspepsia from the perspective of traditional Iranian medicine as described in the following text.

8.1. Study sample size

Since there was no similar study, in the first stage, a sample size of 30 people for each group was considered with the provision that this number would be increased if necessary. Since the results of data analyses indicate the achievement of the study objectives, the study was completed with 60 people.

8.2. Sampling method

Sampling was done by available samples to achieve desired sample size.

Target population: All patients 20–55 years old having the study inclusion criteria.

Study population: Patients 20–55 years old admitted to neurosurgery clinic.

8.2.1. Inclusion criteria for the study

Men and women 20–55 years old having had symptoms of low back pain for more than 3 months and having pain at the time of inclusion, dyspepsia symptoms according to the signs of ROME III (valid questionnaires to diagnose dyspepsia) [33], consistent symptoms from 3 months prior to inclusion in the study, and onset of low back pain at least 6 months prior to inclusion in the study.

Symptoms of patients who were diagnosed comprised

1. One or more of the following:

   a. Bothersome postprandial fullness after a normal-sized meal occurred at least several times a week.

   b. Early satiation that prevented ending a regular feeding and occurred at least several times a week.

2. No evidence of structural disease (including at upper endoscopy) that is likely to explain the symptoms.

8.2.2. Exclusion criteria

Patients who reported the following symptoms were excluded from the study:

- Intensified pain at night or at rest, previous history of cancer, history of chronic infection, history of stroke, urinary incontinence, age over 50 years, age below 20 years, intravenous drug abuse, history of corticosteroid use, history of progressive neurological deficit, unexplained fever, unexplained weight loss, percussion pain in the spine, abdominal, rectal, and pelvic mass, percussion or Patrick heel mark, straight leg raising(SLR), and progressive focal neurological symptoms.

- Symptoms of gastro esophageal reflux disease (GERD) as burning, painful swallowing, history of gastrointestinal surgery, specific symptoms of irritable bowel syndrome (IBS), any abdominal pain, overnight diarrhea and fatty feces, immune system disease, mental abnormality, presence of risk for symptoms such as excessive weight loss, black, tarry, or bloody stools, the presence of uncontrolled severe organ diseases such as cancer or kidney disease, progressive symptoms, use of aspirin or non-steroidal anti-inflammatory drugs (NSAIDs), use of steroids or narcotics, and women who were pregnant or breastfeeding.

In the selection stage, patients who were taking any antibiotics or a proton pump inhibitor (PPI), H2 blockers such as ranitidine, cimetidine, or famotidine, Prokinetic drugs like Dom-

http://dx.doi.org/10.5772/61170

peridone and metoclopramide, consuming lactulose or similar compositions, consuming other herbal drugs, or involved in other research projects were excluded from the study.

Duration of study: Intervention duration and the follow-up period were each 4 weeks, making a total of 8 weeks.

8.3. Study variables and measurement tools

a. Pain intensity due to low back pain was measured by an NRS system that divided the patients into four groups: no pain (0), mild (1), moderate (4-6), and severe (10).

b. Functional disability was measured using the Oswestry questionnaire.

Total score is a fraction of the 50 scores (maximum possible score) multiplied by 100 to get an overall percentage. Patients were divided into the five classes including mild (0–20%), moderate (21–40%), severe (41–60%), crippled (61–80%), and bed bound (81–100%) [34].

c. Severity of dyspepsia was measured by LEEDS questionnaire, and its total score was considered. The results were divided to 4 groups: mild [1-12], moderate [13-24], severe [25-36], very severe [37-4] [35].

Overall body temperament and stomach and back temperaments were examined separately by questionnaire upon arrival.

In this study, pain intensity and functional disability due to low back pain and dyspepsia intensity were measured before intervention, at the end of the second and fourth weeks, and eight weeks after intervention.

9. Intervention

According to the authoritative texts of Iranian traditional medicine, *Mentha longifolia* which is known as an effective herbal medicine for dyspepsia was chosen as the medicinal plant used in this study [23-24]. Aqueous extract of *M. longifolia* was prepared. The medicine was prepared in 500 mg capsules containing 250 mg concentrated *M. longifolia* extract and 250 mg starch as filler.

Medicine standardization

Total phenolic compounds of this extract were determined with Folin–Ciocalteu's reagent [36] that used gallic acid as a standard phenolic compound. The total phenolic contents in the extract was 39.1±1.6 mg GA/g. The contents of flavonoids in the extract was determined with spectrophotometric method [37] using rutin as a standard. The total flavonoids contents in the examined extract was 7.58±1.47mg RU/g.

9.1. Analysis the results

In order to analyze the results in four periods of the variables studied, the Friedman test was used.

9.2. Results

In this study, the mean age of the patients was 41.3±9.6 years. Fourteen patients were male (46.7%) and the rest were female. The mean body mass index (BMI) was 26.3 ± 3.4.

The maximum frequency of general temperament with a frequency of 16 was related to moist and cold temperament; the maximum frequency of the stomach (a frequency of 25) was also consistent with general temperament and was moist and cold. Furthermore, 83.3% of patients had the cold and moist temperament in their back, which is still in line with the general and stomach temperaments indicating a cold and moist temperament.

Table 2 shows the results of functional disability. Results indicate that in the beginning of the study, 14 patients had moderate functional disability resulting from low back pain, 14 patients had severe functional disability due to low back pain, and 2 patients had crippled low back pain. At the end of the eighth week, all patients were placed into the group of minimal disability. Friedman's nonparametric test was used, and the results indicated that the scale had a statistically significant difference (P = 0.001).

Time		Pre	2 weeks	4 weeks	8 weeks
The number of patient		30	30	30	30
Relative frequency percentage of functional disability	MINIMIZE	0	50	100	100
	MODERATE	46.7	50	0	0
	SEVERE	46.7	0	0	0
	CRIPPLED	6.7	0	0	0
	BED-BOUND	0	0	0	0
mean±SD		43.2±8.4	21.3±4.3	6.9±1.4	4.9±1.6
Friedman's nonparametric test		0.001			
SD: Standard deviation					

Table 2. Functional disability (Oswestry disability index) due to chronic low back pain

30 patients in clinical trial with chronic low back pain with functional dyspepsia who used *Mentha longifolia for 4 weeks* Values are expressed as mean (95% confidence interval). Friedman's nonparametric test was used, and the results indicated that the scale had a statistically significant difference (P = 0.001).

Table 3 shows information about severity of pain. At the beginning of the study, 22 patients had moderate low back pain, and 8 of them had severe low back pain. At the end of the eighth week, all patients were placed in the group of minimal low back pain. The Friedman nonparametric test was used, and results indicated that the scale of this group had a statistically significant difference (P = 0.001).

Time		Pre	2 weeks	4 weeks	8 weeks
The number of patient		30	30	30	30
Relative frequency percentage of severity of pain	NO PAIN	0	0	0	0
	MILD	0	33.3	80.0	100
	MODERATE	73.3	66.7	20.0	0
	SEVERE	26.7	0		0
Mean± SD		5.8±0.9	3.9±1.01	2.6±0.9	2.07±0.6
Friedman's nonparametric test			0.001		
SD: Standard deviation					

Table 3. Severity of pain (NRS) due to chronic low back pain

30 patients in clinical trial with **chronic low back pain with functional dyspepsia** who used *Mentha longifolia for 4 weeks.* Values are expressed as mean (95% confidence interval). Friedman's nonparametric test was used, and the results indicated that the scale had a statistically significant difference (P = 0.001).

Table 4 and Diagram 1 show that all patients at the beginning of the study had dyspepsia with different intensity levels, including moderate, severe, and very severe. At the end of the study, all participants had only mild dyspepsia.

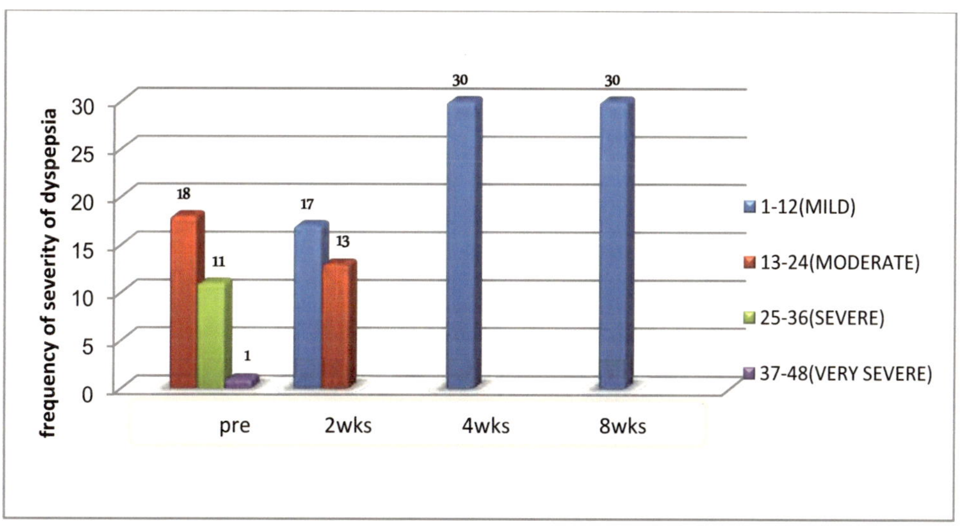

Diagram 1. Severity of dyspepsia at four different times.

30 patients in clinical trial with **chronic low back pain with functional dyspepsia** who used *Mentha longifolia for 4 weeks.* Values are expressed as frequency

Time		Pre	2 weeks	4 weeks	8 weeks
The number of patient		30	30	30	30
Relative frequency percentage of severity of dyspepsia	MILD	0	6.4	100	100
	MODERATE	6.8	4.9	0	0
	SEVERE	4.2	0	0	0
	VERY SEVERE	.4	0	0	0
Mean± SD		22.6±6.45	12±3.6	5.3±2.6	2.7±1.02
Friedman's nonparametric test			0.001		
SD: Standard deviation					

Table 4. Severity of dyspepsia due to functional dyspepsia

30 patients in clinical trial with **chronic low back pain with functional dyspepsia** who used *Mentha longifolia for 4 weeks.* Values are expressed as mean (95% confidence interval). Friedman's nonparametric test was used, and the results for severity of **functional dyspepsia** indicated that the scale had a statistically significant difference (P = 0.001).

In Diagram 2, the results of severity of pain and dyspepsia are shown together. The results of severity of disability and dyspepsia are shown together in Diagram 3.

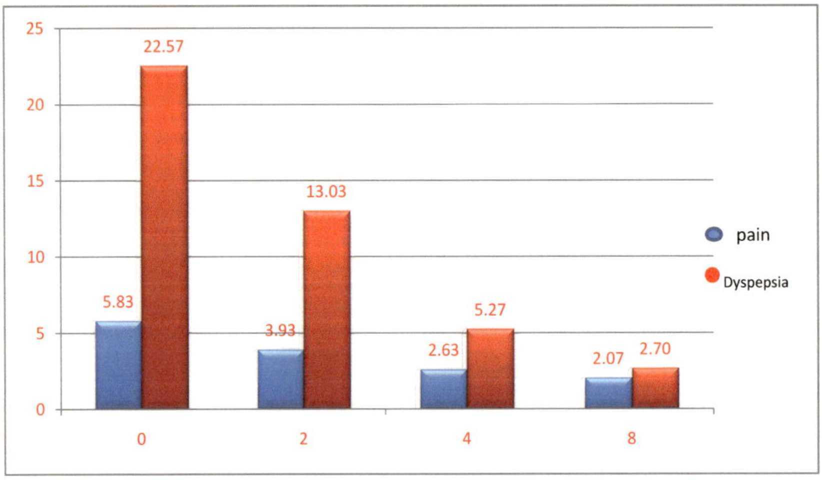

Diagram 2. Severity of pain and dyspepsia at four different times.

Patients in clinical trial with **chronic low back pain with functional dyspepsia** who used *Mentha longifolia for 4 weeks.* Values are expressed as frequency.

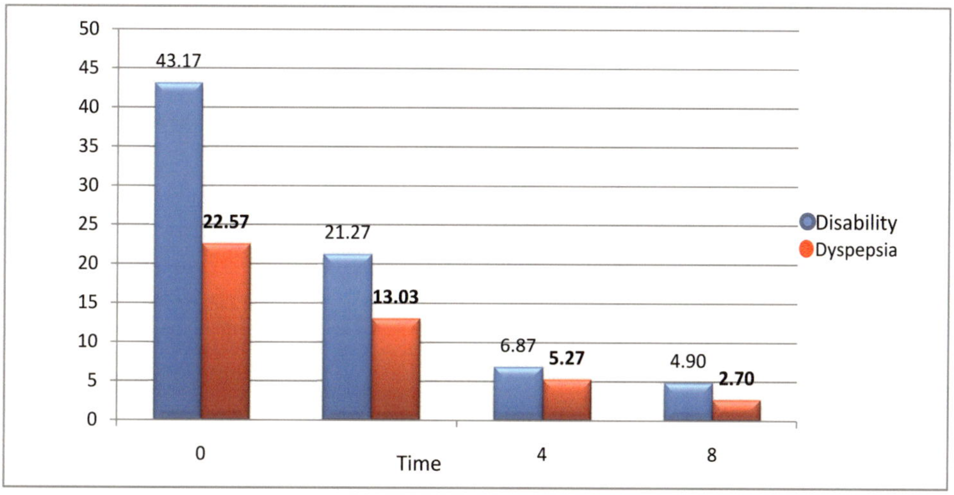

Diagram 3. Severity of disability and dyspepsia at four different times

Patients in clinical trial with **chronic low back pain with functional dyspepsia** who used *Mentha longifolia for 4 weeks.* Values are expressed as frequency.

In order to investigate the correlation severity of pain and dyspepsia, Pearson's correlation coefficient was used. This analysis indicated that in 4 periods there is a direct linear relationship between severity of dyspepsia and pain severity. This result repeated about correlation between severity of dyspepsia and disability due to low back pain. There is a direct linear relationship between them in 4 periods.

10. Discussion and conclusion

The purpose of this trial was to investigate the relationship between dyspepsia and low back pain according to traditional Iranian medicine issue. Although research indicates that dyspepsia and low back pain are synchronized [38-39], so far no trial has been conducted to examine the relationship between them. The results of this trial indicate that intervention was effective on dyspepsia and low back pain simultaneously. Reduction in symptoms of gastrointestinal problems leads to decrease in symptoms associated with low back pain (pain and disability). Although a positive Pearson coefficient did not show a causal relationship between them, it did indicate a direct relationship between dyspepsia and back pain. Of course, more extensive research with a larger number of participants would achieve more accurate results.

Author details

Mohammad Reza Vaez Mahdavi[1*], Mohsen Naseri[1], Nafiseh Hoseini Yekta[1], Younes Roohany[2], Fatemeh Emadi[1,3] and Soghrat Faghihzadeh[4]

*Address all correspondence to: mh_mahdavi@yahoo.com

1 Traditional Medicine Clinical Trial Research Center, Shahed University, Tehran, Iran

2 School of Medicine, Shahed University, Tehran, Iran

3 Department of Iranian Traditional Medicine, Faculty of Medicine Shahed University, Tehran, IR, Iran

4 Epidemiology and Biostatistics Department, Statistics-Faculty, Zanjan, University of Medical Sciences, Zanjan, Iran

References

[1] Arzani, M. A.; Mofarah-ol-Gholoub, editing and research Nazem, E., Baghbani, M., almaee Publications, Tehran, 2011: 101-130.

[2] Arzani, M. A.; Mizan-O-Teb, Revision by Hadi Nasiri, Ehyae-Tebe-Tabiee Publications, Tehran, 2011: 25-28

[3] Chakhmini Kharazmi, M.; Qanuncheh-Fi-Teb, Revision and translation by Esmaiel Nazem, Abej Publications, Tehran, 2010: 89-93

[4] Rodriguez, Nancy R., Nancy M. DiMarco, and Susie Langley. "Nutrition and athletic performance." *Medicine and Science in Sports and Exercise* 41.3 (2009): 709-731.

[5] Bernard, Bruce P., ed. *Musculoskeletal disorders and workplace factors: a critical review of epidemiologic evidence for work-related musculoskeletal disorders of the neck, upper extremity, and low back.* No. 97-141. US Department of Health and Human Services, Public Health Service, Centers for Disease Control and Prevention, National Institute for Occupational Safety and Health, 1997:. 510-511.

[6] Spenglerb, D. M. "Lumbar disc herniation." *Campbell's Orthopaedic Surgery. 3rd ed. Philadelphia: Lippincott* (2000): 3765-3774.

[7] Katz, Jeffrey N. "Lumbar disc disorders and low-back pain: socioeconomic factors and consequences." *The Journal of Bone & Joint Surgery* 88.suppl 2 (2006): 21-24.

[8] Walsh, Kevin, Marie Cruddas, and David Coggon. "Low back pain in eight areas of Britain." *Journal of Epidemiology and Community Health* 46.3 (1992): 227-230.

[9] Hart, L. Gary, Richard A. Deyo, and Daniel C. Cherkin. "Physician office visits for low back pain: frequency, clinical evaluation, and treatment patterns from a US national survey." *Spine* 20.1 (1995): 11-19.

[10] Cassidy, J. David, Linda J. Carroll, and Pierre Côté. "The Saskatchewan health and back pain survey: the prevalence of low back pain and related disability in Saskatchewan adults." *Spine* 23.17 (1998): 1860-1866.

[11] Klenerman, L., et al. "The prediction of chronicity in patients with an acute attack of low back pain in a general practice setting." *Spine* 20.4 (1995): 478-484.

[12] Walker, Bruce F. "The prevalence of low back pain: a systematic review of the literature from 1966 to 1998." *Journal of Spinal Disorders & Techniques* 13.3 (2000): 205-217.

[13] Maniadakis, Nikolaos, and Alastair Gray. "The economic burden of back pain in the UK." *Pain* 84.1 (2000): 95-103.

[14] Shekelle, Paul G., Martin Markovich, and Rachel Louie. "Comparing the costs between provider types of episodes of back pain care." *Spine* 20.2 (1995): 221-226.

[15] Frymoyer, J. W., and W. L. Cats-Baril. "An overview of the incidences and costs of low back pain." *The Orthopedic Clinics of North America* 22.2 (1991): 263-271.

[16] Deyo, Richard A., et al. "Overtreating chronic back pain: time to back off?."*The Journal of the American Board of Family Medicine* 22.1 (2009): 62-68.

[17] Malanga, Gerard, and Erin Wolff. "Evidence-informed management of chronic low back pain with nonsteroidal anti-inflammatory drugs, muscle relaxants, and simple analgesics." *The Spine Journal* 8.1 (2008): 173-184.

[18] Layzell, Mandy. "Improving the management of postoperative pain." *Nursing Times* 101.26 (2004): 34-36.

[19] Rossignol, M., et al. "Clinic on low-back pain in interdisciplinary practice (CLIP) guidelines." *Montréal: Direction de santé publique, Agence de la santé et des services sociaux de Montréal* (2007).

[20] Fitzcharles, Mary-Ann, et al. "Patient barriers to pain management may contribute to poor pain control in rheumatoid arthritis." *The Journal of Pain* 10.3 (2009): 300-305.

[21] Núñez, Montserrat, et al. "Patients' perceptions of health-related quality of life in rheumatoid arthritis." *Clinical Rheumatology* 28.10 (2009): 1157-1165.

[22] Paul, Pauline, and Beverly Williams. *Brunner & Suddarth's Textbook of Canadian Medical-surgical Nursing*. Lippincott Williams & Wilkins, 2009: 600-625

[23] Avicenna, H.; Al-Qanun-Fi-Teb., Al-Ama Lelmatbuaat Publications, Beirut, 2005: 850-883.

[24] Azam Khan, M.; Exir-E-Azam., Institute of Historical Studies, Islamic and Complementary Medicine, vol 4, 2008: 223-242

[25] Kermani, N.; Sharhe Asbaab-o-Alaamaat., Ehyae-Tebe-Tabiee Publications, Tehran, 2008: 246-251.

[26] Machado, Luciana A. C., et al. "The McKenzie method for the management of acute non-specific low back pain: design of a randomised controlled trial [ACTRN012605000032651]." *BMC Musculoskeletal Disorders* 6.1 (2005): 50.

[27] Danneels, L. A., et al. "The effects of three different training modalities on the cross-sectional area of the paravertebral muscles." *Scandinavian Journal of Medicine & Science in Sports* 11.6 (2001): 335-341.

[28] Baron, Kelly Glazer, et al. "Hostility, anger, and marital adjustment: concurrent and prospective associations with psychosocial vulnerability." *Journal of Behavioral Medicine* 30.1 (2007): 1-10.

[29] Abenhaim, Lucien, et al. "The role of activity in the therapeutic management of back pain: report of the International Paris Task Force on Back Pain." *Spine* 25.4S (2000): 1S-33S.

[30] Koumantakis, George A., Paul J. Watson, and Jacqueline A. Oldham. "Trunk muscle stabilization training plus general exercise versus general exercise only: randomized controlled trial of patients with recurrent low back pain."*Physical Therapy* 85.3 (2005): 209-225.

[31] Moseley, Lorimer. "Combined physiotherapy and education is efficacious for chronic low back pain." *Australian Journal of Physiotherapy* 48.4 (2002): 297-302.

[32] Oksuz, Ergun. "Prevalence, risk factors, and preference-based health states of low back pain in a Turkish population." *Spine* 31.25 (2006): E968-E972.

[33] Drossman, Douglas A. "The functional gastrointestinal disorders and the Rome III process." *Gastroenterology* 130.5 (2006): 1377-1390.

[34] Mousavi, Sayed Javad, et al. "The Oswestry disability index, the Roland-Morris disability questionnaire, and the Quebec back pain disability scale: translation and validation studies of the Iranian versions." *Spine* 31.14 (2006): E454-E459.

[35] Moayyedi, P., et al. "The Leeds Dyspepsia Questionnaire: a valid tool for measuring the presence and severity of dyspepsia." *Alimentary Pharmacology and Therapeutics* 12.12 (1998): 1257-1262.

[36] Marinova, D., F. Ribarova, and M. Atanassova. "Total phenolics and total flavonoids in Bulgarian fruits and vegetables." *Journal of the University of Chemical Technology and Metallurgy* 40.3 (2005): 255-260.

[37] Beketov, E. V., V. P. Pakhomov, and O. V. Nesterova. "Improved method of flavonoid extraction from bird cherry fruits." *Pharmaceutical Chemistry Journal* 39.6 (2005): 316-318.

http://dx.doi.org/10.5772/61170

[38] Smith, Michelle D., Anne Russell, and Paul W. Hodges. "How common is back pain in women with gastrointestinal problems?." *The Clinical Journal of Pain* 24.3 (2008): 199-203.

[39] Smith, Michelle D., Anne Russell, and Paul W. Hodges. "Do incontinence, breathing difficulties, and gastrointestinal symptoms increase the risk of future back pain?." The Journal of Pain 10.8 (2009): 876-886.

Chapter 5

Anticancer Plants in Islamic Traditional Medicine

Behjat Javadi, Milad Iranshahy and
Seyed Ahmad Emami

Additional information is available at the end of the chapter

http://dx.doi.org/10.5772/61111

Abstract

Islamic Traditional Medicine (ITM) is a holistic and comprehensive medical school that has antecedents over 12 centuries ago.

In ITM, cancer was a known disease with many options for treatment. Razi (Razhes; 865-925 AD), Ahwazi (Haly Abbas; 930-994 AD), Avicenna (980-1037AD), Jorjani (1042-1136 AD), and Aqili Khorasani (18th century) are among eminent physicians who discussed different types of cancers and their management in their books. They used a large number of plant species for treatment of different tumors.

Although modern medicine has made tremendous advances in cancer control, the effectiveness of its therapeutic approach is often limited by toxic effects on other organs. Moreover, a large number of people in the world have limited or no access to cancer treatment services. Accordingly, benefiting from traditional medicine schools and effective natural medicines to prevent and control cancer would be valuable. In addition, using the teachings of such schools can lead to the discovery of new bioactive compounds and therapeutic methods.

In this chapter, a brief history of Islamic medicine and its approach to treat cancer as well as anticancer medicinal plants have been discussed. Out of 107 ITM suggested plant species, 59 plants or their chemical compounds have proven to possess cytotoxic and antitumor activities using pharmacological investigations. These findings show the profound insight of ITM physicians into cancer treatment.

Keywords: Anticancer Plants, Cancer treatment

1. Introduction

Islamic Traditional Medicine (ITM) is a holistic system of medicine which flourished during the Islamic Golden Age (750-1258 AD). It was practiced and taught throughout the Islamic territory. In that era, Muslim and non-Muslim medical scholars, especially Iranian physicians and pharmacists, translated the scientific knowledge which they inherited from ancient Greece and Iran. They endeavored to revive and develop this medical knowledge, remove superstitious ideas and faults from it, and establish an authentic medical school. Although most ITM scientists were not Arabs, the majority of their books are written in Arabic, the lingua franca of the Islamic civilization. Razi (Razhes; 865-925 AD), Ahwazi (Haly Abbas; 930-994 AD), Avicenna (980-1037AD), Jorjani (1042-1136 AD), and Aqili Khorasani (18th century) are eminent Iranian physicians who had the most contributions to ITM promotion.

Although significant progress has been made in cancer control in the last few decades, the effectiveness of modern therapeutic approach is often limited by toxic effects on other organs. Moreover, a large number of people in the world have limited or no access to cancer treatment services. Accordingly, utilizing information from traditional medicine systems to identify alternative methods to prevent and control cancer would be desirable. Furthermore, use of traditional medicine can lead to the discovery of new bioactive compounds as well as available, safe and affordable drugs.

In Islamic medicine, cancer was a known disease with many options for treatment. In the majority of ITM textbooks there is a chapter dedicated to cancer definition, symptoms, etiology, diagnosis, prevention, and management.

In this chapter we will discuss cancer, its etiology and management in the view of Islamic Traditional Medicine. In addition, ITM medicinal plants used to treat different types of cancers and modern pharmacological data confirming their traditional usage will be inserted in tables.

2. Cancer definition from ITM point of view

ITM is based on the theory of humorism which posits that the human body consists of four basic fluids, namely humors. The four humors are blood, phlegm, yellow bile, and black bile and each one corresponds to paired qualities: blood is hot and wet, phlegm is cold and wet, yellow bile is hot and dry, and black bile is cold and dry. A proper balance between humors is essential to maintaining health. Accordingly, all diseases and disabilities including cancer result from an excess or putridity of these humors.

According to ITM, cancer is a kind of black bile swelling which is accompanied by pain, pulsation, inflammation, and angiogenesis [1]. Blood vessels surrounding a tumor are overfilled and stiff and contain a dark and black blood [2]. The reason for the appellation "cancer" is due to the similarity between the shape of a cancerous tumor affecting an organ and a crab grasping its prey. It may also due to the spherical shape and darkness of tumor and origination of blood vessels from its milieu which resembles crab's feet [3]. Cancer frequently affects soft and porous organs and for this reason, it mainly involves breast and innervated organs (such as uterus) in females, and throat, larynx, testicles and penis in males [1].

Initially, cancer is the size of a broad bean or smaller, hard, spherical, mobile, dark, and slightly warm [3]. It will then begin to grow gradually and reach to the size of a walnut or larger. It might be curable during its early stages of development, but diagnosis is difficult in these stages. On the other hand, upon progression and appearance of clinical manifestations, treatment of cancer would be difficult or even impossible [1].

Ocular, nasal cavity, breast, uterine, liver, and other visceral organs and skin cancers are among the most frequently mentioned cancers in ITM texts. Cancers are divided into two main types: ulcerative and nonulcerative cancers.

Some cancerous tumors are easily ulcerated but some others are not. Cancerous wounds usually spread centripetally and their discharges are purulent. Use of appropriate medications can prevent the ulceration of susceptible tumors. In contrast, some cancerous tumors that are not prone to ulceration would be ulcerated following the administration of improper drugs [1].

Advanced and large tumors are very sensitive and painful, with a distinctive red to yellow color and a caustic and burning pain. Such tumors might erupt spontaneously and a purulent and bloody discharge may appear on wound surface. The resulting wounds are very sensitive and can produce corrosion in surrounding tissues [2].

3. Cancer etiology

According to ITM, excessive accumulation of abnormal black bile in a body site is the main cause of cancer. Aging, prolonged stress exposure, consuming cold and dry food items and hardwork are leading causes of increasing black bile production [1]. In some cases, hemorrhage (such as menstruation, abnormal uterine hemorrhage, or hemorrhoids bleeding) is a defending mechanism against the accumulation of bad humors in the body. Therefore, completely stopping the bleeding by surgical procedures and other medications can result in a black bile accretion and consequently increasing the risk of cancer and other diseases originating from excessive black bile (including cancer, melancholia, liver problems, psoriasis, etc.) [2].

4. Cancer management

Islamic traditional medicine suggested multiple strategies to the control and treatment of cancer. Surgical manipulation, venesection, diet adjustment, and use of natural medicines including solid, semisolid, and liquid dosage forms with oral and external route of administration are among these methods.

4.1. Surgery and manipulation

Surgery is used to eradicate tumors in their early stages of development. Small tumors which are distant from vital organs are good candidates for surgery. The tumor should be cut from its origin and some parts of adjacent nonaffected tissues should be excised as well. In addition, bleeding should be allowed until large blood volumes come out and surrounding tissue should be pressed in order to expel blood mixed with black bile thoroughly. Afterwards, the injured site should be salved or cauterized. However, if the cancerous tumor is located in the vicinity of sensitive and vital organs, surgical procedure and cauterization would be very dangerous and may change the cancer to a nonhealing ulcer [2, 4].

Regular venesection is also suggested during the initial phases of cancer, to withdraw black bile blood from body.

4.2. Nutrition therapy

In Islamic traditional medicine, dietary recommendations have been proposed to slow the progression of advanced tumors that cannot be manipulated due to metastasis concerns. In these cases, nutritional care would increase the longevity of patients. Food items with wet temperament which produce high-quality blood like beer, almond oil, fresh small fishes, soft-boiled egg yolk, lamb, bird meat, ripe and sweet apples, sweet plums, bananas, raisin, black gram (*Vigna mungo* (L.) Hepper), spinach (*Spinacia oleracea* L.), pumpkin, light wine, and fresh cow's milk and dough are administered [1]. On the other hand, excessive intake of foodstuffs which induce black bile production in the body (such as eggplant (*Solanum melongena* L.), lentil (*Lens esculenta* Moench), date (*Phoenix dactylifera* L.), cabbage (*Brassica oleracea* L.), beef, black and thick wine, and salt-cured meat) is severely restricted [5].

4.3. Pharmacotherapy

As mentioned above, from the Islamic Traditional Medicine point of view, an excess of abnormal black bile in various body sites can lead to cancer formation. In order to treat cancer, black bile should be expelled from the body by using an appropriate purgative, and then preventing the generation and accumulation of black bile in vessels as far as possible [2]. For this purpose, many single and compound medications of herbal, animal, and mineral origin have been recommended.

The essential point in pharmacotherapy of cancers and tumors is avoiding the use of caustic and irritant medications to prevent further stimulation and ulceration [2].

Cancer medications can be administered internally (oral, enemas, vaginal douches, etc.) or applied topically (cataplasms, topical oils, liniments, lotions, dusting powders, etc.) [1, 3]. Administration of local anticancer drugs has the following purposes: cancer eradication, metastasis prevention, preventing ulceration, and healing ulcerated tumors.

5. Mechanisms of action of anticancer drugs

Anticancer drugs act through different mechanisms:

i. **Black bile purgatives** are common anticancer drugs which can facilitate elimination of abnormal black bile from whole body. Purgatives should be administered frequently. From the ITM point of view, clover dodder (*Cuscuta epithymum* Murr.) is the most valuable black bile purgative, which is commonly used to treat diseases caused by a surplus or imbalance of this humor such as all types of cancer, melancholia, leprosy, vitiligo, etc. For this purpose, a mixture of clover dodder with cheese whey or hydromel should be administered frequently. A decoction of the plant in oxymel is also prescribed [3]. Common polypody (*Polypodium vulgare* L.), French lavender (*Lavandula stoechas* L.), colocynth [*Citrullus colocynthis* (L.) Schrad.], and black hellebore (*Helleborus niger* L.) are other potent black bile purgatives.

ii. **Antiulcer drugs** can inhibit ulceration of tumors. *Urtica pilulifera* L. and *Aloe vera* (L.) Burm.f. are examples of such plants.

iii. **Wound-healing medications** accelerate healing of cancerous wounds. *Althaea officinalis* L., *Brassica oleracea* L., and *Viola odorata* L. have wound-healing activity.

iv. **Analgesic drugs** relieve cancer pain. *Parietaria officinalis* L. and *Solanum nigrum* L. are plants with analgesic effect.

6. Anticancer plants

One hundred and seven plant species from 53 families have been mentioned to be effective in the management and curing of different types of cancers. Plants Latin and Arabic names, their families, medicinal parts, dosage forms, and routes of administration are given in Table 1.

Scientific name	Family	Arabic common name	Part used	Cancer type	Administration and locality	Ref.
Acacia nilotica (L.) Delile syn. *Acacia arabica* (Lam.) Willd.	Fabaceae	samgh	G	eye	ocular suppository	[3]
Allium ampeloprasum L. syn. *Allium porrum* L.	Liliaceae	korrath	Le	all types	decoction(O)	[6]
Aloe vera (L.) Burm.f.	Liliaceae	sabr	Sa	uterus ulcerating tumor internal organs	unguent powder(E) decoction(O) pill(O)	[1, 3]
Alpinia officinarum Hance	Zingiberaceae	khawlanjan	Rh	all types	electuary(O)	[8, 9]
Althaea officinalis L.	Malvaceae	khatmi	R	all types uterus	liniment cataplasm vaginal bath	[1, 3] [2, 7]
Alyssum homalocarpum (Fisch. & C. A.Mey.) Boiss.	Brassicaceae	tudari urisimun	Se	internal organs skin	cataplasm	[2, 5, 9-11]

Scientific name	Family	Arabic common name	Part used	Cancer type	Administration and locality	Ref.
Amaranthus blitum L.	Amaranthaceae	baghlat al-yamaaniah	Ap	uterus	cataplasm	[7]
Anchusa azurea Mill. syn. *Anchusa italica* Retz.	Boraginaceae	lesan al-thawr	Le	all types	syrup	[7]
Anethum graveolens L.	Apiaceae	shebeth	Ap	uterus	unguent topical oil	[1, 3]
Beta vulgris L.	Chenopodiaceae	salq	Le	all types	decoction(O)	[6]
Boswellia sacra Flueck. syn. *Boswellia carteri* Birdw.	Burseraceae	kondor	Ogr	eye	condensed smoke as collyrium	[2, 3, 5, 8, 9]
Brassica oleracea L.	Brassicaceae	karnab	Le Fl	uterus all types skin	unguent decoction(E) vaginal bath cooked(O) cooked (E)	[1, 3, 7] [6, 8, 9]
Capparis spinosa L.	Capparaceae	kabar	Rb	uterus all types	unguent cataplasm	[3] [1, 5]
Carthamus tinctorius L.	Asteraceae	moasfar	Se	all types	raw seeds(O)	[6]
Carum carvi L.	Apiaceae	kerawia	Se	all types	raw seeds(O)	[6]
Cassia fistula L.	Fabaceae	khiar shanbar	Lg	tongue ulcerated cancer uterine	extract (E)	[3] [12]
Chamaemelum nobile (L.) All.syn. *Anthemis nobilis* L.	Asteraceae	babunaj	Fl	uterus	unguent topical oil decoction(E)	[1, 3, 7, 12]
Cicer arietinum L.	Fabaceae	homs	Se	skin all types ulcerating tumor	cooked(O) infusion(E) cataplasm	[8, 9] [2]
Cichorium intybus L.	Asteraceae	hindeba	Le	uterus all types ulcerating tumor	extract(E) cataplasm extract(O) cataplasm	[1, 6, 8] [7]
Cinnamomum cassia (L.) J.Presl	Luraceae	salikhah	Br	liver	electuary	[2]
Cistus creticus L. syn. *Cistus ladaniferus* Curtis	Cistaceae	ladan	Fl	all types	oil (E)	[3]

Scientific name	Family	Arabic common name	Part used	Cancer type	Administration and locality	Ref.
Citrullus colocynthis (L.) Schrad.	Cucurbitaceae	hanzal	Fr	internal organs	decoction(O) pill(O)	[1]
Commiphora mukul (Hook. ex Stocks) Engl.	Burseraceae	moql	Ogr	uterus	unguent	[1, 3, 7]
Convolvulus pseudoscammonia C. Koch	Convolvulaceae	saqmunia	Rdj	internal organs	decoction(O) pill(O)	[1]
Cordia myxa L.	Boraginaceae	debgh	Fr	uterine cancer	decoction(O)	[12]
Coriandrum sativum L.	Apiaceae	kozborah	Le Se	eye uterus skin all types	extract(E) cataplasm vaginal douche cataplasm extract (E)	[1] [1, 3] [2, 7, 9] [8, 9] [6, 7]
Crocus sativus L.	Iridaceae	za`afaran	St	eye uterus metastatic ulcerating tumor liver	cataplasm cataplasm cataplasm electuary	[3] [1, 2, 11, 13] [12] [2]
Cucurbita maxima Duchartre, *Cucurbita pepo* L.	Cucurbitaceae	qar`a	Fr	internal organs	cooked (O) extract lotion	[1, 6-8]
Cuscuta epithymum (L.) L.	Cuscutaceae	aftimun	Ap	all types ulcerating tumor	powder(O) decoction(O)	[1-4, 6, 8-10]
Cymbopogon schoenanthus (L.) Spreng.	Poaceae	ezkher	Fl	liver	electuary	[2]
Cynara scolymus L.	Asteraceae	kankarzad	G		cataplasm	[2]
Dorema ammoniacum D. Don	Apiaceae	oshaq	Ogr	all types	unguent	[3, 8, 14]
Dracunculus vulgaris Schottsyn. *Arum dracunculus* L.	Araceae	luf al-hayyah	Be Se	nose breast testicle	extract decoction(E)	[2, 3, 5, 8-10] [2]
Ecballium elaterium (L.) A. Rich.	Cucurbitaceae	qetha al-hemar	Fr	all types	liniment(E)	[1, 3]
Erysimum × cheiri (L.) Crantz syn. *Cheiranthus ×cheiri* L.	Brassicaceae	kheiri	Fl	all types uterus	oil(E)	[3, 7] [12]
Ferula gummosa Boiss.	Apiaceae	ghennah	Ogr	all types	unguent	[8]
Ficus carica L.	Moraceae	teen	Fr	tongue all types	cooked(E) cooked (O)	[3] [6]

Scientific name	Family	Arabic common name	Part used	Cancer type	Administration and locality	Ref.
				ulcerating tumor uterus	cataplasm cataplasm	[12, 13] [7]
Glycyrrhiza glabra L.	Fabaceae	sous	R	all types uterus	syrup vaginal douche	[7, 15]
Helleborus niger L.	Ranunculaceae	kharbaq aswad	R	internal organs	decoction(O) pill(O)	[1, 7, 10]
Hordeum vulgare L.	Poaceae	sha`eer	Se	all types	decoction(O)	[1, 3, 6, 7]
Inula helenium L.	Asteraceae	rasan	R	skin	lotion	[14]
Iris × germanica L. syn. *Iris ×florentina* L.		irsa	R	uterus	unguent	[3]
Jasminum sambac (L.) Aiton *Aegle marmelos* (L.) Corrêa ex Roxb.		razeqi	Fl	uterus	unguent topical oil	[3]
Juglans regia L.	Juglandaceae	Jawz	G	ulcerating tumor	dusting powder(E)	[2, 14]
Lactuca sativa (L.) Mill.	Asteraceae	khas	Le	all types uterus	extract(E) cataplasm	[1, 3] [6, 7]
Laurus nobilis L.	Lauraceae	hab al-ghar	Se	tongue uterus	cataplasm cataplasm	[1, 3] [7]
Lavandula stoechas L.	Lamiaceae	ostokhoddus	Ap	internal organs	decoction(O) pill(O)	[1]
Lawsonia inermis L	Lythraceae	henna	Le	uterus	unguent oil(E)	[3]
Lens culinaris Medik. syn. *Lens esculenta* Moench	Fabaceae	adas	Se	uterus ulcerating tumor	vaginal douche cataplasm	[3] [7]
Lilium candidum L.	Liliaceae	susan	Fl	uterus	unguent oil (E)	[1, 3]
Linum usitatissimum L.	Linaceae	katan	Se Mu	all types uterus	unguent oil (E) vaginal bath decoction (E)	[3] [1, 2, 7]
Liquidambar orientalis Mill.	Altingiaceae	mi`a	Ba	all types	unguent	[3]
Lycium afrum L	Solanaceae	hozoz	Le Fs	uterus	extract vaginal douche	[15]
Malva pusilla Sm. syn. *Malva rotundifolia* L.	Malvaceae	khabaazi	Fl	uterus	vaginal bath cataplasm	[7]
Melilotusofficinalis (L.) Pall.	Fabaceae	eklil al-malek	pod	eye	cataplasm	[1, 3]

Scientific name	Family	Arabic common name	Part used	Cancer type	Administration and locality	Ref.
				uterus		[2]
Melissa officinalis L.	Lamiaceae	badranjbuyeh	Le	all types	syrup	[7]
Myrtus communis L.	Myrtaceae	as	Se Le	all types	topical oil extract enema	[14]
Narcissus tazetta L.	Amaryllidaceae	narjes	Fl	uterus	unguent topical oil	[1, 3]
Olea europaea L.	Oleaceae	zeytun	Fr	uterus metastatic cancerous wounds	topical oil oil sediment (E) cataplasm	[1, 3] [13]
Opopanax chironium W.D.J.Koch	Apiaceae	jawshir	Ogr	all types	unguent	[3, 14]
Origanum syriacum L. syn. *Origanum maru* L.	Lamiaceae	mormahur	Ap	metastatic cancerous wounds	cataplasm	[13]
Papaver somniferum L. var. *album* (Mill.) M.A. Veselovskaya	Papaveraceae	khashkhash	Se Sa	eye uterus	ocular suppository cataplasm	[3] [1-3, 5, 12]
Parietaria officinalis L.	Urticaceae	hashishatah al-zojaj	Le	all types	extract(E)	[5]
Phoenix dactylifera L.	Arecaceae	tamr	Fr	tongue	decoction(E)	[3]
Physalis alkekengi L	Solanaceae	kaknaj	Fr	all types uterus	extract(E) unguent	[7] [15]
Pinus gerardiana Wall. ex D.Don	Pinaceae	jalghuzah	N	all types		[6]
Pinus spp.	Pinaceae	ratinaj	Re	uterus	cataplasm	[7]
Pistacia atlantica Desf. *Pistacia terebinthus* L.	Anacardiaceae	elk al-anbat	Ogr	uterus all types	unguent	[1, 3, 6, 8]
Pistacia lentiscus L.	Anacardiaceae	mastaki	Ogr	all types	unguent oil(E)	[1, 3] [6]
Plantago indica L. syn. *Plantago psyllium* L.	Plantaginaceae	bazr qotuna	Se Mu	ulcerating tumor intestine all types	liniment enema	[3, 8] [14]
Plantago major L.	Plantaginaceae	lesan al-hamal	Se Mu Le	uterus ulcerating tumor	vaginal douche cataplasm	[1-3, 7, 12]
Plantago ovata Forssk.	Plantaginaceae	isbaghul	Se Mu	all types uterus	vaginal douche	[1, 6] [7]

Scientific name	Family	Arabic common name	Part used	Cancer type	Administration and locality	Ref.
syn, *Plantago ispaghula* Roxb. ex Fleming						
Platanus orientalis L.	Plantanaceae	dolb	Le	skin	decoction (E) vaginal bath	[2]
Polygonum aviculare L	Polygonaceae	asa al-ra`ee	Ap	uterus	unguent extract (E)	[7, 15]
Polypodium vulgare L.	Polypodiaceae	basfayaj	Rh	internal organs	decoction(O) pill(O)	[1, 7]
Polyporus officinalis (Vill.) Fr.	Polyporaceae	ghariqun		all types	decoction(O)	[4, 7]
Portulaca oleracea L.	Portulaceae	rejlah	Le	ulcerating tumor all types uterus	extract liniment enema extract(O)	[3, 8] [1] [6] [7]
Prunus dulcis (Mill.) D.A.Webb	Rosaceae	samgh al-llawz	G So Se	uterus all types	unguent oil (O)	[1, 3, 6, 12]
Punica granatum L.	Punicaceae	romman	Fr Fp	nose ulcerating tumor	juice(O)	[1] [7]
Raphanus raphanistrum subsp. *sativus* (L.) Domin syn. *Raphanus sativus* L.	Brassicaceae	fojl	tro	all types	decoction(O)	[6]
Rhus coriaria L.	Anacardiaceae	sumaagh				
Ricinus communis L.	Euphorbiaceae	kherwa`a	Se	uterus	unguent oil (E)	[1, 3]
Rosa × damascena Herrm.	Rosaceae	ward	Fl	eye uterus ulcerating tumor	oil(E) cataplasm vaginal douche oil	[1] [2, 3, 7, 12]
Salix aegyptiaca L.	Salicaceae	khelaf	W	skin	dusting powder(E)	[2]
Sempervivum tectorum L.	Crassulaceae	hay al-alam	Fl	all types	extract liniment	[3, 7]
Sesbania bispinosa (Jacq.) W. Wight	Fabaceae	sisban	Le		cataplasm	[9]
Sisymbrium officinale (L.) Scop. syn. *Erysimum officinale* L.	Brassicaceae	arismun, khabbe	Se	hard swelling cancer nonulcerating tumor	cataplasm cataplasm cataplasm cataplasm	[8, 9] [2]

Scientific name	Family	Arabic common name	Part used	Cancer type	Administration and locality	Ref.
				ear breast testicle		
Smilax china L.	Smilacaceae	khashab sini	R	skin	decoction(O)	[8]
Solanum americanum Mill. syn. *Solanum nigrum* L.	Solanaceae	enab al-tha`alab	Le	uterus all types skin	cataplasm extract cataplasm	[1-3, 6, 7] [7] [5, 8-10]
Spinacia oleracea L.	Chenopodiaceae	esfanakh	Le	internal organs	cooked (O)	[1, 6]
Tamarix gallica L.	Tamaricaceae	tarfa	Le R Sh	all types spleen	decoction(O)	[5]
Tanacetum parthenium (L.) Sch.Bip.	Asteraceae	oqhowan	Fl	skin uterus	extract cataplasm unguent oil(E)	[9] [1, 3]
Terminalia bellirica (Gaertn.) Roxb.	Combretaceae	amolaj	Fr	all types	liniment	[7]
Terminalia chebula Retz.	Combretaceae	ehalilaj kaboli	Fr	internal organs	decoction(O) pill(O)	[1]
Trigonella foenum-graecum L.	Fabaceae	holbah	Se mu	tongue uterus all types	infusion(E) oil(E) decoction(E)	[3] [1, 6, 7]
Triticum spelta L.	Poaceae	khondorus	Se	all types	baked(O)	[6]
Urtica pilulifera L.	Urticaceae	anjorah	Se Le	all types skin ulcerating tumor	cataplasm ash dusting powder(E)	[3, 8, 9, 11, 13] [2]
Valeriana celtica L.	Valerianaceae	sonbol	R	liver	electuary	[2]
Vigna mungo (L.) Heppersyn. *Phaseolus mungo* L.	Fabaceae	maash	Se	internal organs	cooked(O)	[1, 6]
Viola odorata L.	Violaceae	banafsaj	Ap	uterus	decoction(E) vaginal bath	[7, 15]
Vitis vinifera L.	Vitaceae	enab	Urf verjuice Rf Fr Fl	all types tongue all types skin	cataplasm concentrated juice(O) raw Fr(O) cataplasm	[3, 6, 7] [6] [6, 10] [10] [12]

Scientific name	Family	Arabic common name	Part used	Cancer type	Administration and locality	Ref.
				ulcerating tumor uterine cancer uterus	decoction(E) unguent	
Zingiber officinale Roscoe	Zingiberaceae	zanjabil	Rh	liver skin	electuary lotion	[2] [14]
Ziziphus jujuba Mill. syn. *Ziziphus vulgaris* Lam.	Rhamnaceae	onnab	Fr	ulcerating tumor uterus	decoction(O)	[12]

Use: E = external use, O = oral use. Part used Ap = aerial parts, Ba = balsam, Be = berries, Br = bark, Ff = fresh fruit, Fl = flowers, Fp = fruit pericarp, Fr = fruit, G = gum, Gre = gum resin, Le = leaves, Mu: mucilage, N = nuts, O = oil, Ogr = oleo-gum resin, Ore = oleoresin, R = root, Rb = root bark, Re = resin, Rdj = Root dry juice, Rf = Ripe fruit, Rh = rhizome, Se = seeds, Sh =shoots, So = seed oil, St = stigma, Tap root = Tro, Sa = sap, Urf = Unripe fruit, W = wood, Wp = whole plant.

Table 1. Medicinal plants mentioned in Islamic Traditional Medicine textbooks effective in the management of cancer.

7. Anticancer and cytotoxic activities of ITM plant species

Many ITM-suggested plants have been shown to exert anticancer activities with different mechanisms such as cytotoxic, antitumor, antiproliferative, cytostatic, and cell-migration-inhibiting effects. Pharmacological data reinterpreting ITM evidence of cancer phytotherapy are given in Table 2.

Species	Plant part(s)/compound	Solvent	Activity	Cell line	Ref.
Aegle marmelos (L.) Corrêa ex Roxb.	Stem bark	ethanol	cytotoxic	K-562, Raji, Jurkat, HEL, Colo38, HL-60, CEM, B-16, MCF-7 and MDA-MB-231	[16-18]
		methanol, ethyl acetate and n-hexane		Brine shrimp	[19]
	Stem bark, roots and leaves/Zeorin, dustanin, aegeline, epilupeol, lupenone and marmin	-		CEM-SS	[20]
	1-hydroxy-5,7-dimethoxy-2-naphthalene-carboxaldehyde (marmelin)	-	antitumor	HCT-116 colon cancer cell tumor xenograft in nude mice	[21]
Allium porrum L.	Bulbs/12-keto-porrigenin and 2,3-seco-porrigenin	-	antiproliferative	J774, WEHI 164, P388 and K3R-1	[22]

Species	Plant part(s)/compound	Solvent	Activity	Cell line	Ref.
	Bulbs/Porrigenins A and B	-		IGR-1, J774, WEHI 164 and P388	[23]
	Saponins	-		J774 and WEHI 164	[24]
	Leaves	aqueous ethanolic extract (70%)	cytotoxic	K562	[25]
	Flavonoids	-		MCF-7	[26]
	Di(2-ethylhexyl)phthalate	-		K562, HL60 and U937	[27]
Aloe vera (L.) Burm.f.	Aloe-emodin	-	cytotoxic and antitumor	Neuroblastoma cells (IMR-32, IMR-5, AF8, and SJ-N-KP), pPNET cells (TC32) and Ewing's sarcoma cells (TC106)	[28]
				PC3	[29]
			cytotoxic	MCC	[30]
				U-373MG and U87 glioma cells	[31, 32]
				T24 human bladder cancer cells	[33]
				Gastric cancer cells	[34]
				MCF-7	[35]
			antitumor	Ehrlich ascitis carcinoma (EAC)	[36]
Anthemis nobilis L.	Sesquiterpene lactones	-	cytotoxic	HeLa and KB	[37]
Beta vulgris L.	Root extract and betanin	water	cytotoxic and antitumor	MCF-7, PC3 and HepG2	[38-41]
Boswellia carteri Birdw.	α and β-boswellic acid acetate from resin	-	cytostatic-inhibits cell migration	KB, HCT-8, A2780 and B16F10	[42]
			cytotoxic	HT-1080	
	Triterpene acids from resin			IMR-32, NB-39 and SK-N-SH	[43]
	Frankincense oil			The bladder carcinoma J82	[44]
	Verticilla-4(20),7,11-triene			Hep-G2	[45]
Brassica oleracea L.	Sulforaphane	-	cytotoxic	MDAH 2774 and SkOV-3	[46]
	Erucin			CACO-2, HL60, K562 and LNCaP	[47]
	Leaves	acidified methanol		HeLa and HepG2	[48]
	2-Pyrrolidinone reach extract			PC3 and HeLa	[49]
	Brassinin	-		PC3	[50]

Species	Plant part(s)/compound	Solvent	Activity	Cell line	Ref.
Capparis spinosa L.	Polysaccharides and alkaloids from fruits	water	cytotoxic and antitumor	HepG2 and transplanted ascites tumor H22	[51, 52]
Carthamus tinctorius L.	*Carthamus tinctorius* and *Panax ginseng*	-	cytotoxic and antitumor	MDA-MB-231 breast cancer cell and normal human mammary gland cell lines	[53]
	Polysaccharide	-	antitumor	T739 lung cancer and S180 Sarcoma in mice	[54]
	Not mentioned	methanol	cytotoxic	HT-29	[55]
Carum carvi L.	Thymoquinone from seeds	-	cytotoxic	TNBC cells	[56]
Cassia fistula L.	Rhein from flowers	-	cytotoxic	COLO 320 DM	[57]
	Stem bark	methanol			[58]
	Furanoflavones from stem bark	-		NB4, A549, SHSY5Y, PC3, and MCF7	[59]
	Fistulaquinone A from fruits			NB4 and PC3	[60]
Cicer arietinum L.	C-25 protein	-	cytotoxic	KB cell line	[61]
Cichorium intybus L.	Leaves	chloroform	antiproliferative	HeLa, MCF7 and A431	[62]
	Lactucin and 13,14-seco-stigma 9(11),14(15)-dien-3alpha-ol	-	cytotoxic	A2780	[63]
Cinnamomum cassia (L.) J.Presl	Cinnamaldehyde	-	cytotoxic	HL60	[64]
	Bark	methanol/hexane/ethyl acetate		HeLa, A549, SK-OV-3, SK-MEL-2, XF-498 and HCT-15	[65]
		aqueous		SiHa	[66]
	2'-Benzoyloxycinnamaldehyde	-		LNCaP, PC-3 and DU145	[67]
	Coumacasia			HL60 and A549	[68]
Cistus creticus L.	Labdane-type diterpenoids from leaves	-	cytotoxic	KB, P-388; and NSCLC-N6	[69]
				CCRF-CEM, MOLT3, H33AJ-JA-13, HUT78, H9, KM3, NAMALWA, JIYOYE, DAUDI, SDK, K562, HL60 and U973	[70-72]
	Shoot	ethanol		HeLa, MDA-MB-453 and FemX	[73]
Commiphora mukul Engl.	Guggulsterones	-	cytotoxic	PC3, HL60 and U973	[74]
Coriandrum sativum L.	Linalool	-	antitumor	Sarcoma-180 solid tumor	[75]
	Leaves	ethanol	cytotoxic	HT-29	[76]

Species	Plant part(s)/compound	Solvent	Activity	Cell line	Ref.
Crocus sativus L.	Stigma	ethanol	antitumor	Sarcoma-180 (S-180), Ehrlich ascites Carcinoma (EAC) and Dalton's lymphoma ascites (DLA)	[77]
			cytotoxic	HeLa, A549 and HepG2	[78, 79]
	Crocin, crocetin, safranal and picrocrocin	-		HeLa, MCF-7, PC3, k562 and HepG2	[80-86]
	Crocin		antitumor	C26 colon carcinoma	[87]
Cucurbita maxima Duchartre,	Seeds	methanol	cytotoxic	Brine shrimp	[88]
	Aerial parts		antitumor	Ehrlich ascites Carcinoma	[89]
	Triterpenes	-	cytotoxic	HL60 and P388	[90]
Cucurbita pepo L.	Leaves	hydroalcoholic	cytotoxic	HepG2 and CT26	[91]
Cuscuta epithymum Mur.	Aerial parts	chloroform and hydroalcoholic	cytotoxic	HeLa, HT29 and MDA-MB-46	[92]
Ecballium elaterium (L.) A. Rich.	Cucurbitacin E	-	cytotoxic	ZR-75-1, COLO 679, OV_95_CC3 and PC-3	[93, 94]
	Fruits	water		AGS and KYSE30	[95]
	Cucurbitacin-D	-		NSCLC-N6	[96]
Ficus carica L.	Leaves, fruits and latex	ethanol, ethyl acetate and dichloromethane	cytotoxic	HeLa	[97]
Glycyrrhiza glabra L.	Root		cytotoxic	4T1	[98]
Inula helenium L.	Root	methanol	cytotoxic	HT-29, MCF-7, Capan-2 and G1	[99]
		ethanol	cytotoxic	MDA-MB-23	[100]
Jasminum sambac (L.) Aiton	Leaves	ethanol	cytotoxic	Brine shrimp	[101]
Juglans regia L.	Juglanin A and B	-	cytotoxic	Hep G2	[102]
	Leaves	chloroform		BHY, MCF7, and HT-29	[103]
	Juglanones A and B	-		A549, MCF-7, BEL-7402, HeLa, COLO205, BGC-823, and SK-OV-3	[104]
	5,7-Dihydroxy-3,4′-dimethoxyflavone and regiolone			MCF-7 and BHY	[105]
Lactuca sativa (L.) Mill.	Sesquiterpene lactones	-	cytotoxic	HeLa and HCT-116	[106]
Laurus nobilis L.	Leaves	n-hexane	cytotoxic	Brine shrimp	[107]
	Sesquiterpene lactones	-		Jurkat	[108]

Species	Plant part(s)/compound	Solvent	Activity	Cell line	Ref.
				, HL-60 and LoVo	
				A2780	[109]
	Essential oil	-		C32, ACHN, LNCaP, and MCF-7	[110]
Lawsonia inermis L.	Bicoumarin, biflavonoid, and biquinone compounds from flowers	-	cytotoxic	MCF-7, Hela, HCT-116, and HT-29	[111]
Linum usitatissimum L.	Secoisolariciresinol and anhydrosecoisolariciresinol	-	cytotoxic	MCF-7 and MDA-MB-231	[112]
Melissa officinalis L.	Essential oil	-	cytotoxic	A549, MCF-7, Caco-2, HL-60, K562 and B16F10	[113]
	Aerial parts	ethanol		HCT-116	[114]
	Leaves	water	cytotoxic and antitumor	MCF-7, MDA-MB-468 and MDA-MB-231; DMBA-induced mammary tumors	[115]
	Citral and essential oil	-	cytotoxic	GBM	[116]
Myrtus communis L.	Phloroglucinols	-	cytotoxic	MT-4 cells, HepG2 and DU145	[117]
Narcissus tazetta L.	Alkaloids	-			[118]
	Stems and leaves	alkaloid extraction	cytotoxic	HL-60, K562, KT1/A3, and A3	[119]
Olea europaea L.	Erythrodiol	-	cytotoxic	HL-60	[120]
	Hydroxytyrosol rich extract from leaves	methanol/water		MCF-7	[121]
	Maslinic acid	-		HT29	[122]
	Tyrosol esters			MCF10A	[123]
Papaver somniferum L. var. *album* (Mill.) M.A.	Noscapine	-	anticancer	Refractory Multiple Myeloma, Non-Hodgkin's Lymphoma and Chronic Lymphocytic Leukemia	[124]
Physalis alkekengi L.	5α-Hydroxy-25,27-dihydro-4,7-didehydro-7-deoxyneophysalin A	-	cytotoxic	PC-3 and LNCaP	[125]
	Physalin			HT1080 and A375-S2	[126, 127]
Pistacia atlantica Desf.	Polyphenol-rich extract	ethanol/water	cytotoxic	HT29	[128]
Pistacia lentiscus L.	Gum extract	hexane	cytotoxic	HCT116	[129]
Plantago major L.	Leaves	hot water	cytotoxic	Antileukemia and anticarcinoma	[130]

Species	Plant part(s)/compound	Solvent	Activity	Cell line	Ref.
	Luteolin-7-*O*-β-glucoside	-		TK-10, MCF-7 and UACC-62	[131]
Platanus orientalis L.	Flavonoids	-	cytotoxic	Human leukemic cell lines and skin cancer cell lines	[132-136]
Polygonum aviculare L	Aerial parts	methanol	cytotoxic	MCF-7	[137]
Portulaca oleracea L.	Triterpenoids	-	cytotoxic	HepG2	[138]
	Not mentioned	methanol	cytotoxic	CNE-1, HeLa and HT-29 and MCF-7	[139]
	Seed	methanol	cytotoxic	HepG2	[140]
	Alkaloids	-	cytotoxic	K562, A549, MCF-7 and MDA-MB-435	[141]
Punica granatum L.	Genistein and extract	not mentioned	cytotoxic	MCF-7, MMTV-Wnt-1,	[142]
	Polyphenols	juice	cytotoxic and antitumor	BT-474 and MDA-MB-231	[143]
	Fruit rind extract and fowers	methanol	cytotoxic	A549 and MCF-7	[144-146]
	Galactomannan polysaccharide	-	cytotoxic and antitumor	A375, HCT116, and HepG2; DLA and EAC murine ascites and EAC solid tumor mouse models	[147]
Raphanus sativus L.	4-(Methylthio)-3-butenyl isothiocyanate	-	cytotoxic	murine leukaemia cell line (L1210)	[148]
	4-Methylthio-butanyl derivatives	-	cytotoxic	A549, SK-OV-3, SK-MEL-2, and HCT-15	[149]
Ricinus communis L.	Leaves	volatile oil	cytotoxic	SK-MEL-28 and HeLa	[150]
Rosa × damascena Mill.	Flowers	volatile oil	cytotoxic	SW742	[151]
Smilax china L.	Phenylpropanoid glycosides	-	cytotoxic	KB, HeLa, DLD-1, MCF-7, A-549 and Med	[152]
	Kaempferol-7-O-beta-D-glucoside	-	cytotoxic	A375 and HL60	[153]
	Polyphenols	-	cytotoxic	MCF-7 and MDA-MB-231	[154]
Solanum nigrum L.	Steroidal glycosides	-	cytotoxic	HT-29, HCT-15, LNCaP, PC-3, T47D, HepG2, NCI-H460, MCF-7, SF-268 and MDA-MB-231	[155, 156]
	Glycoprotein	-	cytotoxic	MCF-7, HCT-116 and HT-29	[157-160]
	Aerial parts	methanol	cytotoxic	HeLa and Vero	[161]
	Leaves	water	cytotoxic	AU565	[162]
	Not mentioned	hydro-alcoholic	cytotoxic	HepG2 and CT26	[91]

Species	Plant part(s)/compound	Solvent	Activity	Cell line	Ref.
	Solamargine	-		K562	[163]
	Polyphenol rich extract	water		PZ-HPV-7	[164]
	Berries	ethanol		Jurkat and HL-60	[165]
Tanacetum parthenium L.	Parthenolide	-	anticancer	Leukemia	[166]
Terminalia chebula Willd. ex Flem.	Tannins	-	cytotoxic	A-549, SK-OV-3, SK-MEL-2, XF-498 and HCT-15	[167]
	Fruits	methanol		HOS-1	[168]
Trigonella foenum-graecum L.	Seeds	water	cytotoxic	HL-60	[169]
				TCP, B-cell lymphomas, FRO and MCF7	
	Diosgenin	-		A549	
Viola odorata L.	Cyclotides	-	cytotoxic	MCF-7 and MCF-7/ADR	[170]
Vitis vinifera L.	Resveratrol	-	cytotoxic	3T6 and HL60	[171]
	Seed extract	methanol		KB cells	[172]
	Viniferin-enriched extracts	ethanol/water		HCC1954, HCC1500 and MCF7	[173, 174]
Zingiber officinale Roscoe	[6]-Paradol and structurally related compounds	-	cytotoxic	KB	[175]
	Gingerols and diarylheptanoids	-		HL-60, A431, K562, HeLa, HCT-116, HT-29 and K562/ADR	[176-181]

Table 2. Anticancer activities of ITM plant species.

8. Conclusion

Taken together, it can be concluded that what physicians of Islamic medicine used for cancer treatment is proven through modern research. Out of 107 plant species which are introduced in Islamic Iranian medicine for cancer treatment, 59 plants or their chemical compounds have proven to possess cytotoxic and antitumor activity in recent investigations and some have entered clinical trials and their effectiveness has been evaluated on humans.

These findings show the profound insight of Islamic physicians on cancer treatment. In spite of the lack of modern facilities and developed equipment, they introduced anticancer plants that have shown cytotoxic properties in new researches. The correlation between these findings signifies the originality of past experiences and studies, representing a worthwhile fund and valuable science dating back more than twelve centuries. This heritage is based on the experiences of thousands years of Greek, Indian and ancient Iranian physicians and relies on immense number of clinical trials on thousands of people. Furthermore, the application of traditional medicinal knowledge reinterpreted by modern data can lead to more effective and evidence-based use of medicinal plants, which can contribute to therapeutic decisions on different illnesses.

Author details

Behjat Javadi[1], Milad Iranshahy[2] and Seyed Ahmad Emami[2*]

*Address all correspondence to: emamia@mums.ac.ir

1 Department of Traditional Pharmacy, School of Pharmacy, Mashhad University of Medical Sciences, Mashhad, Iran

2 Department of Pharmacognosy, School of Pharmacy, Mashhad University of Medical Sciences, Mashhad, Iran

References

[1] Jorjâni SI. *Zakhireh Khârazmshâhi* (*Treasure of Khârazmshâh*). Photoprint of the manuscript dated 1206 AD, edited with Introduction by A.A. Saeedi Sirjani. Tehran: The Iranian Culture Foundation; 1977. pp. 358, 562-563, 585-586 (in Persian)

[2] Razi MZ. *Al-Hâwi fi al-Tibbe* (*Continens*). Toaymi H K (ed). Vol.4. Beirut: Dar Ihya al-Turath al-Arabi; 2002. pp. 5-16 (in Arabic)

[3] Ibn Sina HA. *Al-Qanun fi al-Tibb* (*The Canon of Medicine*). Vol.4. New Delhi: Jamia Hamdard; 1998. pp. 195-197(in Arabic)

[4] Ahwazi Arjani AA. *Kamel al-Sina'ah al-Tibbiyah* (*The Perfect Art of the Medicine*) (in Arabic). Al-Dassuqi I (ed). Saadat Press; 1877. P.190-191 (in Arabic)

[5] Qarshi I. *Al-Shamel fi al-Sinaat al-Tibbiah* (*Comprehensive Book on the Art of Medicine*). Ziedan Y (ed). Vol. 7. Abu Dhabi: al-Majma' al-Thaqafi (Publications of the Cultural Centre); 1999. pp. 943-944 (in Arabic)

[6] Jorjâni SI. *Al-Aghrâz al-Tibbiah wa al-Mabâhethi al-Alâiiah* (*Medical goals and Alaâii's discussions*). Photoprint of the manuscript dated 1399 AD, edited with Introduction by P.N. Khanlari. Tehran: The Iranian Culture Foundation; 1966. pp. 555-558 (in Persian)

[7] Chashti MAK. *Exir-e-Azam*. 2 edn., Delhi: Nami Monshi Nolkshur; 1884. pp. 308-313 (in Persian)

[8] Tonekaboni, M.M. *Tohfat al-Momenin* (*Rarity of the Faithful*). Qum: Nour Vahy Press; 2011. pp.126-278, 328-423 (in Persian)

[9] Aqili Khorasani MH. *Makhzan al-Adwiah (Drug Treasure)*. Reprinted from a copy which was printed in Calcutta dated in 1844. Tehran: Enqelab-e Eslami Publishing and Educational Organization; 1992. pp. 530-797 (in Persian)

[10] Ibn Beytar Z. *Al-Jamee Le-Mofradaat al-Adwiah wal-Aghziyah (Comprehensive Book in Simple Drugs and Foods)*. Beirut: Dar- Al-Kotob Al-ilmiyah; 2001. pp. 160-185 (in Arabic)

[11] al-Ghassani A. *Hadiqat Al-Azhar fi Mahiyat Al-'Ushb wa Al-'Uqar (Garden of Flowers in the Explanation of the Character of Herbs and Drugs)*. Beirut: Dar Al-Gharb Al-Islami; 1990. p.10 (in Arabic)

[12] Razi MZ. *Taqasim Al-'Ilal (Kitab At-Taqsim Wa at-Tasgir)*. Hamami SM (ed). Aleppo: Aleppo University Publications, Institute for the History of Arabic Science; 1992. pp. 416-582 (in Arabic)

[13] Ibn Beytar Z. *Al-Moghni fi-al-Tebb*. Digital photo of a handwritten manuscript dated 1834 AD. pp. 210-213 (in Arabic)

[14] Tabari A. *Ferdows al-Hekmah fi al-Tibb (Paradise of Wisdom on Medicine)*. Al-Seddiqi (ed). Berlin: Aftab Press; 1928. pp.228-230 (in Arabic)

[15] Akhawayni Bukhari AB. *Hedayat al-Mota'allemin fi al-Tibb (An Educational Guide for Medical Students)*. Matini J (ed). Mashhad: Ferdowsi University of Mashhad Publication; 1992. pp. 606-607 (in Arabic)

[16] Lampronti I, Martello D, Bianchi N, Borgatti M, Lambertini E, Piva R, et al. In vitro antiproliferative effects on human tumor cell lines of extracts from the Bangladeshi medicinal plant *Aegle marmelos* Correa. *Phytomedicine.* 2003;10(4):300-8. PMID: 12809360

[17] Costa-Lotufo LV, Khan MTH, Ather A, Wilke DV, Jimenez PC, Pessoa C, et al. Studies of the anticancer potential of plants used in Bangladeshi folk medicine. *J Ethnopharmacol.* 2005;99(1):21-30. PMID: 15848015

[18] Khan MT, Lampronti I, Martello D, Bianchi N, Jabbar S, Choudhuri MS, et al. Identification of pyrogallol as an antiproliferative compound present in extracts from the medicinal plant *Emblica officinalis*: effects on in vitro cell growth of human tumor cell lines. *Int J Oncol.* 2002;21(1):187-92. PMID: 12063567

[19] Hamid K, Diba F, Urmi KF, Uddin ME, Zohera FT, Habib MR. In vitro antioxidant and cytotoxicity screening of different bark extracts of *Aegle marmelos* L. *J Appl Pharmaceut Sci.* 2012;2(3):92-5.

[20] Mustahil NA, Riyanto S, Sukari MA, Rahmani M, Mohd Nor SM, Ali AM. Antileukemic activity of extracts and constituents of *Aegle marmelos. Res J Chem Environ.* 2013;17(1):62-7.

[21] Subramaniam D, Giridharan P, Murmu N, Shankaranarayanan NP, May R, Houchen CW, et al. Activation of apoptosis by 1-hydroxy-5,7-dimethoxy-2-naphthalene- car-

boxaldehyde, a novel compound *from Aegle marmelos. Canc Res*. 2008;68(20):8573-81. doi: 10.1158/0008-5472.CAN-08-2372.

[22] Abdullaev FI. Cancer chemopreventive and tumoricidal properties of saffron (*Crocus sativus* L.). *Exper Biol Med*. 2002;227(1):20-5. PMID: 11788779

[23] Carotenuto A, Fattorusso E, Lanzotti V, Magno S, De Feo V, Carnuccio R, et al. Porrigenins A and B, novel cytotoxic and antiproliferative sapogenins isolated from *Allium porrum*. *J Natural Prod*. 1997;60(10):1003-7. PMID: 9358643

[24] Fattorusso E, Lanzotti V, Taglialatela-Scafati O, Di Rosa M, Ianaro A. Cytotoxic saponins from bulbs of *Allium porrum* L. *J Agric Food Chem*. 2000;48(8):3455-62. PMID: 10956133

[25] Lee KH, Kang HG, Cho CH, Lee MJ, Lee JH, Kim CH. Antimutagenic and antileukemic activities of *Aloe vera* L. *Natural Prod Sci*. 2000;6(2):56-60.

[26] Jose J, Sudhakaran S, Sumesh Kumar TM, Jayaraman S, Jayadevi Variyar E. A comparative evaluation of anticancer activities of flavonoids isolated from *Mimosa pudica, Aloe vera* and *Phyllanthus niruri* against human breast carcinoma cell line (MCF-7) using MTT assay. *Int J Pharmacy Pharmaceut Sci*. 2014;6(2):319-22.

[27] Lee KH, Kim JH, Lim DS, Kim CH. Anti-leukaemic and anti-mutagenic effects of di(2-ethylhexyl)phthalate isolated from *Aloe vera* Linne. *J Pharmacy Pharmacol*. 2000;52(5):593-8. PMID: 10864149

[28] Pecere T, Gazzola MV, Mucignat C, Parolin C, Vecchia FD, Cavaggioni A, et al. Aloe-emodin is a new type of anticancer agent with selective activity against neuroectodermal tumors. *Canc Res*. 2000;60(11):2800-4. PMID:10850417

[29] Liu K, Park C, Li S, Lee KW, Liu H, He L, et al. Aloe-emodin suppresses prostate cancer by targeting the mTOR complex 2. *Carcinogenesis*. 2012 Jul;33(7):1406-11. PMID: 22532249. PMCID: 3405653.

[30] Wasserman L, Avigad S, Beery E, Nordenberg J, Fenig E. The effect of aloe emodin on the proliferation of a new Merkel carcinoma cell line. *Am J Dermatopathol*. 2002;24(1):17-22. PMID: 11803275

[31] Acevedo-Duncan M, Russell C, Patel S, Patel R. Aloe-emodin modulates PKC isozymes, inhibits proliferation, and induces apoptosis in U-373MG glioma cells. *Int Immunopharmacol*. 2004;4(14 SPEC.ISS.):1775-84. PMID:15531293

[32] Ismail S, Haris K, Abdul Ghani ARI, Abdullah JM, Johan MF, Amohamed Yusoff AA. Enhanced induction of cell cycle arrest and apoptosis via the mitochondrial membrane potential disruption in human U87 malignant glioma cells by aloe emodin. *J Asian Natural Prod Res*. 2013;15(9):1003-12.

[33] Lin JG, Chen GW, Li TM, Chouh ST, Tan TW, Chung JG. Aloe-Emodin induces apoptosis in T24 human bladder cancer cells through the p53 dependent apoptotic pathway. *J Urol.* 2006;175(1):343-7. PMID:16406939

[34] Guo J, Xiao B, Liu Q, Gong Z, Le Y. Suppression of C-myc expression associates with anti-proliferation of aloe-emodin on gastric cancer cells. *Canc Invest.* 2008;26(4): 369-74. doi: 10.1080/07357900701788130.

[35] Hosseini J, Mahmoodi M, Jalili A, Hosseini S, Hosseini-Zijoud SM, Khoshdel A, et al. Aloe-emodin induces apoptosis through the up-regulation of fas in the human breast cancer cell line MCF-7. *Life Sci J.* 2014;11(SPEC.ISS.2):47-53.

[36] Naveena, Bharath BK, Selvasubramanian. Antitumor activity of *Aloe vera* against Ehrlich ascitis carcinoma (EAC) in Swiss albino mice. *Int J Pharma Bio Sci.* 2011;2(2): 400-9.

[37] Grabarczyk H, Drozdz B, Hladon B, Wojciechowska J. Sesquiterpene lactones. Part XV. New cytostatic active sesquiterpene lactone from herb of *Anthemis nobilis* L. *Polish J Pharmacol Pharmacy.* 1977;29(4):419-23. PMID: 905207

[38] Kapadia GJ, Azuine MA, Rao GS, Arai T, Iida A, Tokuda H. Cytotoxic effect of the red beetroot (*Beta vulgaris* L.) extract compared to doxorubicin (adriamycin) in the human prostate (PC-3) and breast (MCF-7) cancer cell lines. *Anti-Canc Agents Medic Chem.* 2011;11(3):280-4. PMID: 21434853

[39] Kapadia GJ, Rao GS, Ramachandran C, Iida A, Suzuki N, Tokuda H. Synergistic cytotoxicity of red beetroot (*Beta vulgaris* L.) extract with doxorubicin in human pancreatic, breast and prostate cancer cell lines. *J Complement Integ Med.* 2013;10. doi: 10.1515/jcim-2013-0007

[40] Haroun AA, Taie HAA. Cytotoxicity and antioxidant activity of beta vulgaris extract released from grafted carbon nanotubes based nanocomposites. *Macromol Symp.* 2014;337(1):25-33. DOI: 10.1002/masy.201450303

[41] Lee EJ, An D, Nguyen CTT, Patil BS, Kim J, Yoo KS. Betalain and betaine composition of greenhouse- or field-produced beetroot (*beta vulgaris* L.) and inhibition of HepG2 cell proliferation. *J Agric Food Chem.* 2014;62(6):1324-31. doi: 10.1021/jf404648u.

[42] Zhao W, Entschladen F, Liu H, Niggemann B, Fang Q, Zaenker KS, et al. Boswellic acid acetate induces differentiation and apoptosis in highly metastatic melanoma and fibrosarcoma cells. *Canc Detect Prevention.* 2003;27(1):67-75. PMID: 12600419

[43] Akihisa T, Tabata K, Banno N, Tokuda H, Nishihara R, Nakamura Y, et al. Cancer chemopreventive effects and cytotoxic activities of the triterpene acids from the resin of *Boswellia carteri.* Biol Pharmaceut Bull. 2006;29(9):1976-9. PMID: 16946522

[44] Frank MB, Yang Q, Osban J, Azzarello JT, Saban MR, Saban R, et al. Frankincense oil derived from *Boswellia carteri* induces tumor cell specific cytotoxicity. *BMC Complement Alt Med.* 2009;9. doi: 10.1186/1472-6882-9-6.

[45] Ali SI, Zhang CR, Mohamed AA, El-Baz FK, Hegazy AK, Kord MA, et al. Major constituents of *Bosweilla carteri* resin exhibit cyclooxygenase enzyme inhibition and antiproliferative activity. *Natural Prod Commun.* 2013;8(10):1365-6. PMID: 24354175

[46] Bryant CS, Kumar S, Chamala S, Shah J, Pal J, Haider M, et al. Sulforaphane induces cell cycle arrest by protecting RB-E2F-1 complex in epithelial ovarian cancer cells. *Mol Canc.* 2010;9. doi: 10.1186/1476-4598-9-47

[47] Melchini A, Traka MH. Biological profile of erucin: A new promising anticancer agent from cruciferous vegetables. *Toxins.* 2010;2(4):593-612. doi: 10.3390/toxins2040593.

[48] Hafidh RR, Abdulamir AS, Abu Bakar F, Jalilian FA, Jahanshiri F, Abas F, et al. Novel anticancer activity and anticancer mechanisms of *Brassica oleracea* L. var. capitata f. rubra. *Eur J Integ Med.* 2013;5(5):450-64.

[49] Thangam R, Suresh V, Rajkumar M, Vincent JD, Gunasekaran P, Anbazhagan C, et al. Antioxidant and in vitro anticancer effect of 2-pyrrolidinone rich fraction of *Brassica oleracea* var. capitata through induction of apoptosis in human cancer cells. *Phytother Res.* 2013;27(11):1664-70. doi: 10.1002/ptr.4908.

[50] Kim SM, Park JH, Kim KD, Nam D, Shim BS, Kim SH, et al. Brassinin induces apoptosis in PC-3 human prostate cancer cells through the suppression of PI3K/Akt/mTOR/S6K1 signaling cascades. *Phytother Res.* 2014;28(3):423-31. doi: 10.1002/ptr.5010.

[51] Ji YB, Dong F, Ma DB, Miao J, Jin LN, Liu ZF, et al. Optimizing the extraction of antitumor polysaccharides from the fruit of *Capparis spionosa* L. by response surface methodology. *Molecules.* 2012;17(6):7323-35. PMID: 22699566.

[52] Yu L, Mo K, Wang W, Cui RT, Zou X, Ji YB. Relationship between apoptosis and [Ca2+]i in HepG2 induced by *Capparis spinosa* alkaloid. *Chin Tradition Herbal Drugs.* 2009;40(2):255-8.

[53] Loo WTY, Cheung MNB, Chow LWC. The inhibitory effect of a herbal formula comprising ginseng and *Carthamus tinctorius* on breast cancer. *Life Sci.* 2004;76(2):191-200. PMID: 15519364

[54] Shi X, Ruan D, Wang Y, Ma L, Li M. Anti-tumor activity of safflower polysaccharide (SPS) and effect on cytotoxicity of CTL cells,NK cells of T739 lung cancer in mice. *Zhongguo Zhongyao Zazhi.* 2010;35(2):215-8. PMID: 20394298

[55] Son ES, Lee JM, Choi JU, Park HR. Selective cytotoxicity of Carthamus tinctorius against glucose-deprived HT-29 human colon carcinoma cells. *J Medic Plant Res.* 2011;5(19):4931-7.

[56] Sutton KM, Greenshields AL, Hoskin DW. Thymoquinone, a bioactive component of black caraway seeds, causes G1 phase cell cycle arrest and apoptosis in triple-negative breast cancer cells with mutant p53. *Nutri Canc.* 2014;66(3):408-18. doi: 10.1080/01635581.2013.878739.

[57] Duraipandiyan V, Baskar AA, Ignacimuthu S, Muthukumar C, Al-Harbi NA. Anticancer activity of Rhein isolated from *Cassia fistula* L. flower. *Asian Pac J Trop Dis.* 2012;2(SUPPL.1):S517-S23. doi:10.1016/S2222-1808(12)60213-8

[58] Linu M, Shankar S. In vitro cytotoxic activity of methanolic extract of stem bark of *Cassia fistula* L. *Res J Biotechnol.* 2012;7(4):141-8.

[59] Gao XM, Shen YQ, Huang XZ, Yang LY, Shu LD, Hu QF, et al. 2''-ethyl-furanoflavone derivatives from the stems of *Cassia fistula* and their cytotoxicity. *J Brazil Chem Soc.* 2013;24(4):685-9.

[60] Yang J, Wang H, Liu G, Lou J, Li L, Hu Q, et al. A new anthraquinone from the fruit of *Cassia fistula* and its cytotoxicity. *Asian J Chem.* 2014;26(14):4519-20.

[61] Kumar S, Kapoor V, Gill K, Singh K, Xess I, Das SN, et al. Antifungal and antiproliferative protein from *Cicer arietinum*: A bioactive compound against emerging pathogens. *BioMed Res Int.* 2014;2014. doi: 10.1155/2014/387203. In Press.

[62] Csupor-Löffler B, Hajdú Z, Réthy B, Zupkó I, Máthé I, Rédei T, et al. Antiproliferative activity of Hungarian asteraceae species against human cancer cell lines. Part II. *Phytother Res.* 2009;23(8):1109-15. doi: 10.1002/ptr.2755.

[63] Zhou CX, Zou L, Zhao ZZ, Zhu H, He QJ, Yang B, et al. Terpenoids from *Cichorium intybus*. *Natural Prod Commun.* 2012;7(8):971-2. PMID: 22978206

[64] Ka H, Park HJ, Jung HJ, Choi JW, Cho KS, Ha J, et al. Cinnamaldehyde induces apoptosis by ROS-mediated mitochondrial permeability transition in human promyelocytic leukemia HL-60 cells. *Canc Lett.* 2003;196(2):143-52. PMID: 12860272

[65] Lee HS, Kim SY, Lee CH, Ahn YJ. Cytotoxic and mutagenic effects of *Cinnamomum cassia* bark-derived materials. *J Microbiol Biotechnol.* 2004;14(6):1176-81. doi: 10.1186/1471-2407-10-210.

[66] Koppikar SJ, Choudhari AS, Suryavanshi SA, Kumari S, Chattopadhyay S, Kaul-Ghanekar R. Aqueous Cinnamon Extract (ACE-c) from the bark of *Cinnamomum cassia* causes apoptosis in human cervical cancer cell line (SiHa) through loss of mitochondrial membrane potential. *BMC Cancer.* 2010;10.

[67] Kang HS, Ock J, Lee HJ, Lee YJ, Kwon BM, Hong SH. Early growth response protein 1 upregulation and nuclear translocation by 2'-benzoyloxycinnamaldehyde induces prostate cancer cell death. *Canc Lett.* 2013;329(2):217-27. doi: 10.1016/j.canlet.2012.11.006.

[68] Ngoc TM, Nhiem NX, Khoi NM, Son DC, Hung TV, Kiem PV. A new coumarin and cytotoxic activities of constituents from *Cinnamomum cassia*. *Natural Prod Commun*. 2014;9(4):487-8. PMID: 24868863

[69] Chinou I, Demetzos C, Harvala C, Roussakis C, Verbist JF. Cytotoxic and antibacterial labdane-type diterpenes from the aerial parts of *Cistus incanus* subsp. *creticus*. *Planta Medica*. 1994;60(1):34-6. PMID: 8134413

[70] Dimas K, Demetzos C, Marsellos M, Sotiriadou R, Malamas M, Kokkinopoulos D. Cytotoxic activity of labdane type diterpenes against human leukemic cell lines in vitro. *Planta Medica*. 1998;64(3):208-11. PMID: 9581515

[71] Dimas K, Demetzos C, Mitaku S, Vaos B, Marselos M, Tzavaras T, et al. Cytotoxic activity and antiproliferative effects of a new semi-synthetic derivative of Ent-3β-hydroxy-13-epi-manoyl oxide on human leukemic cell lines. *Anticanc Res*. 1999;19(5 B): 4065-72. PMID: 11582537

[72] Demetzos C, Dimas K, Hatziantoniou S, Anastasaki T, Angelopoulou D. Cytotoxic and anti-inflammatory activity of labdane and cis-clerodane type diterpenes. *Planta Medica*. 2001;67(7):614-8. PMID: 11582537

[73] Skorić M, Todorović S, Gligorijević N, Janković R, Živković S, Ristić M, et al. Cytotoxic activity of ethanol extracts of in vitro grown *Cistus creticus* subsp. *creticus* L. on human cancer cell lines. *Indus Crops Prod*. 2012;38(1):153-9. doi:10.1016/j.indcrop.2012.01.017

[74] Shah R, Gulati V, Palombo EA. Pharmacological properties of guggulsterones, the major active components of gum guggul. *Phytother Res*. 2012;26(11):1594-605. doi: 10.1002/ptr.4647.

[75] Jana S, Patra K, Sarkar S, Jana J, Mukherjee G, Bhattacharjee S, et al. Antitumorigenic potential of linalool is accompanied by modulation of oxidative stress: An in vivo study in sarcoma-180 solid tumor model. *Nutri Canc*. 2014;66(5):835-48. doi: 10.1080/01635581.2014.904906.

[76] Nithya TG, Sumalatha D. Evaluation of invitro anti-oxidant and anticancer activity of *Coriandrum Sativum* against human colon cancer HT- 29 cell lines. *Int J Pharmacy Pharmaceut Sci*. 2014;6(2):421-4.

[77] Nair SC, Pannikar B, Panikkar KR. Antitumour activity of saffron (*Crocus sativus*). *Canc Lett*. 1991;57(2):109-14. PMID: 2025883

[78] Tavakkol-Afshari J, Brook A, Mousavi SH. Study of cytotoxic and apoptogenic properties of saffron extract in human cancer cell lines. *Food Chem Toxicol*. 2008;46(11): 3443-7. doi: 10.1016/j.fct.2008.08.018.

[79] Samarghandian S, Boskabady MH, Davoodi S. Use of in vitro assays to assess the potential antiproliferative and cytotoxic effects of saffron (*Crocus sativus* L.) in human

lung cancer cell line. *Pharmacognosy Mag.* 2010;6(24):309-14. doi: 10.4103/0973-1296.71799.

[80] Escribano J, Alonso GL, Coca-Prados M, Fernández JA. Crocin, safranal and picrocrocin from saffron (*Crocus sativus* L.) inhibit the growth of human cancer cells in vitro. *Canc Lett.* 1996;100(1-2):23-30. PMID: 8620447

[81] Noureini SK, Wink M. Antiproliferative effects of crocin in HepG2 cells by telomerase inhibition and hTERT down-regulation. *Asian Pac J Canc Prevention.* 2012;13(5): 2305-9. PMID: 22901211

[82] Malaekeh-Nikouei B, Mousavi SH, Shahsavand S, Mehri S, Nassirli H, Moallem SA. Assessment of cytotoxic properties of safranal and nanoliposomal safranal in various cancer cell lines. *Phytother Res.* 2013;27(12):1868-73. doi: 10.1002/ptr.4945.

[83] Samarghandian S, Shabestari MM. DNA fragmentation and apoptosis induced by safranal in human prostate cancer cell line. *Ind J Urol.* 2013;29(3):177-83. doi: 10.4103/0970-1591.117278.

[84] Geromichalos GD, Papadopoulos T, Sahpazidou D, Sinakos Z. Safranal, a *Crocus sativus* L constituent suppresses the growth of K-562 cells of chronic myelogenous leukemia. In silico and in vitro study. *Food Chem Toxicol.* 2014;74:45-50. doi: 10.1016/j.fct. 2014.09.001.

[85] Kim SH, Lee JM, Kim SC, Park CB, Lee PC. Proposed cytotoxic mechanisms of the saffron carotenoids crocin and crocetin on cancer cell lines. *Biochem Cell Biol.* 2014;92(2):105-11. doi: 10.1139/bcb-2013-0091.

[86] Rezaee R, Jamialahmadi K, Zanjani BR, Mahmoudi M, Abnous K, Rabe SZT, et al. Crocin effects on human myeloma cells regarding intracellular redox state, DNA fragmentation, and apoptosis or necrosis profile. *Jundishapur J Natural Pharmaceut Prod.* 2014;9(4). PMID: 25625054

[87] Rastgoo M, Hosseinzadeh H, Alavizadeh H, Abbasi A, Ayati Z, Jaafari MR. Antitumor activity of PEGylated nanoliposomes containing crocin in mice bearing C26 colon carcinoma. *Planta Medica.* 2013;79(6):447-51. doi: 10.1055/s-0032-1328363.

[88] Begum Y, Hossen F, Rahman MM. In vitro cytotoxic properties of methanol extracts of the seeds of *benincasa hispida* and *cucurbita maxima. Eur J Sci Res.* 2011;54(2):193-7.

[89] Saha P, Mazumder UK, Haldar PK, Naskar S, Kundu S, Bala A, et al. Anticancer activity of methanol extract of *Cucurbita maxima* against Ehrlich as-cites carcinoma. *Int J Res Pharmaceut Sci.* 2011;2(1):52-9.

[90] Kikuchi T, Takebayashi M, Shinto M, Yamada T, Tanaka R. Three new multiflorane-type triterpenes from pumpkin (*Cucurbita maxima*) seeds. *Molecules.* 2013;18(5): 5568-79. doi: 10.3390/molecules18055568.

[91] Shokrzadeh M, Azadbakht M, Ahangar N, Hashemi A, Saeedi Saravi SS. Cytotoxicity of hydro-alcoholic extracts of *Cucurbita pepo* and *Solanum nigrum* on HepG2 and CT26 cancer cell lines. *Pharmacognosy Mag*. 2010;6(23):176-9. doi: 10.4103/0973-1296.66931

[92] Jafarian A, Ghannadi A, Mohebi B. Cytotoxic effects of chloroform and hydroalcoholic extracts of aerial parts of *Cuscuta chinensis* and *Cuscuta epithymum* on Hela, HT29 and MDA-MB-468 tumor cells. *Res Pharmaceut Sci*. 2014;9(2):115-22.

[93] Attard E, Cuschieri A. Cytotoxicity of Cucurbitacin E extracted from *Ecballium elaterium* in vitro. *J Natural Remedies*. 2004;4(2):137-44.

[94] Attard E, Cuschieri A, Brincat MP. Morphological effects induced by Cucurbitacin E on ovarian cancer cells in vitro. *J Natural Remedies*. 2005;5(1):70-4.

[95] Bohlooli S, Jafari N, Jahed S. Cytotoxic effect of freeze-dried extract of *Ecballium elaterium* fruit on gastric adenocarcinoma (AGS) and esophageal squamous cell carcinoma (KYSE30) cell lines. *J Gastrointest Canc*. 2012;43(4):579-83. doi: 10.1007/s12029-012-9383-4.

[96] Jacquot C, Rousseau B, Carbonnelle D, Chinou I, Malleter M, Tomasoni C, et al. Cucurbitacin-D-induced CDK1 mRNA up-regulation causes proliferation arrest of a non-small cell lung carcinoma cell line (NSCLC-N6). *Anticanc Res*. 2014;34(9):4797-806. PMID: 25202060

[97] Khodarahmi GA, Ghasemi N, Hassanzadeh F, Safaie M. Cytotoxic effects of different extracts and latex of *ficus carica* L. on HeLa cell line. *Iranian J Pharmaceut Res*. 2011;10(2):273-7. PMID: 24250354

[98] Hamta A, Shariatzadeh SMA, Soleimani Mehranjani M, Fallah Huseini H, Hosseinabadi F. The cytotoxic effects of *Glycyrrhiza glabra* L. root extract on 4T1 cell line derived from BALB/c mice mammary tumors. *J Medic Plants*. 2014;13(50):92-103.

[99] Dorn DC, Alexenizer M, Hengstler JG, Dorn A. Tumor cell specific toxicity of *Inula helenium* extracts. *Phytother Res*. 2006;20(11):970-80. PMID: 16912983

[100] Mazzio E, Badisa R, Mack N, Deiab S, Soliman KFA. High throughput screening of natural products for anti-mitotic effects in MDA-MB-231 human breast carcinoma cells. *Phytother Res*. 2014;28(6):856-67. doi: 10.1002/ptr.5065.

[101] Rahman MA, Hasan MS, Hossain MA, Biswas NN. Analgesic and cytotoxic activities of *Jasminum sambac* (L.) Aiton. *Pharmacologyonline*. 2011;1:124-31.

[102] Liu JX, Di DL, Wei XN, Han Y. Cytotoxic diarylheptanoids from the pericarps of walnuts (*Juglans regia*). *Planta Medica*. 2008;74(7):754-9. doi: 10.1055/s-2008-1074536.

[103] Salimi M, Majd A, Sepahdar Z, Azadmanesh K, Irian S, Ardestaniyan MH, et al. Cytotoxicity effects of various *Juglans regia* (walnut) leaf extracts in human cancer cell lines. *Pharmaceut Biol*. 2012;50(11):1416-22. doi: 10.3109/13880209.2012.682118.

[104] Li CY, Du HJ, Su XH, Zhong YJ, Yuan ZP, Li YF, et al. Juglanones A and B: Two novel tetralone dimers from walnut pericarp (*Juglans regia*). *Helvetica Chim Acta.* 2013;96(6):1031-5. DOI: 10.1002/hlca.201200525

[105] Salimi M, Ardestaniyan MH, Mostafapour Kandelous H, Saeidnia S, Gohari AR, Amanzadeh A, et al. Anti-proliferative and apoptotic activities of constituents of chloroform extract of *Juglans regia* leaves. *Cell Prolifer.* 2014;47(2):172-9.

[106] Han YF, Cao GX, Gao XJ, Xia M. Isolation and characterisation of the sesquiterpene lactones from *Lactuca sativa* L var. *anagustata.* Food Chemistry. 2010;120(4):1083-8. doi:10.1016/j.foodchem.2009.11.056

[107] Kivçak B, Mert T. Preliminary evaluation of cytotoxic properties of *Laurus nobilis* leaf extracts. *Fitoterapia.* 2002;73(3):242-3. PMID: 12048018

[108] Dall'Acqua S, Viola G, Giorgetti M, Loi MC, Innocenti G. Two new sesquiterpene lactones from the leaves of *Laurus nobilis. Chem Pharmaceut Bull.* 2006;54(8):1187-9. PMID:16880666

[109] Barla A, Topçu G, Öksüz S, Tümen G, Kingston DGI. Identification of cytotoxic sesquiterpenes from *Laurus nobilis* L. *Food Chem.* 2007;104(4):1478-84. doi:10.1016/j.foodchem.2007.02.019

[110] Loizzo MR, Tundis R, Menichini F, Saab AM, Statti GA. Cytotoxic activity of essential oils from Labiatae and Lauraceae families against in vitro human tumor models. *Anticanc Res.* 2007;27(5 A):3293-9. PMID: 17970073

[111] Li Q, Gao W, Cao J, Bi X, Chen G, Zhang X, et al. New cytotoxic compounds from flowers of *Lawsonia inermis* L. *Fitoterapia.* 2014;94:148-54.

[112] Lehraiki A, Attoumbré J, Bienaimé C, Matifat F, Bensaddek L, Nava-Saucedo E, et al. Extraction of lignans from flaxseed and evaluation of their biological effects on breast cancer MCF-7 and MDA-MB-231 cell lines. *J Medic Food.* 2010;13(4):834-41. doi: 10.1089/jmf.2009.0172.

[113] de Sousa AC, Alviano DS, Blank AF, Barreto Alves P, Alviano CS, Gattass CR. *Melissa officinalis* L. essential oil: Antitumoral and antioxidant activities. *J Pharmacy Pharmacol.* 2004;56(5):677-81. PMID:15142347

[114] Encalada MA, Hoyos KM, Rehecho S, Berasategi I, de Ciriano MGI, Ansorena D, et al. Anti-proliferative Effect of *Melissa officinalis* on Human Colon Cancer Cell Line. *Plant Foods Human Nutri.* 2011;66(4):328-34. doi: 10.1007/s11130-011-0256-y.

[115] Saraydin SU, Tuncer E, Tepe B, Karadayi S, Özer H, Şen M, et al. Antitumoral effects of *Melissa officinalis* on breast cancer in vitro and in vivo. *Asian Pac J Canc Prevention.* 2012;13(6):2765-70. PMID: 22938456

[116] De Queiroz RM, Takiya CM, Guimarães LPTP, Rocha GDG, Alviano DS, Blank AF, et al. Apoptosis-inducing effects of *Melissa officinalis* L. essential oil in glioblastoma multiforme cells. *Canc Invest*. 2014;32(6):226-35. doi: 10.3109/07357907.2014.905587

[117] Cottiglia F, Casu L, Leonti M, Caboni P, Floris C, Busonera B, et al. Cytotoxic phloroglucinols from the leaves of *Myrtus communis*. *J Natural Prod*. 2012;75(2):225-9. doi: 10.1021/np2009219.

[118] Youssef DTA, Khalifa AA. Cytotoxic quaternary alkaloids from the flowers of *Narcissus tazetta*. *Pharmazie*. 2001;56(10):818-22. PMID: 11683132

[119] Liu J, Li Y, Ren W, Hu WX. Apoptosis of HL-60 cells induced by extracts from *Narcissus tazetta* var. chinensis. *Canc Lett*. 2006;242(1):133-40. PMID: 16427186

[120] Juan ME, Wenzel U, Daniel H, Planas JM. Erythrodiol, a natural triterpenoid from olives, has antiproliferative and apoptotic activity in HT-29 human adenocarcinoma cells. *Mol Nutri Food Res*. 2008;52(5):595-9. doi: 10.1002/mnfr.200700300.

[121] Bouallagui Z, Han J, Isoda H, Sayadi S. Hydroxytyrosol rich extract from olive leaves modulates cell cycle progression in MCF-7 human breast cancer cells. *Food Chem Toxicol*. 2011;49(1):179-84. doi: 10.1016/j.fct.2010.10.014.

[122] Reyes-Zurita FJ, Pachón-Peña G, Lizárraga D, Rufino-Palomares EE, Cascante M, Lupiáñez JA. The natural triterpene maslinic acid induces apoptosis in HT29 colon cancer cells by a JNK-p53-dependent mechanism. *BMC Cancer*. 2011;11. doi: 10.1186/1471-2407-11-154.

[123] Busnena BA, Foudah AI, Melancon T, El Sayed KA. Olive secoiridoids and semisynthetic bioisostere analogues for the control of metastatic breast cancer. *Bioorg Medic Chem*. 2013;21(7):2117-27. doi: 10.1016/j.bmc.2012.12.050.

[124] University of Southern California. *Study of Noscapine for Patients With Low Grade Non Hodgkin's Lymphoma or Chronic Lymphocytic Leukemia Refractory to Chemotherapy*. In: ClinicalTrials.gov [Internet]. Bethesda (MD): National Library of Medicine (US). 2015 Jan 25. Available from: http://clinicaltrials.gov/ct2/results?term=noscapine&Search=Search.

[125] Zhang CH, Wang ZT, Yang YP, Sun QS. A novel cytotoxic neophysalin from *Physalis alkekengi* var. francheti. *Chin Chem Lett*. 2009;20(11):1327-30.

[126] He H, Zang LH, Feng YS, Chen LX, Kang N, Tashiro SI, et al. Physalin A induces apoptosis via p53-Noxa-mediated ROS generation, and autophagy plays a protective role against apoptosis through p38-NF-κB survival pathway in A375-S2 cells. *J Ethnopharmacol*. 2013;148(2):544-55. doi: 10.1016/j.jep.2013.04.051.

[127] He H, Zang LH, Feng YS, Wang J, Liu WW, Chen LX, et al. Physalin a induces apoptotic cell death and protective autophagy in HT1080 human fibrosarcoma cells. *J Natural Prod*. 2013;76(5):880-8. doi: 10.1021/np400017k.

[128] Rezaei PF, Fouladdel S, Hassani S, Yousefbeyk F, Ghaffari SM, Amin G, et al. Induction of apoptosis and cell cycle arrest by pericarp polyphenol-rich extract of Baneh in human colon carcinoma HT29 cells. *Food Chem Toxicol*. 2012;50(3-4):1054-9. doi: 10.1016/j.fct.2011.11.012.

[129] Balan KV, Demetzos C, Prince J, Dimas K, Cladaras M, Han Z, et al. Induction of apoptosis in human colon cancer HCT116 cells treated with an extract of the plant product, chios mastic gum. *In Vivo*. 2005;19(1):93-102. PMID: 15796160

[130] Chiang LC, Chiang W, Chang MY, Lin CC. In vitro cytotoxic, antiviral and immunomodulatory effects of *Plantago major* and *Plantago asiatica*. *Am J Chin Med*. 2003;31(2): 225-34. PMID: 12856861

[131] Gálvez M, Martín-Cordero C, López-Lázaro M, Cortés F, Ayuso MJ. Cytotoxic effect of *Plantago spp*. on cancer cell lines. *J Ethnopharmacol*. 2003;88(2-3):125-30. PMID: 12963131

[132] Mitrocotsa D, Bosch S, Mitaku S, Dimas C, Skaltsounis AL, Harvala C, et al. Cytotoxicity against human leukemic cell lines, and the activity on the expression of resistance genes of flavonoids from *Platanus orientalis*. *Anticanc Res*. 1999;19(3 A):2085-8. PMID:10470152

[133] Mitrokotsa D, Mitaku S, Demetzos C, Harvala C, Mentis A, Perez S, et al. Bioactive compounds from the buds of *Platanus orientalis* and isolation of a new kaempferol glycoside. Planta Medica. 1993;59(6):517-20. PMID: 8302950

[134] Dimas K, Demetzos C, Mitaku S, Marselos M, Tzavaras T, Kokkinopoulos D. Cytotoxic activity of kaempferol glycosides against human leukaemic cell lines in vitro. *Pharmacol Res*. 2000;41(1):85-8. PMID: 10600274

[135] Afifi-Yazar FU, Kasabri V, Abu-Dahab R. Medicinal plants from jordan in the treatment of cancer: Traditional uses vs in vitro and in vivo evaluations part 1. *Planta Medica*. 2011;77(11):1203-9. doi: 10.1055/s-0030-1270832.

[136] Khan I, Sangwan PL, Dar AA, Rafiq RA, Farrukh MR, Dhar JK, et al. A validated high-performance thin-layer chromatography method for the identification and simultaneous quantification of six markers from *Platanus orientalis* and their cytotoxic profiles against skin cancer cell lines. *J Separ Sci*. 2013;36(16):2602-10. doi: 10.1002/jssc.201300380.

[137] Habibi Roudkenar M, Mohammadi Roushandeh A, Delazar A, Halabian R, Soleimani Rad J, Mehdipour A, et al. Effects of polygonum aviculare herbal extract on proliferation and apoptotic gene expression of MCF-7. DARU, *J Pharmaceut Sci*. 2011;19(5): 326-31. PMID:

[138] Xin HL, Xu YF, Hou YH, Zhang YN, Yue XQ, Lu JC, et al. Two novel triterpenoids from *Portulaca oleracea* L. *Helvetica Chim Acta*. 2008;91(11):2075-80.

[139] Tan GCS, Wong KM, Pearle-Wong GQ, Yeo SL, Yeap SK, Yiap BC, et al. In vitro cytotoxic and antiproliferative effects of *portulaca oleracea* methanol extract on breast, cer-

vical, colon and nasopharyngeal cancerous cell lines. *Sains Malaysiana*. 2013;42(7): 927-35.

[140] Farshori NN, Al-Sheddi ES, Al-Oqail MM, Musarrat J, Al-Khedhairy AA, Siddiqui MA. Cytotoxicity assessments of *Portulaca oleracea* and *Petroselinum sativum* seed extracts on human hepatocellular carcinoma cells (HepG2). *Asian Pac J Canc Prevention*. 2014;15(16):6633-8. PMID: 25169500

[141] Tian JL, Liang X, Gao PY, Li DQ, Sun Q, Li LZ, et al. Two new alkaloids from *Portulaca oleracea* and their cytotoxic activities. *J Asian Natural Prod Res*. 2014;16(3):259-64. doi: 10.1080/10286020.2013.866948.

[142] Jeune MAL, Kumi-Diaka J, Brown J. Anticancer activities of pomegranate extracts and genistein in human breast cancer cells. *J Medic Food*. 2005;8(4):469-75. PMID: 16379557

[143] Banerjee N, Talcott S, Safe S, Mertens-Talcott SU. Cytotoxicity of pomegranate polyphenolics in breast cancer cells in vitro and vivo: Potential role of miRNA-27a and miRNA-155 in cell survival and inflammation. *Breast Canc Res Treat*. 2012;136(1): 21-34. doi: 10.1007/s10549-012-2224-0.

[144] Jayakumar S, Haridass S, Krishnamurthy V. Anticancer activity of *Punica Granatum* rind extracts against human lung cancer cell line. *Asian J Pharmaceut Clin Res*. 2012;5(SUPPL 2):204-10.

[145] Joseph MM, Aravind SR, Varghese S, Mini S, Sreelekha TT. Evaluation of antioxidant, antitumor and immunomodulatory properties of polysaccharide isolated from fruit rind of *Punica granatum*. *Mol Med Rep*. 2012;5(2):489-96. doi: 10.3892/mmr. 2011.638.

[146] Bekir J, Mars M, Vicendo P, Fterrich A, Bouajila J. Chemical composition and antioxidant, anti-inflammatory, and antiproliferation activities of pomegranate (*Punica granatum*) flowers. *J Medic Food*. 2013;16(6):544-50. doi: 10.1089/jmf.2012.0275.

[147] Joseph MM, Aravind SR, George SK, Varghese S, Sreelekha TT. A galactomannan polysaccharide from *Punica granatum* imparts in vitro and in vivo anticancer activity. *Carbohyd Polymers*. 2013;98(2):1466-75. doi: 10.1016/j.carbpol.2013.07.023.

[148] Salah-Abbes JB, Abbès S, Abdel-Wahhab MA, Oueslati R. In-vitro free radical scavenging, antiproliferative and anti-zearalenone cytotoxic effects of 4-(methylthio)-3-butenyl isothiocyanate from Tunisian *Raphanus sativus*. *J Pharmacy Pharmacol*. 2010;62(2):231-9. PMID: 20487203

[149] Kim KH, Moon E, Kim SY, Choi SU, Lee JH, Lee KR. 4-Methylthio-butanyl derivatives from the seeds of *Raphanus sativus* and their biological evaluation on anti-inflammatory and antitumor activities. *J Ethnopharmacol*. 2014;151(1):503-8. doi: 10.1016/j.jep.2013.11.003.

[150] Zarai Z, Chobba IB, Mansour RB, Békir A, Gharsallah N, Kadri A. Essential oil of the leaves of *Ricinus communis* L.: In vitro cytotoxicity and antimicrobial properties. *Lipids Health Dis*. 2012;11. doi: 10.1186/1476-511X-11-102.

[151] Rezaie-Tavirani M, Fayazfar S, Heydari-Keshel S, Rezaee MB, Zamanian-Azodi M, Rezaei-Tavirani M, et al. Effect of essential oil of *Rosa damascena* on human colon cancer cell line SW742. *Gastroenterol Hepatol Bed to Bench*. 2013;6(1):25-31. PMID: 24834241

[152] Kuo YH, Hsu YW, Liaw CC, Lee JK, Huang HC, Kuo LMY. Cytotoxic phenylpropanoids glycosides from the stems of *Smilax china*. *J Natural Prod*. 2005;68(10):1475-8. PMID: 16252910

[153] Li YL, Gan GP, Zhang HZ, Wu HZ, Li CL, Huang YP, et al. A flavonoid glycoside isolated from *Smilax china* L. rhizome in vitro anticancer effects on human cancer cell lines. *J Ethnopharmacol*. 2007;113(1):115-24. PMID: 17606345

[154] Wu LS, Wang XJ, Wang H, Yang HW, Jia AQ, Ding Q. Cytotoxic polyphenols against breast tumor cell in *Smilax china* L. *J Ethnopharmacol*. 2010;130(3):460-4. PMID: 20669365

[155] Hu K, Kobayashi H, Dong A, Jing Y, Iwasaki S, Yao X. Antineoplastic agents III: Steroidal glycosides from *solanum nigrum*. *Planta Medica*. 1999;65(1):35-8. PMID: 10083842

[156] Zhou X, He X, Wang G, Gao H, Zhou G, Ye W, et al. Steroidal saponins from *Solanum nigrum*. *J NaturProd*. 2006;69(8):1158-63. PMID: 16933867:

[157] Heo KS, Lee SJ, Ko JH, Lim K, Lim KT. Glycoprotein isolated from *Solanum nigrum* L. inhibits the DNA-binding activities of NF-κB and AP-1, and increases the production of nitric oxide in TPA-stimulated MCF-7 cells. *Toxicol In Vitro*. 2004;18(6):755-63. PMID: 15465640

[158] Heo KS, Lee SJ, Lim KT. Cytotoxic effect of glycoprotein isolated from *Solanum nigrum* L. through the inhibition of hydroxyl radical-induced DNA-binding activities of NF-kappa B in HT-29 cells. *Environ Toxicol Pharmacol*. 2004;17(1):45-54. doi: 10.1016/j.etap.2004.02.003.

[159] Lee SJ, Oh PS, Ko JH, Lim K, Lim KT. A 150-kDa glycoprotein isolated from *Solanum nigrum* L. has cytotoxic and apoptotic effects by inhibiting the effects of protein kinase C alpha, nuclear factor-kappa B and inducible nitric oxide in HCT-116 cells. *Canc Chemother Pharmacol*. 2004;54(6):562-72. PMID: 15349752

[160] Lim KT. Glycoprotein isolated from *Solanum nigrum* L. kills HT-29 cells through apoptosis. *J Medic Food*. 2005;8(2):215-26. PMID: 16117614

[161] Patel S, Gheewala N, Suthar A, Shah A. In-vitro cytotoxicity activity of *Solanum nigrum* extract against Hela cell line and Vero cell line. *Int J Pharmacy Pharmaceut Sci*. 2009;1(SUPPL. 1):38-46.

[162] Huang HC, Syu KY, Lin JK. Chemical composition of *Solanum nigrum* linn extract and induction of autophagy by leaf water extract and its major flavonoids in AU565 breast cancer cells. *J Agric Food Chem*. 2010;58(15):8699-708. doi: 10.1021/jf101003v.

[163] Sun L, Zhao Y, Li X, Yuan H, Cheng A, Lou H. A lysosomal-mitochondrial death pathway is induced by solamargine in human K562 leukemia cells. *Toxicol In Vitro*. 2010;24(6):1504-11. doi: 10.1016/j.tiv.2010.07.013. Epub 2010 Jul 18.

[164] Akbar N, Thakur VS, Yunus M, Mahdi AA, Gupta S. Selective cell cycle arrest and induction of apoptosis in human prostate cancer cells by a polyphenol-rich extract of *Solanum nigrum*. *Int J Mol Med*. 2012;29(2):277-84. PMID: 22076244

[165] Gabrani R, Jain R, Sharma A, Sarethy IP, Dang S, Gupta S. Antiproliferative effect of *Solanum nigrum* on human leukemic cell lines. *Ind J Pharmaceut Sci*. 2012;74(5):451-3. PMID: 23716874

[166] Mathema VB, Koh YS, Thakuri BC, Sillanpää M. Parthenolide, a sesquiterpene lactone, expresses multiple anti-cancer and anti-inflammatory activities. *Inflammation*. 2012;35(2):560-5. PMID: 21603970

[167] Lee SH, Ryu SY, Choi SU, Lee CO, No Z, Kim SK, et al. Hydrolysable tannins and related compound having cytotoxic activity from the fruits of Terminalia chebula. *Arch Pharmacal Res*. 1995;18(2):118-20.

[168] Saleem A, Husheem M, Härkönen P, Pihlaja K. Inhibition of cancer cell growth by crude extract and the phenolics of *Terminalia chebula* retz. fruit. *J Ethnopharmacol*. 2002;81(3):327-36. PMID: 12127233

[169] Alsemari A, Alkhodairy F, Aldakan A, Al-Mohanna M, Bahoush E, Shinwari Z, et al. The selective cytotoxic anti-cancer properties and proteomic analysis of *Trigonella Foenum-Graecum*. *BMC Complement Alt Med*. 2014;14. PMID: 24679057

[170] Gerlach SL, Rathinakumar R, Chakravarty G, Göransson U, Wimley WC, Darwin SP, et al. Anticancer and chemosensitizing abilities of cycloviolacin 02 from *Viola odorata* and psyle cyclotides from Psychotria leptothyrsa. *Biopolymers*. 2010;94(5):617-25. PMID: 20564026

[171] Berardi V, Ricci F, Castelli M, Galati G, Risuleo G. Resveratrol exhibits a strong cytotoxic activity in cultured cells and has an antiviral action against polyomavirus: Potential clinical use. *J Exper Clin Canc Res*. 2009;28(1). PMID:19570215

[172] Aghbali A, Hosseini SV, Delazar A, Gharavi NK, Shahneh FZ, Orangi M, et al. Induction of apoptosis by grape seed extract (*Vitis vinifera*) in oral squamous cell carcinoma. *Bosnian J Basic Med Sci*. 2013;13(3):186-91. PMID: 23988171

[173] Giovannelli L, Innocenti M, Santamaria AR, Bigagli E, Pasqua G, Mulinacci N. Antitumoural activity of viniferin-enriched extracts from *Vitis vinifera* L. cell cultures. *Natur Prod Res*. 2014;28(22):2006-16. PMID: 24949881

[174] Hamadani SF, Pourseyedi S, Esmaeili-Mahani S. Cytotoxic effect of Rishbaba grape (*Vitis vinifera*) seed extract on human breast cancer cell line (MCF-7) and its interaction with the anticancer drug doxorubicin. *Physiol Pharmacol*. 2014;18(2):170-8.

[175] Keum YS, Kim J, Lee KH, Park KK, Surh YJ, Lee JM, et al. Induction of apoptosis and caspase-3 activation by chemopreventive [6]-paradol and structurally related compounds in KB cells. *Canc Lett*. 2002;177(1):41-7. PMID: 11809529

[176] Wang CC, Chen LG, Lee LT, Yang LL. Effects of 6-Gingerol, an antioxidant from ginger, on inducing apoptosis in human leukemic HL-60 cells. *In Vivo*. 2003;17(6):641-5. PMID:14758732

[177] Wei QY, Ma JP, Cai YJ, Yang L, Liu ZL. Cytotoxic and apoptotic activities of diarylheptanoids and gingerol-related compounds from the rhizome of Chinese ginger. *J Ethnopharmacol*. 2005;102(2):177-84. PMID: 16024193

[178] Nigam N, Bhui K, Prasad S, George J, Shukla Y. [6]-Gingerol induces reactive oxygen species regulated mitochondrial cell death pathway in human epidermoid carcinoma A431 cells. *Chemico-Biol Interact*. 2009;181(1):77-84. PMID: 19481070

[179] Yang L, Zhou C, Huang K, Song L, Zheng Q, Yu R, et al. Antioxidative and cytotoxic properties of diarylheptanoids isolated from Zingiber officinale. Zhongguo Zhongyao Zazhi. 2009;34(3):319-23. PMID: 19445158

[180] Liu Q, Peng YB, Qi LW, Cheng XL, Xu XJ, Liu LL, et al. The cytotoxicity mechanism of 6-shogaol-treated HeLa human cervical cancer cells revealed by label-free shotgun proteomics and bioinformatics analysis. Evidence-based Complementary and Alternative Medicine. 2012;2012. PMID: 23243437

[181] Lv L, Chen H, Soroka D, Chen X, Leung T, Sang S. 6-gingerdiols as the major metabolites of 6-gingerol in cancer cells and in mice and their cytotoxic effects on human cancer cells. J Agric Food Chem. 2012;60(45):11372-7. PMID: 23066935

Section 2

Mind

Chapter 6

Animal Assisted Intervention for Rehabilitation Therapy and Psychotherapy

Okjin Kim, Sunhwa Hong, Hyun-A Lee,
Yung-Ho Chung and Si-Jong Lee

Additional information is available at the end of the chapter

http://dx.doi.org/10.5772/61117

Abstract

Animal-assisted Intervention (AAI) is a goal-oriented intervention that intentionally includes or incorporates animals in health, education, and human service for the purpose of therapeutic gains in humans. AAI incorporates human-animal teams in formal human service such as Animal-assisted Therapy (AAT) or Animal-assisted Education (AAE). Animal-assisted Activity (AAA) is the informal AAI often conducted on a volunteer basis by the human-animal team for motivational, educational, and recreational purposes. AAI could be used for rehabilitation therapy and psychotherapy for patients with various symptoms. AAI uses animals, mostly dogs, to aid in healing patients holistically. Dogs have an overwhelming gratitude and exuberance for life and this effect on people is astounding. Furthermore, AAI has been researched and its effectiveness on patients' outcomes and healing is documented. With a soaring trend of the incorporation of complementary therapies into the mainstream of therapy and health care, animal-facilitated therapy has become a popular interest for the therapy team to integrate into a patient's plan of therapy.

The purpose of this manuscript is to raise awareness about AAI and to familiarize readers with the concepts surrounding AAI so that they can be informed aids to clients who might benefit from the technique.

Keywords: Animal-assisted Intervention, Animal-assisted Therapy, Animal-assisted Education, Rehabilitation, Psychotherapy

1. Introduction

1.1. Definition of animal-assisted intervention

Animal-assisted Intervention (AAI) is a goal-oriented intervention that intentionally includes or incorporates animals in health, education and human service for the purpose of therapeutic gains in humans (Table 1). AAI incorporates human-animal teams in formal human service such as Animal-assisted Therapy (AAT) or Animal-assisted Education (AAE) [1].

AAT is a goal-oriented, planned, and structured therapeutic intervention directed and/or delivered by health, education, and human service professionals. Intervention progress is measured and included in professional documentation. AAT is delivered and/or directed by a formally trained professional with expertise within the scope of the professionals' practice. AAT focuses on enhancing physical, cognitive, behavioral and/or socio-emotional functioning of the particular human client [1]. Figure 1 shows the scheme of animal-assisted therapy.

AAE is a goal-oriented, planned, and structured intervention directed and/or delivered by educational and related service professional. AAE is conducted by qualified general and special education teachers. Regular education teachers who conduct AAE must have knowledge of the animals involved. An example of AAE delivered by a regular education teacher is an educational visit that promotes responsible pet ownership. AAE, when done by special education teachers, is also considered therapeutic and a goal-oriented intervention. The focus of the activities is on academic goals, pro-social skills, and cognitive functioning. The student's progress is measured and documented. An example of AAE delivered by a special education teacher is a dog-assisted reading program [1].

Animal-assisted activity (AAA)	Provide opportunities for motivational, educational, and/or recreational benefits in order to enhance the quality of life of humans. AAA is delivered in a variety of environments by specially trained professionals and/or volunteers in association with animals that meet specific criteria of safety.
Animal-assisted therapy (AAT)	Are goal-directed interventions in which a specifically trained animal is an integral part of the treatment process. AAT is delivered and/or directed by a health/human service provider working within the scope of his or her profession. AAT is designed to promote improvement in human physical, social, emotional, and/or cognitive functioning. They are provided in a variety of settings and involve the individual. This process needs to be documented and evaluated throughout.
Animal-assisted education (AAE)	Relies on the use of animals for specific educational purposes, as is the case with problematic children characterized by behavioral problems.

*Source: Cirulli et al. [2]

Table 1. Animal-assisted interventions (AAIs): Definitions

Animal-assisted Activity (AAA) is the informal interactions/visitations often conducted on a volunteer basis by the human-animal team for motivational, educational, and recreational purposes. There are no treatment goals for the interactions. AAAs are generally facilitated by individuals who do not have a health, education, or human service degree. Human-animal teams have received at least introductory training, preparation, and assessment to participate in informal visitations. Human-animal teams who provide AAA may also work formally and directly with a healthcare, educator, and/or human service provider on specific documentable goals. In this case, they are participating in AAT or AAE that is conducted by a specialist in his/her profession. Examples of AAA include animal-assisted crisis response that focuses on providing comfort and support for trauma, crisis, and disaster survivors, and visiting companion animals for 'meet and greet' activities with residents in nursing homes [1].

Table 2 shows the characteristics of therapy animals for animal-assisted interventions. We can select an appropriate therapy animal for an AAI program.

Kinds	Breed	Move	Contact	Emotional communication	Safety	Exercise	Pleasure of animal	Infectivity
Fish	★	▽	▽	◊	★	▽	◊	☆
Reptiles	◊	◊	◊	◊	☆	▽	◊	☆
Avian	★	◊	☆	◊	★	▽	◊	☆
Hamster	★	★	◊	◊	☆	◊	◊	☆
Guinea pig	★	★	★	◊	★	◊	◊	☆
Rabbit	★	★	★	☆	★	◊	◊	☆
Sheep, Goat	◊	◊	★	☆	☆	☆	◊	☆
Cattle	◊	◊	☆	☆	☆	☆	◊	☆
Pig	◊	◊	☆	☆	☆	☆	☆	☆
Cat	☆	☆	★	★	☆	☆	★	☆
Dog	☆	☆	★	★	☆	★	★	☆
Horse	◊	▽	☆	★	☆	★	☆	☆
Dolphin	▽	▽	☆	☆	☆	★	◊	☆
Pet insect	★	★	▽	▽	★	▽	▽	★
Monkey	▽	◊	◊	☆	▽	☆	☆	▽

★= Excellent, ☆= good, ◊ = Medium, ∇= Bad

Table 2. Characteristics of therapy animals for animal-assisted interventions (AAIs)

2. History of animal-assisted intervention

Animals and humans have existed in therapeutic relationships with each other for more than 12,000 years. In 1790 in York, England, rabbits and chickens were used in therapies with

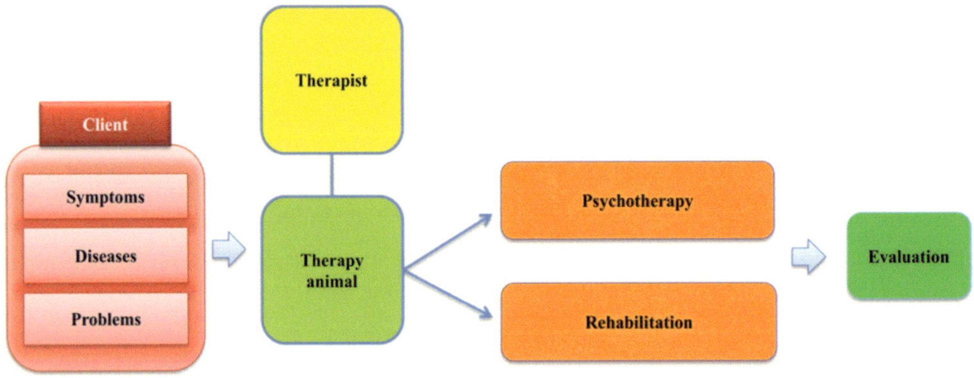

Figure 1. Scheme of animal-assisted therapy (AAT)

mentally ill patients learning self-control [3]. During the 1830s, the British charity commissioner recommended that mental institutions have animals on the grounds to create a more pleasing and less prison-like atmosphere [4]. Florence Nightingale observed that a small pet is often an excellent companion for the sick, especially for the chronic cases [4]. In 1867, epilepsy patients at Bethel in Bielefield, West Germany had farm animals and horses incorporated into their treatment plans [5]. In 1942, the U.S. Army Air Corps Convalescent Hospital in Pawling, New York considered working with farm animals restful for some patients in comparison to traditional medical treatment [5].

In the 1960s, a New York psychologist, Dr. Boris Levinson, incorporated his dog, Jingles, in the treatment plan of an adolescent and then discussed his findings in a published paper titled "The Dog as the Co-therapist" in *Mental Hygiene* [6].

In 1980, McCulloch, Bustad, and Katcher founded the Delta Society, an international nonprofit organization focused on the "human-animal bond" (Delta Society; recently, changed as 'Pet Partners') [7]. This organization declared that its mission was "to promote animals helping people improve their health, independence, and quality of life" [3]. The goals of the organization include "expanding awareness of the positive effects animals can have on human health; removing the barriers that prevent involvement of animals in everyday life; and expanding the therapeutic role of animals in human health, service, and education." The mission statement has now evolved to read simply "Improving human health through service and therapy animals" (Delta Society; recently, changed as 'Pet Partners') [7]. In 2008, the Korean Association of Animal Assisted Psychotherapy was founded in Korea (http://www.kaaap.org/). In 2012, Delta Society changed its name to Pet Partners.

We summarized the historical perspective of human and animal relationships and development of research in Table 3.

12,000 years ago	A human skeleton holding a puppy was found in northern Israel.
Ninth century	Animals were incorporated in treatment of the handicapped in Gheel, Belgium.
1790	Rabbits and chickens were used in therapy with the mentally ill in York, England.
1830	British charity commissioner recommended animals for mental institutions.
1867	Farm animals and horses were used in treatment of epilepsy patients at Bethel in Bielefield, West Germany.
1942	Patients at U.S. Army Air Corps Convalescent Hospital, Pawling, New York worked with farm animals and considered treatment "restful".
1944	Sociologist James Bossad's publication "The Mental Hygiene of Owning a Dog" discussed beneficial relationships between pets and their owners.
1962	Psychologist Borris Levinson used his dog, Jingles, in the treatment of an adolescent; he published his findings in "The Dog as the Co-therapist".
1970s	A visiting therapy dog, Skeezer, became a permanent resident at Children's Psychiatric Hospital, Ann Arbor, Michigan. Psychiatrist Michael McCulloch prescribed pets to patients. Veterinarian Leo Bustad started "Bustad Buddies" at Pullman Memorial Hospital and Tacoma Lutheran Nursing Home in Washington.
1972	Psychotherapist Boris Levinson conducted a survey and found that one third of New York psychotherapists used pets in treatment
1973	Humane Society's "pet mobile" program brought animals to visit nursing homes in Pikes Peak region, Colorado.
1977	Dr. Dean Katcher and Erika Friedmann conducted early research on effects of pets on blood pressure and mortality rates.
1980	Delta Society, a nonprofit organization focused on the human–animal bond, was founded.
2008	Korean Association of Animal Assisted Psychotherapy was founded in Korea.
2012	Delta Society changed its name to Pet Partners.

*Modified source: Morrison [8]

Table 3. Historical perspective of human and animal relationships and development of research

3. Benefits of human-animal bond

Animals and humans have existed in therapeutic relationships with each other for more than 12,000 years. One of the earliest cited findings is the skeletal remains, found in northern Israel, of a human holding a puppy. In Gheel, Belgium, in the ninth century, animals were used in treatment plans with handicapped persons [4]. In 1790 in York, England, rabbits and chickens were used in therapies with mentally ill patients learning self-control [3].

The American Veterinary Medical Association's Committee on the Human-Animal Bond defines the human-animal bond as, "a mutually beneficial and dynamic relationship between people and other animals that is influenced by behaviors that are essential to the health and well-being of both. This includes, but is not limited to, emotional, psychological, and physical interactions of people, other animals, and the environment". [9].

The human-animal bond has been described as the mutually beneficial and dynamic relationship between people and other animals that is influenced by behaviors essential to the health and well-being of both. This includes, but is not limited to, emotional, psychological, and physical interactions of people, other animals, and the environment [9].

Fiure 2 shows an animal-assisted therapy program for the children with autism in Korea. We summarized the benefits of animal-assisted interventions in Figure 3.

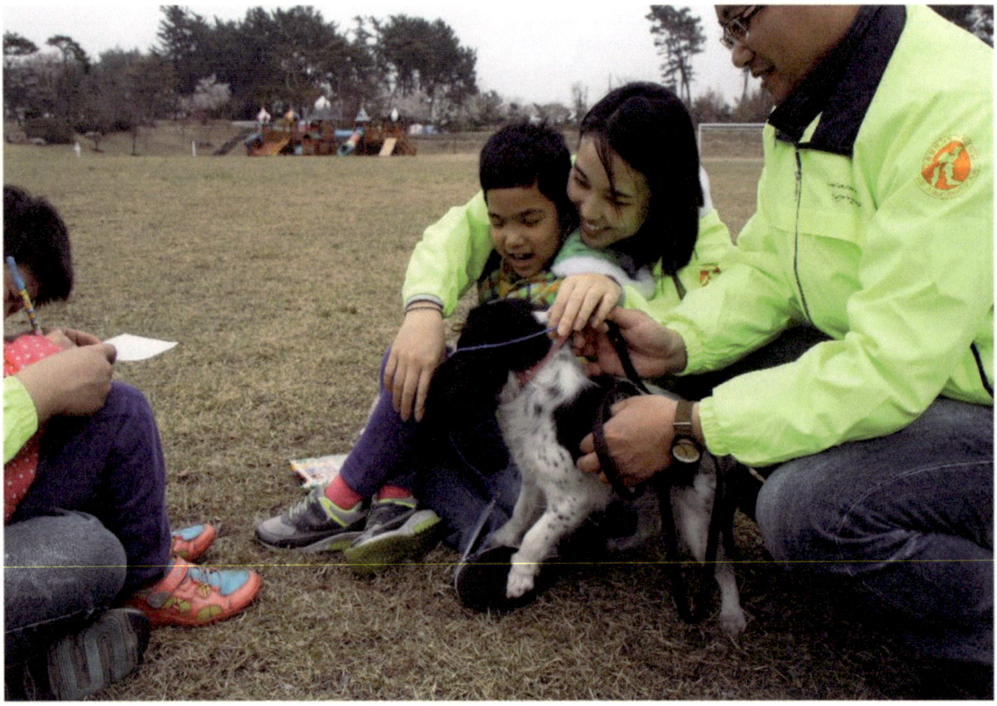

Figure 2. Animal-assisted therapy program for the children with autism

4. Animal-assisted intervention for rehabilitation therapy

AAI is the utilization of animals as a therapeutic modality to facilitate healing and rehabilitation of patients with acute or chronic ailments [10]. Many elderly and lonely individuals have discovered that pets satisfy their needs and enable them to hold on to the world of reality, of care, of human toil and sacrifice, and of intense emotional relationships. The incorporation of animal services for the benefit of human health has been establish and implemented in various countries such as the United States and the United Kingdom for many years.

http://dx.doi.org/10.5772/61117

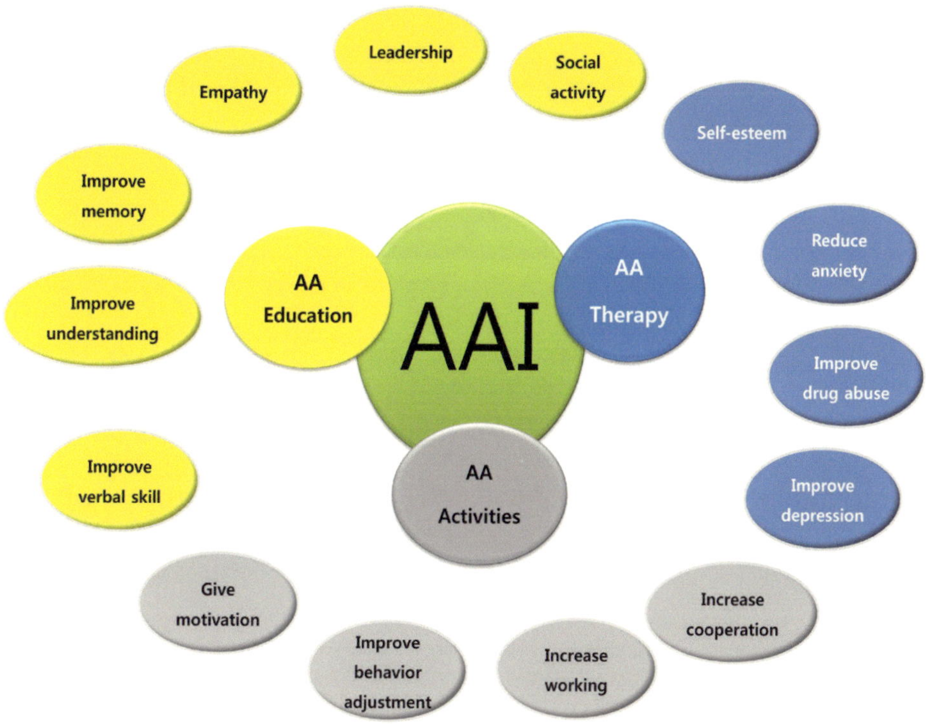

Figure 3. Benefits of animal-assisted interventions

Animal assisted intervention has been used with people of all ages from the elderly to young children. Programs span a wide range of situations and conditions, including older people with Alzheimer's disease; the emotionally and mentally ill; developmentally delayed children and adults; and children with Down's syndrome, cerebral palsy, brain damage, and learning disabilities. The key factor of all such programs that can be called AAT is that animals are utilized not just as entertainment or for companionship but in a goal-directed way that is assessed and evaluated for its impact. They also involve trained workers and suitably selected animals.

Animals can assist the physically handicapped in a variety of ways. Therapeutic riding is being used for persons with cerebral palsy, muscular dystrophy, multiple sclerosis, and others with diminished motor control. It helps to improve their posture, balance, mobility, and function. It also provides significant emotional and cognitive benefits. Figure 4 shows an animal-assisted therapy program for the elderly with dementia in Korea.

5. Animal-assisted intervention for psychotherapy

Animals tend to focus and absorb people's attention in non-threatening ways and are also known to exert a calming or de-arousing influence [11–13]. Moreover, the ability of domesti-

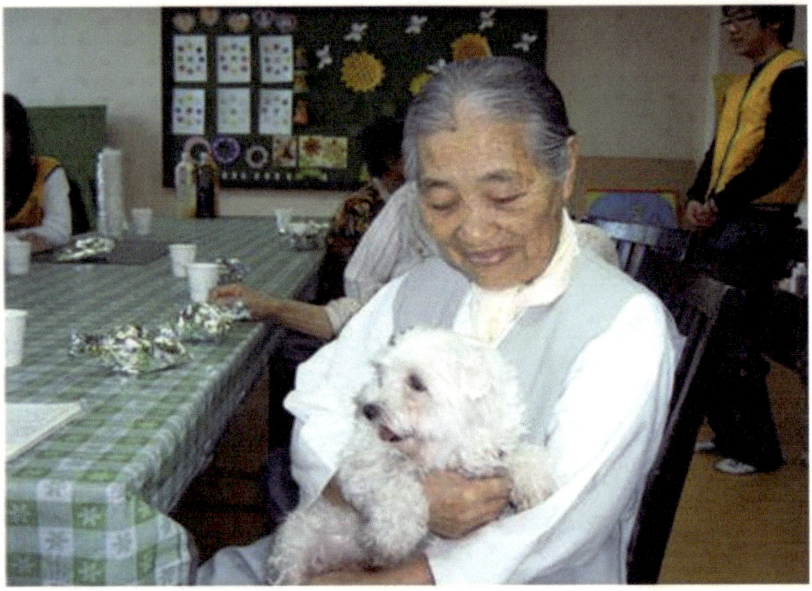

Figure 4. Animal-assisted therapy program for the elderly with dementia

cated animals to respond affectionately to human attentions and to elicit pro-social behavior and positive effect may serve as an emotional bridge to mediate interactions in therapeutic contexts [14].

There is increasing evidence suggesting that a close relationship with a pet animal is associated with significant health effects in people. The presence of an animal, or even the mere observation of animals [12, 15], can buffer physiological and psychological responses to stress and anxiety; as an example, a transient decrease in blood pressure and heart rate has been observed in adults and children in the presence of a companion dog as well as while interacting with friendly but unknown dogs [16, 17]. The presence of an animal, particularly a dog, is able to act as an "ice-breaker"; it catalyzes communication and enhances opportunities for social exchange and shared interests who, in turn, can promote a feeling of social integration [18]. Different animals are purposely included in various therapeutic/activity programs also known as AAIs, which are receiving growing attention in the fields of nursing, medicine, and psychotherapy because of their potential to influence a large number of health-related problems in different clinical populations. Figure 5 shows Animal-assisted therapy program for children with depression in Korea.

6. Field studies of animal-assisted intervention

Based on the research to date, AAIs may be indicated for but not limited to patients of all ages who need improvement in mood, motivation, self-esteem, and physical and psychological

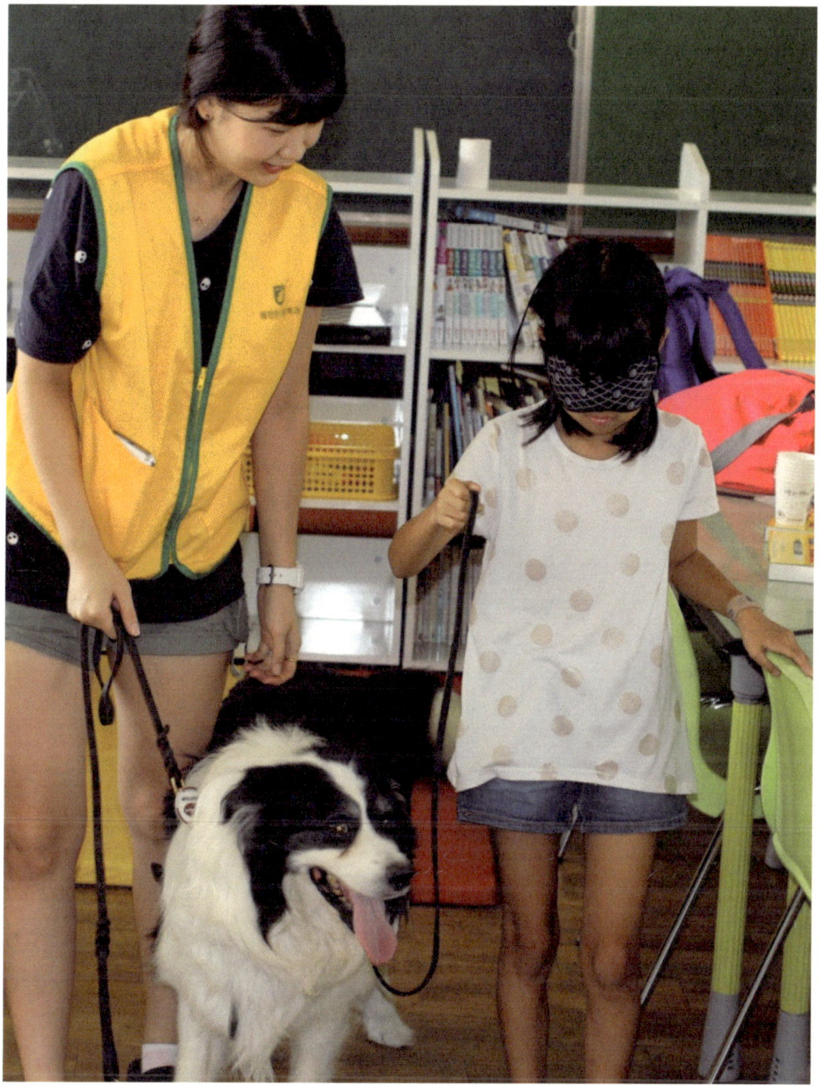

Figure 5. Animal-assisted therapy program for children with depression

well-being. This includes men, women, and children of all ages who have had pertinent precautions and safety issues addressed. Specific medical indications include but are not limited to autism, dementia, chronic diseases, mental disorders, and neurological disorders including aphasia and epilepsy [19–24].

Settings that are appropriate for AAIs may include, but are not limited to, institutional settings such as hospitals, nursing homes, hospice care, mental health facilities, schools, and correctional facilities. Other settings may include the home, farm, or alternative locations with access to therapeutic animals such as dolphins [25].

Animals involved in AAI include, but are not limited to, dogs, cats, horses, donkeys, dolphins, birds, gerbils, hamsters, rabbits, and fish. Most commonly used in previous research is AAI that involves dogs and is the most common type of AAI. AAI with dogs is used with a wide variety of populations and is found in both group and individual therapy settings. The interaction between dogs and clients is an important aspect in canine-assisted therapy [26, 27].

We summarized the research publications in the field of animal-assisted interventions in Table 4.

Human disorders	Researches of animal-assisted interventions
Senile dementia, Alzheimer's disease	[23, 28–33]
Psychiatric disorders, schizophrenia	[34–40]
Autism	[24, 42–45]
Cancer	[45–47]
Chronic heart failure	[48, 49]
Spinal cord injury	[50]
Cerebral palsy	[51]
Multiple sclerosis	[52]
Language disorders, aphasia	[53–56]

*Source: Cirulli et al. (2011)

Table 4. Research publications in the field of animal-assisted interventions

7. Vision and prospects of animal-assisted intervention

In AAI, the activity performed by the "animal therapist" towards the "human patient" is very complex and to be successful, above all, should entail the contribution of many professional figures. For this reason, a combined effort of a cross-disciplinary team made up of various professional categories should always characterize an AAI program. These categories interact and bring their own specific contribution in a complementary way.

The "therapeutic potential" of AAI could vary according to the animal species involved. As an example, dogs' ability to develop a complex communication system with humans, enhanced by the domestication process, makes these animals particularly able to increase responsiveness and willingness to communicate. By and large, domesticated animals should be used as they have been selected for their ability to interact socially (and emotionally) with humans.

8. Conclusion

AAIs, which include both AAA and AAT, have historically been beneficial to human health. AAIs are modalities that offer an integrative approach to enhance the treatment of various health concerns. Although many healthcare professionals and facilities use AAIs in the treatment of patients or clients, extensive opportunities are still available for further implementation into healthcare.

In Korea, the Korean Association of Animal Assisted Psychotherapy (KAAAP) was founded in 2008 (http://www.kaaap.org/). KAAAP has performed a lot of research projects and archived positive functioning outcomes for various clients following AAI using human-animal interaction. The use of AAI appears to provide a valuable addition to clinical treatment practices and therefore are worthy of further investigation.

Acknowledgements

This research was supported by the Basic Science Research Program through the National Research Foundation of Korea (NRF) funded by the Ministry of Education, Science, and Technology (2010-0021940).

Author details

Okjin Kim[1,2*], Sunhwa Hong[3], Hyun-A Lee[1], Yung-Ho Chung[4] and Si-Jong Lee[1]

*Address all correspondence to: kimoj@wku.ac.kr

1 Korean Association of Animal Assisted Psychotherapy, Republic of Korea

2 Graduate School of Animal Assisted Psychotherapy, Wonkwang University, Republic of Korea

3 Center for Animal Resources Development, Wonkwang University, Republic of Korea

4 Department of Companion Animal and Animal Resources Science, Joongbu University, Republic of Korea

References

[1] IAHAIO. White paper. The IAHAIO definitions for animal-assisted intervention and animal-assisted activity and guidelines for wellness of animals involved. 2014.

[2] Cirulli F, Borgi M, Berry A, Francia N and Alleva E. Animal-assisted interventions as innovative tools for mental health. *Ann. Ist. Super. Sanità*. 2011; 47: 341-348.

[3] Salotto P. Pet-assisted therapy: A loving intervention and an emerging profession: Leading to a friendlier, healthier, and more peaceful world. Norton, MA: D. J. Publications. 2001.

[4] Serpell JA. Animal-assisted interventions in historical perspective. In A. H. Fine (Ed.), Handbook on animal-assisted therapy: Theoretical foundations and guidelines for practice (2nd ed., Chap. 1). New York: Academic Press. 2006.

[5] Bustad L. Animals, aging and the aged. Minneapolis: University of Minnesota Press. Levinson, B. (1962). The dog as co-therapist. *Mental.Hygiene*. 1980;46:59-65.

[6] Levinson BM. The dog as a "co-therapist". Ment Hyg. 1962;46:59-65.

[7] Delta Society. Introduction to animal assisted activities and therapies. 2005; Retrieved December 10, 2006, from *http://www.deltasociety.org/AnimalsAAAAbout.htm.*

[8] Morrison ML. Health Benefits of Animal-assisted Interventions. Complementary Health Practice Review 2007;12:51-62. DOI: 10.1177/1533210107302397.

[9] Olson PN. The modern working dog—a call for interdisciplinary collaboration. *J. Am. Vet. Med. Assoc.* 2002;352-355.

[10] Curran G. Role animals take with therapy modalities for rehabilitation patients. *Community Medicine*. 1996;6:29-36.

[11] DeSchriver M, Riddick C. Effects of watching aquariums on elders' stress. *Anthrozoös*. 1990;4:44-48.

[12] Katcher AH, Friedmann E, Beck AM, Lynch JJ. Looking, talking and blood pressure: The physiological consequences of interaction with the living environment. In: Katcher AH, Beck AM (Ed.). New perspectives on our lives with companion animals. Philadelphia: University of Pennsylvania Press; 1983.

[13] Wilson CC. The pet as an anxiolytic intervention. *J. Nerv. Ment. Dis*. 1991;179:482-489.

[14] Serpell J. In the company of animals: A study of human-animal relationships. Cambridge: Cambridge University Press; 1996.

[15] Wells D. The effect of videotapes of animals on cardiovascular responses to stress. *Stress Health* 2005;21:209-213.

[16] Friedmann E, Thomas S, Cook L, Tsai C, Picot S. A friendly dog as potential moderator of cardiovascular response to speech in older hypertensives. *Anthrozoös*. 2007;20:51-63.

[17] Allen K, Blascovich J, Mendes WB. Cardiovascular reactivity and the presence of pets, friends, and spouses: The truth about cats and dogs. *Psychosom. Med.* 2002;64:727-739.

[18] Knight S, Edwards V. In the company of wolves: The physical, social, and psychological benefits of dog ownership. *Journal of Aging and Health*. 2008;20:437-455.

[19] Allen K, Shykoff B, Izzo JL. Pet ownership, but not ACE inhibitor therapy, blunts home blood pressure responses to mental stress. *Hypertension.* 2001;38:815-820.

[20] Filan SL, Llewellyn-Jones RH. Animal-assisted therapy for dementia: A review of the literature. *International Psychogeriatric.* 2006;18:597-611.

[21] Kaminski M, Pellino T, Wish J. Play and pets: The physical and emotional impact of child-life and pet therapy and hospitalized children. *Children's Health Care.* 2002;31;321-335.

[22] Macauley BL. Animal-assisted therapy for persons with aphasia: A pilot study. *Journal of Rehabilitation Research and Development.* 2006;43:357-366.

[23] Richeson NE. Effects of animal-assisted therapy on agitated behaviors and social interactions of older adults with dementia. *Am. J. Alzheimers. Dis. Other. Demen.* 2003;18:353-358.

[24] Sams MJ, Fortney EV, Willenbring S. Occupational therapy incorporating animals for children with autism: A pilot investigation. *American Occupational Therapy Association.* 2006;60:268-274.

[25] Arkow P. Animal-assisted therapy and activities: A study, resource guide and bibliography for the use of companion animals in selected therapies (9th ed.). Stratford, NJ: Phil Arkow.2004.

[26] Fine A. (ed.). Handbook on animal-assisted therapy; Theoretical foundations and guidelines for practice (3rd ed.). San Diego, CA: Academic Press.2010.

[27] Thompson MJ. Animal-assisted play therapy: Canines as co-therapist. In G. R. Walz, J. C. Bleuer, & R. K. Yep (Eds.), Compelling counseling interventions: VISTAS 2009 (pp. 199-209). Alexandria, VA: American Counseling Association. 2009.

[28] Kanamori M, Suzuki M, Yamamoto K, Kanda M, Matsui Y, Kojima E. A day care program and evaluation of animal-assisted therapy (AAT) for the elderly with senile dementia. *Am. J. Alzheimers. Dis. Other. Demen.* 2001;16:234-239.

[29] Edwards NE, Beck AM. Animal-assisted therapy and Nutrition in Alzheimer's disease. *West. J. Nurs. Res.* 2002;24:697-712.

[30] Marx MS, Cohen-Mansfield J, Regier NG, Dakheel-Ali M, Srihari A, Thein K. The impact of different dog-related stimuli on engagement of persons with dementia. *Am. J. Alzheimers. Dis. Other. Demen.* 2010;25:37-45.

[31] Motomura N, Yagi T, Ohyama H. Animal assisted therapy for people with dementia. *Psychogeriatrics* 2004;4:40-42.

[32] McCabe BW, Baun MM, Speich D, Agrawal S. Resident dog in the Alzheimer's special care unit. *West. J. Nurs. Res.* 2002;24:684-696.

[33] Kramer SC, Friedmann E, Bernstein PL. Comparison of the effect of human interaction, animal-assisted therapy, and AIBO-assisted therapy on long-term care residents with dementia. *Anthrozoös*. 2009;22:43-57.

[34] Barker SB, Pandurangi AK, Best AM. Effects of animal assisted therapy on patients' anxiety, fear, and depression before ECT. *J. Ect*. 2003;19:38-44.

[35] Prothmann A, Bienert M, Ettrich C. Dogs in child psychotherapy: Effects on state of mind. *Anthrozoös*. 2006;19:265-277.

[36] Berget B, Ekeberg O, Braastad BO. Animal-assisted therapy with farm animals for persons with psychiatric disorders: Effects on self-efficacy, coping ability and quality of life, a randomized controlled trial. *Clin. Pract. Epidemiol. Ment. Health*. 2008;4:9.

[37] Barak Y, Savorai O, Mavashev S, Beni A. Animal-assisted therapy for elderly schizophrenic patients: A one-year controlled trial. *Am. J. Geriatr. Psychiatry*. 2001;9:439-442.

[38] Kovacs Z, Kis R, Rozsa S, Rozsa L. Animal-assisted therapy for middle-aged schizophrenic patients living in a social institution. A pilot study. *Clin. Rehabil.* 2004;18:483-486.

[39] Nathans-Barel I, Feldman P, Berger B, Modai I, Silver H. Animal-assisted therapy ameliorates anhedonia in schizophrenia patients. A controlled pilot study. *Psychother.Psychosom*. 2005;74:31-35.

[40] Chu CI, Liu CY, Sun CT, Lin J. The effect of animal-assisted activity on inpatients with schizophrenia. *J. Psychosoc. Nurs. Ment. Health. Serv*. 2009;47:42-48.

[41] Bizub AL, Joy A, Davidson L. It's like being in another world: Demonstrating the benefits of therapeutic horseback riding for individuals with psychiatric disability. *Psychiatr. Rehabil. J*. 2003;26:377-384.

[42] Silva K, Correia R, Lima M, Magalhaes A, de Sousa L. Can dogs prime autistic children for therapy? Evidence from a single case study. *J. Altern. Complement. Med.* 2011;17:655-659.

[43] Solomon O. What a dog can do: Children with autism and therapy dogs in social interaction. ETHOS, *Journal of the Society for Psychological Anthropology*. 2010;38:143-166.

[44] Bass MM, Duchowny CA, Llabre MM. The effect of therapeutic horseback riding on social functioning in children with autism. *J. Autism. Dev. Disord*. 2009;39:1261-1267.

[45] Bouchard F, Landry M, Belles-Isles M, Gagnon J. A magical dream: A pilot project in animal-assisted therapy in pediatric oncology. *Can. Oncol. Nurs. J*. 2004;14:14-17.

[46] Orlandi M, Trangeled K, Mambrini A, Tagliani M, Ferrarini A, Zanetti L. Pet therapy effects on oncological day hospital patients undergoing chemotherapy treatment. *Anticancer. Res*. 2007;27:4301-4303.

[47] Johnson RA, Meadows RL, Haubner JS, Sevedge K. Animal-assisted activity among patients with cancer: Effects on mood, fatigue, self-perceived health, and sense of coherence. *Oncol. Nurs. Forum.* 2008;35:225-232.

[48] Cole KM, Gawlinski A, Steers N, Kotlerman J. Animal-assisted therapy in patients hospitalized with heart failure. *Am. J. Crit. Care* 2007;16:575-585.

[49] Abate SV, Zucconi M, Boxer BA. Impact of canine-assisted ambulation on hospitalized chronic heart failure patients' ambulation outcomes and Satisfaction: A Pilot Study. *J.Cardiovasc. Nurs.* 2011;26:224-230.

[50] Lechner HE, Kakebeeke TH, Hegemann D, Baumberger M. The effect of hippotherapy on spasticity and on mental well-being of persons with spinal cord injury. *Arch. Phys. Med. Rehabil.* 2007;88:1241-1248.

[51] McGibbon NH, Benda W, Duncan BR, Silkwood-Sherer D. Immediate and long-term effects of hippotherapy on symmetry of adductor muscle activity and functional ability in children with spastic cerebral palsy. *Arch. Phys. Med. Rehabil.* 2009;90:966-974.

[52] Silkwood-Sherer D, Warmbier H. Effects of hippotherapy on postural stability, in persons with multiple sclerosis: A pilot study. *J. Neurol. Phys. Ther.* 2007;31:77-84.

[53] Gee N, Harris S, Johnson K. The role of therapy dogs in speed and accuracy to complete motor skills tasks for preschool children. *Anthrozoös.* 2007;20:375-386.

[54] Macauly B, Gutierrez K. The effectiveness of hippotherapy for children with language-learning disabilities. *Commun. Disord. Q.* 2004;25:205-217.

[55] Martin F, Farnum J. Animal-assisted therapy for children with pervasive developmental disorders. *West J. Nurs. Res.*2002;24:657-670.

[56] LaFrance C, Garcia LJ, Labreche J. The effect of a therapy dog on the communication skills of an adult with aphasia. J. Commun. Disord. 2007;40:215-224.

Chapter 7

Kampo, a Traditional Japanese Medicine, for the Body, Mind, and Soul

Shin Takayama, Takehiro Numata, Natsumi Saito, Soichiro Kaneko and Tetsuharu Kamiya

Additional information is available at the end of the chapter

http://dx.doi.org/10.5772/60702

Abstract

Traditional Japanese (Kampo) medicine is widely used to treat numerous conditions. Kampo medicine includes herbal formulas, acupuncture, moxibustion, and massage. After the Great East Japan Earthquake (GEJE), Kampo medicine was used to treat the imbalances in the body, mind, and soul in severely affected areas. The effects of the Kampo medicine saikokeishikankyoto (SKK) for the treatment of post-traumatic stress disorder (PTSD) have been proven in our clinical study. In this chapter, we have summarized both our reports from the Kampo medical clinics that were set up after the GEJE disaster and our findings of the clinical study on PTSD treatment in disaster survivors.

Keywords: Japan, Kampo, Tsunami, Disaster, Earthquake

1. Introduction

1.1. The history and current status of traditional Japanese (Kampo) medicine

Traditional Japanese medicine, known as Kampo, originated from China and was introduced to Japan via Korea in the sixth century. Kampo medicine is widely used to treat numerous conditions, including imbalances in the body, mind, and soul. Kampo treatment includes herbal formulas, acupuncture, moxibustion, and massage, and treatment is determined based on the diagnosis according to the original Kampo concept. The diagnosis involves obtaining the history of the illness and a physical examination (i.e., tongue examination, pulse examination, and abdominal examination). Kampo education has been conducted at all 80 medical schools in Japan since 2005 [1]. Currently, Kampo is used by approximately 84% of clinical practitioners in Japan [2]. Powdered extract preparations of Kampo formula are used widely in Japan, and 148 formulae are covered by the National Health Insurance [3]. The clinical study of Kampo medicine has gradually been increasing; 378 randomized controlled trials (RCTs) of Kampo medicine were reported in the Evidence Reports of Kampo Treatment by the Special Committee for Evidence-Based Medicine, the Japan Society for Oriental Medicine [4].

1.2. Imbalances of the body, mind, and soul associated with the Great East Japan earthquake (GEJE) and tsunami

The coastal areas of eastern Japan were devastated by a massive earthquake and tsunami on March 11, 2011(Figure 1). Tsunami waves reached a maximum height of approximately 16 m at the Miyagi fishery port of Onagawa, sweeping away people, cars, houses, and entire communities. It was reported that approximately 18,000 people died or were missing, and that at least 400,000 houses were completely or partially destroyed (Figure 2) [5]. More than 400,000 people were forced to evacuate to temporary shelters. Many schools and community centers were converted into evacuation centers. These evacuation centers were isolated due to inundated and severed roads in the Miyagi Prefecture, which prevented communication with other areas of the country. The nuclear power plant in Fukushima Prefecture was also destroyed by the tsunami, causing radiation contamination along the eastern coast of Fukushima. Severe problems with the supply of air, water, food, and shelter emerged due to radiation pollution. The government urged people living within a 20- to 30-km radius of the Fukushima Nuclear Power Plants to evacuate to distant and safer areas (Figure 1) [6]. Everyone in eastern Japan experienced anxiety, irritability, sadness, and despair.

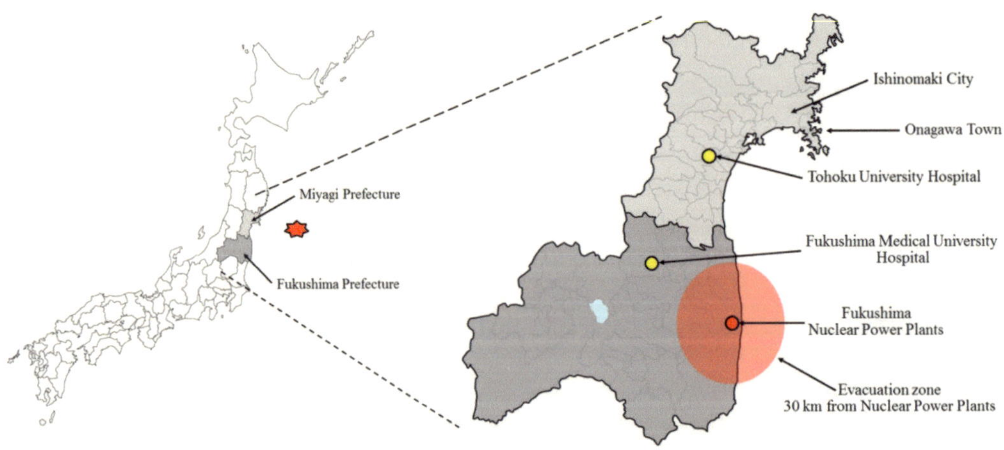

Figure 1. The seismic center of the GEJE and the locations of the Miyagi and Fukushima Prefectures, the Tohoku University Hospital in the Miyagi Prefecture, and the Fukushima Medical University Hospital in the Fukushima Prefecture [6].

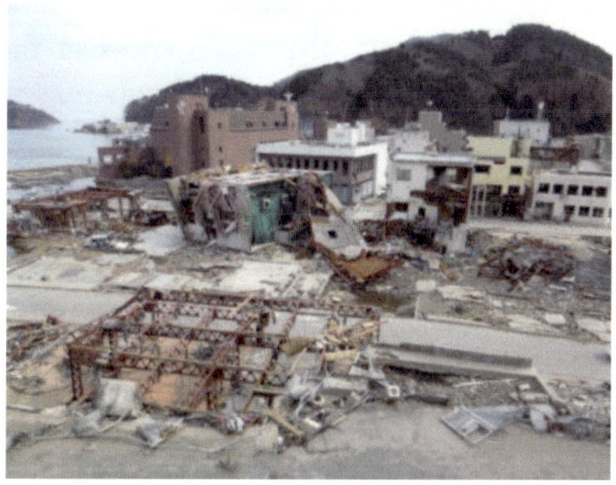

Figure 2. A scene from the Onagawa peninsula after the GEJE and tsunami.

1.3. Purpose

After the GEJE, we provided Kampo treatment to residents in the severely stricken disaster areas of the Miyagi and Fukushima Prefectures. Our experience demonstrated the potential efficacy of traditional medicine after this massive natural disaster [6-10]. We then performed a clinical study of Kampo medicine for the treatment of PTSD in disaster survivors [11]. In this chapter, we have summarized both our reports from the Kampo medical clinics that were set up after the GEJE disaster and our clinical study of PTSD treatment in disaster survivors.

2. Kampo medicine clinics in the Miyagi and Fukushima Prefectures after the GEJE [6-10]

We set up 12 Kampo medicine clinics at the evacuation centers in Onagawa and Ishinomaki in the first 73 days after the disaster. We treated 72 patients during the acute period (1–14 days after the disaster), 117 patients during the subacute period (15–42 days), and 47 patients during the chronic period (43–73 days). Figure 3 shows the treatment operations conducted at one evacuation center [7, 8].

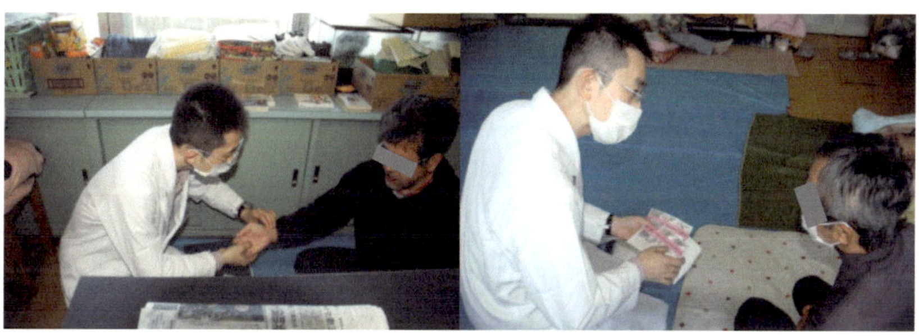

Figure 3. Kampo treatment at an evacuation center [7, 8].

During the acute period, many patients presented with the common cold, hypothermia, and enterocolitis (Figure 4). For patients with acute symptoms of the common cold, Kampo preparations such as kakkonto and keishito were used, whereas ninjinto was used to treat hypothermia (Figure 5). Patients with prolonged symptoms that failed to improve with antibiotic or anti-inflammatory medication were prescribed shosaikoto and other similar Kampo preparations. Goreisan was used to treat enterocolitis accompanied by diarrhea or vomiting that was not relieved by antidiarrheal agents or intestinal regulators.

During the subacute period, allergic symptoms such as persistent cough, pharyngeal pain, runny nose, and itchy eyes were common (Figure 4). Although many patients had already received antihistamines and other antiallergy medications, many complained of decreased efficiency in debris removal activities due to adverse drug reactions such as drowsiness and impaired attention. These patients were prescribed Kampo preparations with antiallergy properties such as shoseiryuto.

During the chronic period, an increase in psychiatric symptoms such as irritability, anxiety, lightheadedness, and insomnia as well as somatoform disorders were observed (Figure 4). For these symptoms, we prescribed Kampo preparations with tranquilizing properties, such as yokukansan and kamikihito. Many patients complained of constipation and were prescribed cathartics such as mashiningan and junchoto.

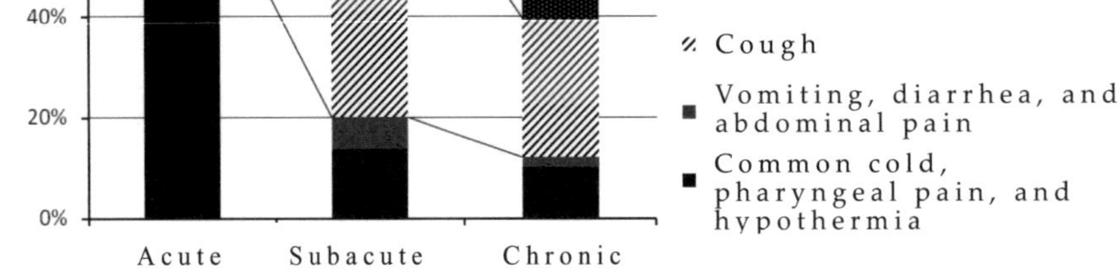

Figure 4. A comparison of symptoms during the acute (1st to 14th day after the disaster, n = 72), subacute (15th to 42nd day, n = 117), and chronic (43rd to 73rd day, n = 47) periods. This figure was modified from [7] and [8].

We also performed massage therapy and acupuncture at seven evacuation centers in the Miyagi and Fukushima Prefectures (Figures 6 and 7, respectively). Massage therapy was performed manually, as shown in Figure 6. Both traditional acupuncture needles and press tack needles were used to administer the acupuncture therapy (Figures 8 and 9, respectively). In total, 553 people were treated (mean age, 54.0 years; 206 men, 347 women). The interview assessments showed that the most common complaint was shoulder/back stiffness (Table 1) (Figures 10 and 11). Many people indicated that they experienced both physical and psycho-

http://dx.doi.org/10.5772/60702

logical relief with therapy, and 92.3% were satisfied with the therapeutic outcome. These findings indicate that massage therapy and acupuncture at the time of a disaster offer both mental and physical relief and may be a therapeutic approach that can be effectively used in combination with Western medical practices [10].

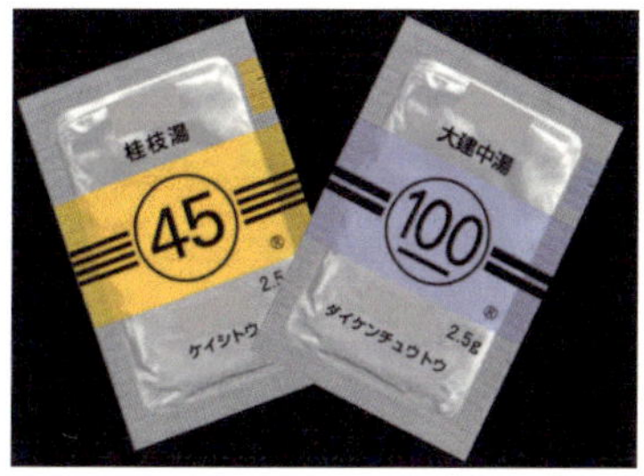

Figure 5. Examples of the extract powders of the Kampo formulae used in the evacuation centers.

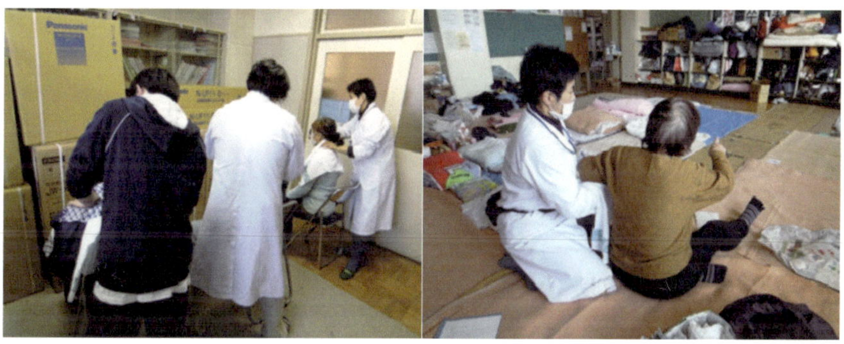

Figure 6. A scene from the massage therapy conducted in one of the evacuation centers in a coastal area of the Miyagi Prefecture [7, 10].

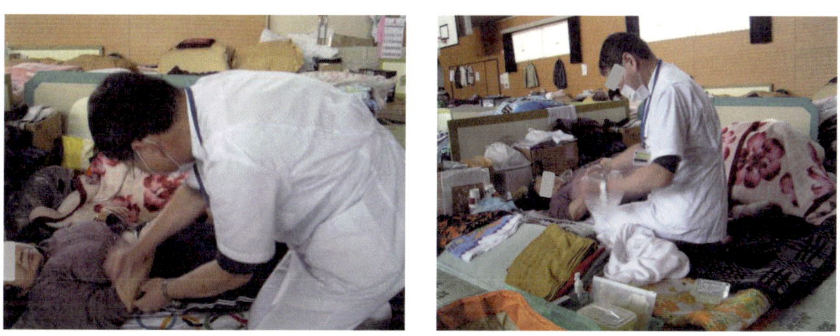

Figure 7. A scene from the acupuncture therapy conducted in the living quarters of an evacuation center in the Fukushima Prefecture.

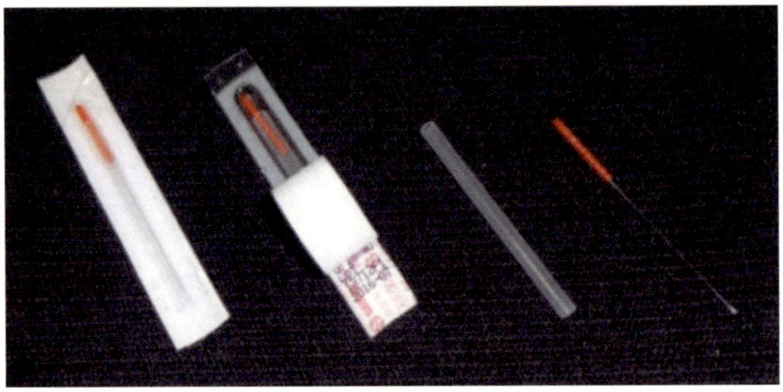

Figure 8. An example of the acupuncture needles used in the acupuncture therapy.

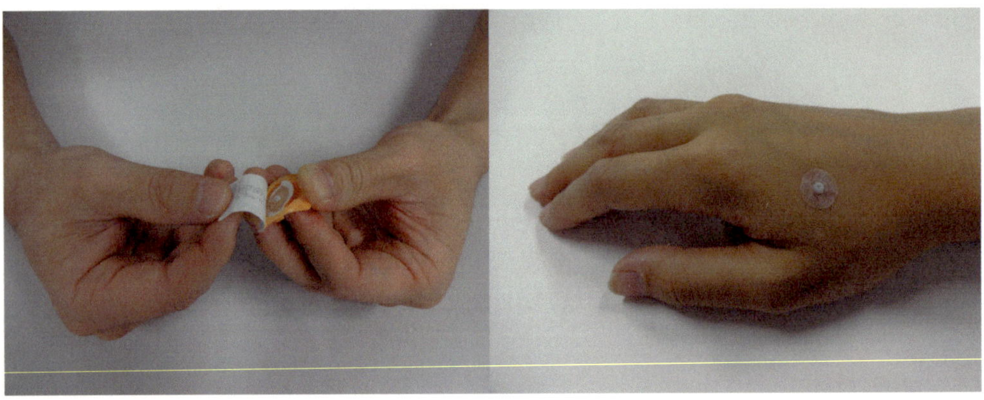

Figure 9. An example of the press tack needles used to administer acupuncture.

Age (year old)	Gender	Symptoms					Affected sites					
		Pain	Stiffness	Numbness	Edema	The others	Head	Shoulder and back	Upper limb	Lumbar	Lower limb	The others
Age < 20	Male (n = 6)		5			1	2	3		2	2	1
	Female (n = 5)	2	3	2				3	2	2	1	
20 ≤ age < 40	Male (n = 6)	3	5					3		5	1	
	Female (n = 13)	2	10	1		1	2	9	1	6	4	
40 ≤ age < 60	Male (n = 17)	7	10	2	1			12		6	5	
	Female (n = 26)	5	17	4	3	1	4	20	6	9	7	
60 ≤ age < 80	Male (n = 11)	3	6	1	2	1		7		6	4	
	Female (n = 34)	25	18	1	2		2	20	5	14	14	1
80 ≤ age	Male (n = 5)	5	3					3	1	3	2	
	Female (n = 5)	1	3		2			2			2	1
Total	N = 128	53	80	11	10	4	10	82	15	53	42	3
	%	41.4	62.5	8.6	7.8	3.1	7.8	64.1	11.7	41.4	32.8	2.3

Table 1. The symptoms and affected sites reported by the evacuees [10].

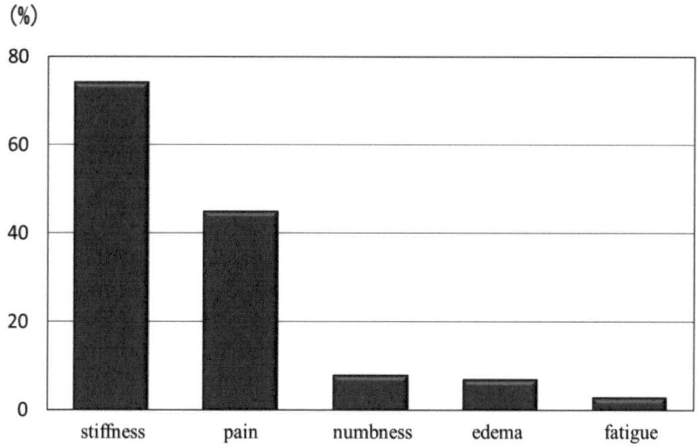

Figure 10. The total number of evacuees that report each symptom [10].

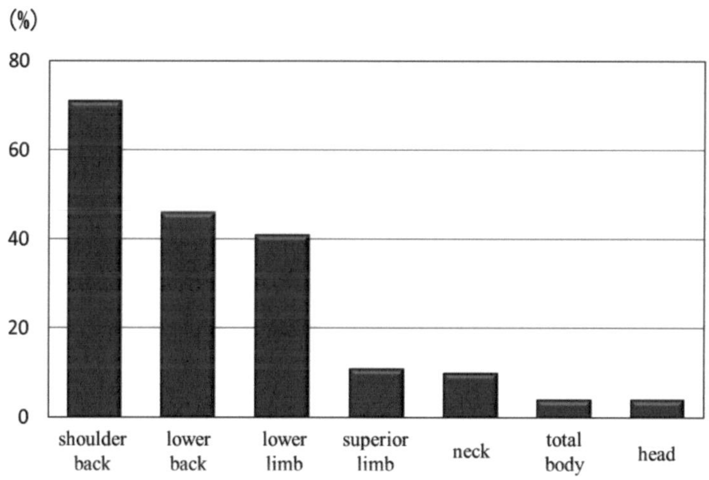

Figure 11. The total number of evacuees with the affected site [10].

3. Clinical study of Kampo medicine for PTSD in GEJE survivors [11]

3.1. Purpose

Many survivors had an elevated risk of developing PTSD after the GEJE and tsunami. Therefore, a randomized, observer-blinded, controlled trial was conducted to examine the efficacy and safety of the traditional Japanese herbal formula SKK in treating PTSD in disaster survivors.

3.2. Methods

3.2.1. Participants

Subjects were recruited from the outpatient clinic at the National Sendai-Nishitaga Hospital in Sendai, Japan. All participants completed an intake assessment that included a medical history, physical examination, and standard blood examination as well as an Impact of Event Scale-Revised (IES-R) to assess the severity of PTSD at baseline. The inclusion criteria were as follows: survivors of the GEJE and tsunami who (1) were older than 20 years, (2) were diagnosed with PTSD according to the Diagnostic and Statistical Manual (DSM)-IV TR, and (3) had an IES-R score $\geq$ 25 (cut-off point). The exclusion criteria were as follows: (1) major medical illness such as neoplastic disease, acute inflammation, or any other disease that would most likely prevent the completion of this study; (2) psychosis due to other disorders such as schizophrenia, depression, and/or dementia; (3) delirium due to drugs, alcohol, metabolic intoxication, or inflammation; and (4) the use of neuroleptics, antianxiety drugs, antiepileptic drugs, antidepressants, or herbal remedies during the past two months.

3.2.2. The study protocol

The study protocol was performed with the intention to treat. The SKK extract was prescribed to the patients in the SKK group. The SKK extract (TJ-11) was processed by Tsumura (Tokyo, Japan), and it contained the following mixture of dried herbs: Radix Bupleuri (6 g), Trichosanthis Kirilowii (3 g), Cinnamomi Cassiae (3 g), Radix Scutellariae Baicalensis (3 g), Concha Ostreae (3 g), Radix Glycyrrhizae (2 g), and Rhizoma Zingiberis (2 g). These herbs are registered in the Japan Pharmacopoeia (15th Edition). Each participant in the SKK group received 2.5 g of SKK powder (1.17 g extract) 3 times per day for 2 weeks. The processes involved in the production and supply of SKK comply with the Good Manufacturing Practices for Kampo products and are also approved by the Ministry of Health, Labour, and Welfare of Japan. Participants understood that those randomized into the control group could receive any treatment after completion of the whole trial if they wanted. Patients were free to withdraw from the study at any time. Clinical assessments were performed at baseline and at the study endpoint.

3.2.3. Outcome measurement

The primary clinical outcome measure was the severity of PTSD symptoms as measured by the total IES-R. The secondary outcome measures were the 3 IES-R subscale scores: avoidance, hyperarousal, and intrusion.

3.2.4. Statistical analysis

The analyses were performed as a modified intention to treat. All statistical analysis was performed using the SPSS software (version 16.0, SPSS Japan Inc., Tokyo, Japan). Measurements (mean and SD) were calculated at baseline and at the endpoint for all continuous primary and secondary measures. A two-way analysis of variance (ANOVA) was conducted to compare outcomes between the SKK and control group. The changes in each group from baseline to the endpoint were compared using a post-hoc paired t-test when the intergroup difference was significant (P < 0.05).

3.2.5. Ethical committee

The study protocol was approved by the Institutional Review Board of Sendai-Nishitaga National Hospital in Sendai, Japan, and registered with the University Hospital Medical Information Network (UMIN) clinical trial registry (UMIN000010890, http://www.umin.ac.jp/ctr/index.htm).

3.2.6. Results

The 43 participants were randomized into the SKK (n = 21) and control (n = 22) groups (Table 2). The magnitude of changes in the total IES-R scores differed significantly between the two groups (p<0.001). A post-hoc analysis showed that the total IES-R score improved significantly in the SKK group, from 49.6 ± 11.9 to 25.5 ± 17.0 (p<0.001) (Figure 12). The subscale scores improved significantly in the SKK group (avoidance, p=0.003; hyperarousal, p<0.001; intrusion, p<0.001) (Figure 13).

	Group		*P* value
	SKK	Control	
n	21	22	
Sex (m/f)	9/12	13/9	0.45
Age (year)	52.3 ± 13.0	48.0 ± 20.9	0.42
IES-R (baseline)	49.6 ± 11.6	43.7 ± 13.7	0.14

Table 2. Characteristics of the SKK and control groups.

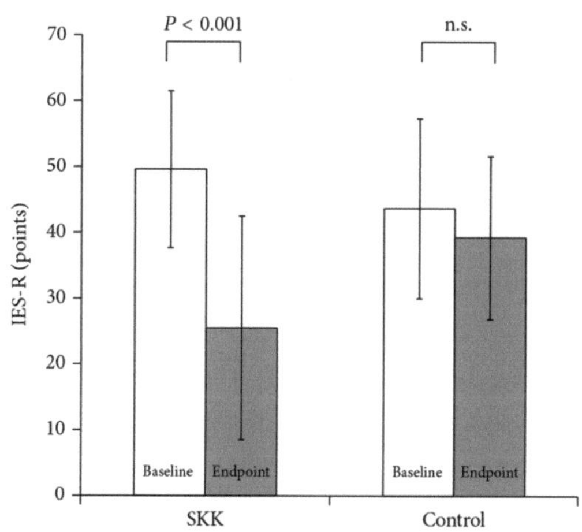

Figure 12. Changes in the total IES-R scores. The two-way ANOVA showed a significant difference between the groups (p<0.001), and a post-hoc analysis showed that the total IES-R scores were significantly improved in the SKK group only.

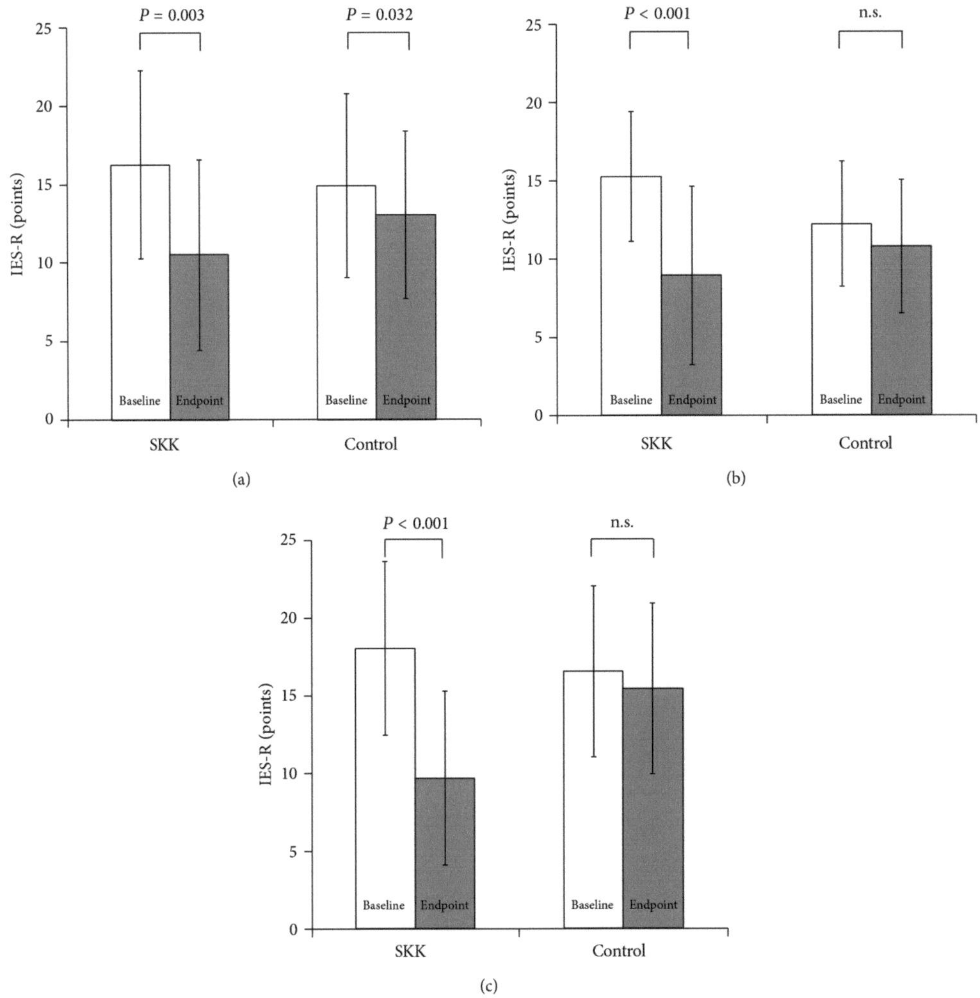

Figure 13. (a) Changes in the IES-R avoidance subscale score. (b) Changes in the IES-R hyperarousal subscale score. (c) Changes in the IES-R intrusion subscale score. The two-way ANOVA showed that each subscale differed significantly between the SKK and control groups ([a] p=0.025, [b] p=0.005, [c] p=0.001). Post-hoc analyses showed that all subscale scores changed significantly from baseline to the endpoint in the SKK group ([a] p=0.003, [b] p<0.001, [c] p<0.001). In the control group, only the avoidance subscale score showed a significant change ([a] p=0.032, [b] n.s., [c] n.s.).

4. Discussion

4.1. Medical operations with Kampo medicine in the Miyagi and Fukushima Prefectures after the GEJE

Approximately one month after the GEJE, an increase in psychiatric symptoms such as insomnia, irritability, lightheadedness, and anxiety as well as somatoform disorders was observed. These symptoms may be attributed to fatigue related to the extended stay of the evacuees at the evacuation centers and to the stress experienced from recurring aftershocks. In addition, patient complaints of constipation may be attributed to the composition of the distributed meals, which consisted mainly of carbohydrates. In this disaster medical operation, we observed that Kampo treatment relieved symptoms in our patients. Kampo treatment is generally applied after taking a history of the patient's illness and conducting a physical examination [5], and was a useful tool for this particular natural disaster when commonly used medical supplies were scarce. The powder extract preparations of Kampo medicine have been used widely in Japan, and their cost is subsidized by the National Health Insurance. There also were occasions in which Kampo preparations were used as treatments for symptoms that emerged during the chronic period, such as psychiatric disorders and constipation. Kampo therapy imparted beneficial effects on both physical and mental/emotional symptoms in patients.

Clinical evidence supports the effectiveness of Kampo medicines administered to patients affected by the GEJE and tsunami. Based on our experience, we find that Kampo treatment can be performed on a wide range of symptoms. In addition, Kampo treatment can be performed concurrent in many patients over a large area similar to the magnitude affected by the recent GEJE and tsunami. It is our vision and hope that Kampo preparations are included in future medical relief supplies for disaster victims and that Kampo treatments are applied for treating a wide range of medical conditions.

Through the medical operation with massage therapy and acupuncture, we realized that Kampo treatments can alleviate various symptoms when given in combination with Western medical practices even under such difficult circumstances as those encountered after the GEJE and tsunami [7-10]. Moreover, the characteristic symptoms of stiffness and pain started to increase approximately one month after the GEJE. It is said that both systemic changes and psychological symptoms contribute to chronic pain [7]. We speculate that complaints of pain increased due to several factors, including the unaccustomed stay at an evacuation center, lying down in a space too small to roll over, the contents of the distributed meals, environmental problems, psychological shock, and stress. In addition to the relief of pain and stiffness, massage therapy and acupuncture can contribute to the early detection of other problems that evacuees might be prone to develop, because the long therapy sessions allow practitioners to listen attentively to their patients. The therapy satisfaction rate of 92.3% may reflect not only the simple effects of the physical treatment but also the relaxing effects derived from the inherent sense of trust and safety generated by the warmth of the manual treatment and conversation during the therapy sessions. In early April, when voluntary massage therapy and acupuncture was started, running water had not yet been restored at any evacuation center. Under these conditions, evacuees could not bathe or even wash their hands properly. During this period, we performed only massage therapy in consideration of infection risks, and started acupuncture therapy only after the evacuees were again able to bathe. However, under such conditions of inadequate sanitation, the use of contact needles that noninvasively stimulate the skin may be an option. Moreover, the circumstances for setting up a treatment room varied among the evacuation centers.

4.2. Clinical study of Kampo medicine for PTSD in survivors after the GEJE

Our clinical study showed that SKK significantly improved PTSD caused by the disaster. A recent study showed that PTSD was strongly suspected in about 10% of all high school students in the city of Sendai 9 months after the GEJE [12]. Both psychological and pharmacological treatments are effective for PTSD, but there is a severe shortage of psychologists and psychotherapists in the disaster-stricken area. General physicians and primary care doctors must routinely care for PTSD patients. Antidepressants, benzodiazepines, and antipsychotics are used to treat PTSD, but these medications have adverse effects. Drug dependency is common with the use of benzodiazepines. Selective serotonin reuptake inhibitors (SSRIs) are also used to treat PTSD, but continuous treatment is often necessary to prevent relapse. Better pharmacological treatments that are both safe and effective are thus needed. Since the disaster, we have tried traditional herbal medicines such as yokukansan that are known to be effective for the treatment of mental disorders [13]. We observed that patients treated with SKK showed very clear improvements in PTSD symptoms. These clinical observations led us to conduct a clinical trial to test the efficacy of SKK on PTSD. This clinical trial showed that SKK treatment resulted in the marked, rapid, and tolerable amelioration of PTSD symptoms in all participants, with no severe adverse events.

Several pharmacological mechanisms underlying the effects of SKK have been investigated [14-16]. Acute moderate to high stress activates serotonergic neurons in the hippocampus to release 5-hydroxytryptamine (5-HT). 5-HT then activates postsynaptic 5-HT1A receptors that inhibit the process of hippocampal long-term potentiation [14]. The repeated administration of SKK significantly increases 5-HT concentrations in the hippocampus and the corpus striatum and the concentrations of norepinephrine (NE) and 5-HT in the hippocampus [15]. SKK also regulates plasma interleukin-6 and soluble interleukin-6 receptor concentrations and improves depressed mood in climacteric women with insomnia [16]. These findings may partially explain the mechanisms of SKK action in the treatment of mental disorders.

5. Conclusion

We summarized our experiences with Kampo medicine in clinics that were set up after the GEJE and in a clinical study of Kampo medicine for PTSD treatment in GEJE survivors. Kampo medicine, which includes herbal formulae, acupuncture, and massage therapy, is a potentially useful treatment for disorders or imbalances of the body, mind, and soul.

Acknowledgements

All authors declare no personal competing financial or nonfinancial interests in this study. Tohoku University Graduate School of Medicine has received a grant from Tsumura Co. Ltd., the manufacturer of SKK.

http://dx.doi.org/10.5772/60702

Author details

Shin Takayama*, Takehiro Numata, Natsumi Saito, Soichiro Kaneko and Tetsuharu Kamiya

*Address all correspondence to: takayama@med.tohoku.ac.jp

Department of Kampo Medicine, Tohoku University Hospital, Japan

References

[1] Motoo Y, Seki T, Tsutani K. Traditional Japanese medicine, Kampo: its history and current status. Chinese Journal of Integrative Medicine 2011; 17(2):85-87.

[2] http://www.nikkankyo.org/topix/news/091209_ad/enquete.pdf

[3] Motoo Y, Arai I, Hyodo I, Tsutani K. Current status of Kampo (Japanese herbal) medicines in Japanese clinical practice guidelines. Complementary Therapies in Medicine 2009; 17(3):147-154.

[4] Motoo Y, Arai I, Tsutani K. Use of Kampo diagnosis in randomized controlled trials of Kampo products in Japan: a systematic review. PLoS One 2014; 9(8): e104422.

[5] Great East Japan Earthquake. National Police Agency 2014.

[6] Takayama S, Watanabe K, Iwasaki K, Numata T, Kuroda H, Ishii T, Yaegashi N. Japanese Kampo medicine after the great East Japan earthquake in Miyagi and Fukushima prefectures. The Journal of Kampo, Acupuncture and Integrative Medicine. In press 2014.

[7] Takayama S, Okitsu R, Iwasaki K, Watanabe M, Kamiya T, Hirano A, Matsuda A, Monma T, Numata T, Kusuyama H, Hirata S, Kikuchi A, Seki T, Takeda T, Yaegashi N. The role of oriental medicine in the great East Japan earthquake disaster. Kampo Medicine 2011; 62(5):621-626.

[8] Takayama S, Okitsu R, Iwasaki K, Watanabe M, Kamiya T, Hirano A, Matsuda A, Monma T, Numata T, Kusuyama H, Hirata S, Kikuchi A, Seki T, Takeda T, Yaegashi N. Role of oriental medicine in the great East Japan earthquake. German Journal of Acupuncture and Related Techniques 2012; 55(2): 15-18.

[9] Takayama S, Numata T, Iwasaki K, Kuroda H, Kagaya Y, Ishii T, Yaegashi N. The role of integrative medicine and Kampo treatment in an aging society: experience with Kampo treatment during a natural disaster. Nihon Ronen Igakkai Zasshi 2014; 51(2): 128-131.

[10] Takayama S, Kamiya T, Watanabe M, Hirano A, Matsuda A, Monma Y, Numata T, Kusuyama H, Yaegashi N. Report on disaster medical operations with acupuncture/

massage therapy after the great East Japan earthquake. Integrative Medicine Insights 2012; 7: 1-5.

[11] Numata T, Gunfan S, Takayama S, Takahashi S, Monma Y, Kaneko S, Kuroda H, Tanaka J, Kanemura S, Nara M, Kagaya Y, Ishii T, Yaegashi N, Kohzuki M, Iwasaki K. Treatment of posttraumatic stress disorder using the traditional Japanese herbal medicine saikokeishikankyoto: a randomized, observer-blinded, controlled trial in survivors of the great East Japan earthquake and tsunami. Evidence-Based Complementary and Alternative Medicine: eCAM 2014; 683293.

[12] Takeda T, Tadakawa M, Koga S, Nagase S, Yaegashi N. Premenstrual symptoms and posttraumatic stress disorder in Japanese high school students 9 months after the great East-Japan earthquake. The Tohoku Journal of Experimental Medicine 2013; 230(3): 151-154.

[13] Iwasaki K, Satoh-Nakagawa T, Maruyama M, Monma Y, Nemoto M, Tomita N, Tanji H, Fujiwara H, Seki T, Fujii M, Arai H, Sasaki H. A randomized, observer-blind, controlled trial of the traditional Chinese medicine Yi-Gan San for improvement of behavioral and psychological symptoms and activities of daily living in dementia patients. The Journal of Clinical Psychiatry 2005; 66(2): 248-252.

[14] Oosthuizen F, Wegener G, Harvey BH. Nitric oxide as inflammatory mediator in post-traumatic stress disorder (PTSD): evidence from an animal model. Neuropsychiatric Disease and Treatment 2005; 1(2): 109-123.

[15] Itoh T, Michijiri S, Murai S, Saito H, Saito H, Itsukaichi O, Fujiwara H. Effects of chai-hu-guizhi-ganjiang-tang on the levels of monoamines and their related substances, and acetylcholine in discrete brain regions of mice. The American Journal of Chinese Medicine 1996; 24(1): 53-64.

[16] Ushiroyama T, Ikeda A, Sakuma K, Ueki M. Chai-hu-gui-zhi-gan-jiang-tang regulates plasma interleukin-6 and soluble interleukin-6 receptor concentrations and improves depressed mood in climacteric women with insomnia. The American Journal of Chinese Medicine 1996; 33(5): 703-711.

Chapter 8

Yoga & Qigong — A Self-reliant Practice for Health of Body & Mind

Ping-chung Leung

Additional information is available at the end of the chapter

http://dx.doi.org/10.5772/60568

Abstract

Yoga originated from India and is becoming popular worldwide. Qigong originated from China and is less known outside China. Interestingly, both Indian Yoga and Chinese Qigong emphasize on three common components in their fundamental practices, viz. (i) stretching of muscles, tendons and ligaments when thousands of proprioceptive receptors which initiate the "gate theory" of neurological control of pain perception are stimulated; (ii) controlled breathing which harmonizes the somatic and autonomic systems of neurological activities; and (iii) the wonderful outcome after such simple voluntary efforts, a state of tranquility of the mind, which could be understood as Meditation. A comprehensive review on the reports on Yoga and Qigong practices affecting the important physiological processes and mental states of the practitioners is completed to provide reliable information about the value of the practices. Result of the review shows that there are sufficient evidences today, after many carefully planned research studies, on the supportive effects of both Yoga and Qigong on not only neuromuscular pathologies but also problems in cardiovascular, pulmonary and most remarkably, mental health. Yoga and Qigong practices are good for both the body and mind.

Keywords: Yoga, Qigong, Body-mind health

1. Introduction

The current concept of Health is not only "a state of complete physical, mental, social and spiritual well-being, and not merely an absence of disease or free from infirmary" as was defined by the World Health Organization [1]. With the increasing complexity of the modern society, the stress and pressure encountered by the individual living in affluent communities could be expected [2]. In the extreme situations, total loss of ability to social adaptation could result in institutionalization in asylum related infrastructures. For the less severely affected, depression and mental stress may significantly affect the activities of daily living of the individual. The rising incidence of psychiatric disorders as a disease therefore appears mandatory [3]. Likewise, apparently normal working individuals may actually suffer from periodical depression in response to fluctuating emotional and work pressure. Psychiatrists and general practitioners are encountering more and more such patients [4]. This group of people under mental stresses may sadly develop into varying degrees of anxiety disorders and depression, or may eventually turn psychiatric. Others, who are either capable of self-care or enjoy good family support, could manage to maintain a reasonably balanced mental stability. The ability to maintain such stability is often the result of special efforts ranging from persistence on bodily exercises, social activities and unique life styles [5, 6].

In this chapter we explore the value of bodily exercises originated in the Orient that require persistent self-practices through which the individual gradually reaches a state of physical and mental stability, esteeming to a higher level of mental serenity which might carry the individual away from the drastic stresses being experienced. Yoga from India and Qigong from China are two popular systems of self-performed bodily exercises that help to maintain the Healthy state of the body and mind [7, 8].

2. Yoga and Qigong

The experts in Yoga or Qigong usually belong to special groups of respectable practitioners and tend to strongly believe that only their own unique stereotyped practices would be able give the best results to guarantee good outcomes. Taking a logical objective view, one could carefully scrutinize the broad framework of the systems of practice to identify the essential components that might be common to the different groups which insist on their limited authorities. Since most of the groups are commanding many enthusiastic followers, there must be commonalities within all the groups in spite of the differences.

With this intension in mind one may identify basic common elements of physical activities in Yoga. They are: special physical postures and stretching exercises; special ways of breathing; and deep relaxation which develops into meditation. For the distinguished experienced expert, a great stress on Indian philosophy is also emphasized [7].

Looking at Qigong: special stretching physical activities with some special postures are also adopted; special ways of breathing are equally stressed, which again lead to deep relaxation and meditation. The philosophical background of Qigong practice is linked with Buddhism, Taoism and Confucianism [9].

Using modern physiological knowledge to conceptualize the special components of activity of both Yoga and Qigong one could link those activities to special stimulations related to

http://dx.doi.org/10.5772/60568

unique neurophysiologic pathways that are capable of bringing about a harmonious state between the somatic and the autonomic components of the neurological system [7].

What does stretching do? Stretching produces tension within the muscles, tendons, ligaments and the components around the joints. Stretching with selected postures produces tension on special groups of muscles, tendons, ligaments and joints that are normally more relaxed, under-used or never extensively used. Muscles, tendons, ligaments and joint capsules are provided with heavy distributions of proprioceptive receptors over their origins and insertions, so as to enable the detection of movements and subsequently, maintain good co-ordinations for the need of functional balance. When the proprioceptive receptions are stimulated, a concerted message is sent up the spinal cord to the mid-brain where cortical messages are converged. According to Melzack who invented the "Gate Theory", the proprioceptive message at the mid-brain, will block off unwanted messages coming in from other brain regions, thus producing a "gate" effect against pain perception, and leading towards a balanced summation of neurological messages from various cortical sources. With every intensional stretch, additional proprioceptive messages are sent up. When muscle groups that are not normally active in day to day activities are activated, they send out massive unusual proprioceptive messages to the mid brain, thus initiating neurological activities pertaining to the "Gate Theory" [10]: a mechanism that blocks pain perception and harmonizes the two indifferent somatic and autonomic neurological systems.

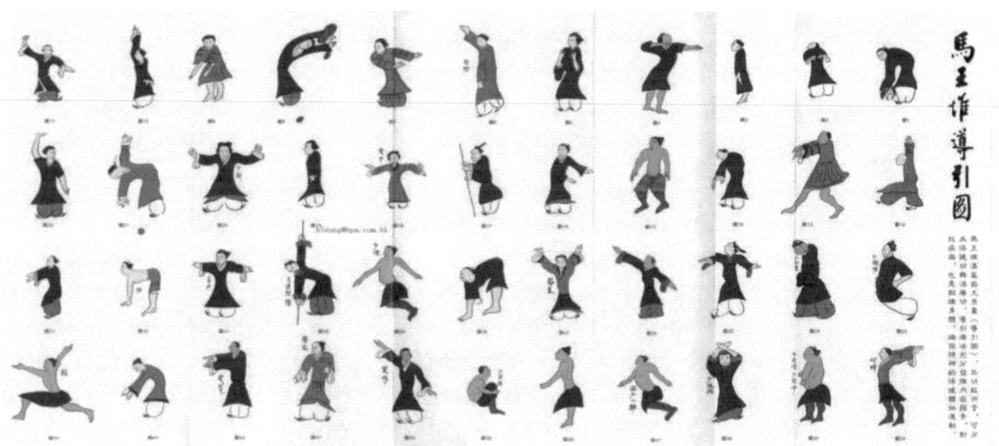

Figure 1. Excavated document showing varieties of stretching exercises recommended over 2000 years ago in China.

What does controlled breathing do? Controlled breathing creates unusual motor activities within the respiratory cycles which are directed to follow a new pattern of activity. The modified rates, intensities and duration of inspiration and expiration, the different groups of muscles mobilized and involved, together compose a totally novel, unusual system of respiratory motor activities. Neurological messages received through these complex unusual motor activities are new to the higher central nervous system. The control of respiratory function is unique in that either the somatic motor system, which allows voluntary activities,

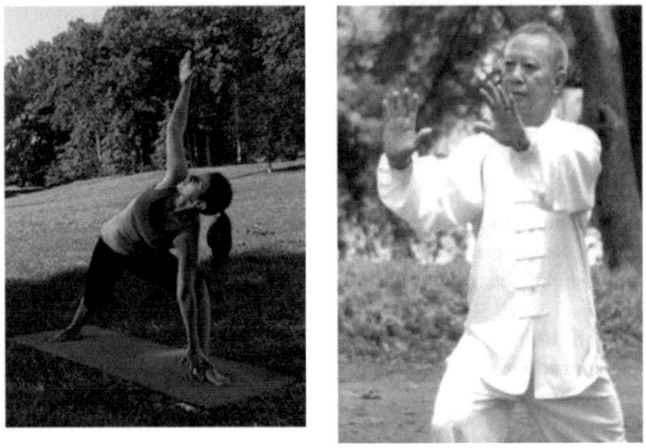

(a) (b)

Figure 2. a. Stretching in Yoga practice **b.** Stretching in Qigong Practice

or the autonomic (parasympathetic) nervous system, which generates automatic regulatory activities of respiration, could be responsible. Intentional controlled breathing therefore is making use of the somatic motor activity to impose stimulations on the autonomic nervous system, which has wide connections with the internal organs. Intentional controlled breathing therefore opens up new channels of communication between the internal organs which otherwise stay independent of the body's voluntary control. These new channels of communication, could explain how Yoga and Qigong practices help to build up a state of physiological harmony through stretching and controlled breathing, and the subsequent feeling of tranquility [11, 12].

What does meditation do? No one is free from the somatic stimulations and cognitive, mental activities culminating into worries and mental disturbances. Busy daily activities may be causes of worries and anxiety. Worldly events straightforward or complicated, may also contribute towards sleep disturbances which seriously affect one's quality of life. Spiritual tranquility is very much adored by those affected. Priests, monks and Buddhists might have special means to achieve a special state of spiritual tranquility. What about ordinary people? Practicing Yoga and Qigong might allow individuals to acquire a mental state like the priest or monk. We have to make postulation according to some basic physiological phenomena so as to understand the mechanisms leading to meditation, when the brain is free from worldly concerns and worries.

The two essential activities that both Yoga and Qigong practice are slow repeated joint stretchings and controlled deep breathings. Joint stretchings initiate the "gate theory" which help to control pain perception. What does deep breathing do?

Normally, lung function, like the heart, the guts and endocrine system, are under the control of the autonomic nervous system. The individual does not need to give any instruction or control; the function of those organs would be automatically maintained. However, the respiratory system enjoys a double favour of either controlled or autonomous function. With this special functional ability, forcing the respiratory processes through the voluntary channel should induce special physiological interactions. The forced inspiratory and extended expiratory movements connect the somatic and autonomic systems, which are normally independent from each other. The bridging effect is probably, a harmonizing process resembling the "gate theory". The "gate" effect removes pain input. The forced respiratory activity removes or harmonizes unfavourable activities in the other autonomic organs. The harmonized situation would be felt somewhere in the brain reaching a state of tranquility, i.e. a vivid experience of "Meditation". Yoga and Qigong, through the synchronized activities of stretching and forced respiratory training, induce a state of meditation, a supreme feeling of tranquility [9, 11, 12].

3. Physiological states

Clinical researches in many institutes have gathered evidences on the effects of Yoga and Qigong on different physiological functions. Improvements in the basic parameters of respiratory functions have been demonstrated [13, 14]. Cardiac functions and related hypertension are also found to improve during the exercises and the effects persist afterwards in both Yoga and Qigong [15-17]. Changes in internal secretions i.e. endocrine adjustments are going along simultaneously with both Yoga and Qigong [18, 19]. The practice of both Yoga and Qigong, and their wide popularity are always linked with satisfactions related to improvements of musculoskeletal strength. Moreover, clear indications are available that muscle strengthening and pain alleviation could be a pleasant result in musculo-skeletal diseases [20, 21].

3.1. Effects of Qigong on separate physiological functions

3.1.1. Qigong and musculoskeletal function

Many carefully planned studies have been carried out to study Qigong's direct effects on musculoskeletal function. One study was completed at the Beijing Sports University in 2004 on a group of people aged 50 to 70. After giving standard Qigong training, the physical fitness was assessed, compared with the pre-training states. Results showed that leg and hand grip strengths improved while body weight, pelvic girdle and fat thickness etc. did not change [14].

3.1.2. Qigong and cardio-respiratory function

The Beijing Sports University study also looked at the cardio pulmonary functions of the participants. The heart rates declined at all stages of Qigong training while the respiratory function improved towards the end of the training [14].

Another study done at Jiangxi University on 70 people, 61 to 68 years of age, given Qigong for six months, showed a general improvement of heart functions, measured with high resolution ultrasonic tools, manifested as stroke volume (SV), early and late diastolic velocities (VE and VA).

The results are shown in Table 1 indicating better stroke volume (SV) and early diastolic velocity (VE) in the trained group compared with the control group. VE-VA showed even a more convincing improvement [22].

	Control Group (n = 31)		**Study Group (n = 39)**	
	Before training	**After six months' training**	**Before training**	**After six months' training**
SV (ml)	57.94 ± 16.01	58.51 ± 16.99	55.72 ± 15.78	67.15 ± 13.67**#
VE (cm/s)	65.95 ± 19.95	66.30 ± 19.75	66.50 ± 18.24	75.05 ± 17.66**#
VA (cm/s)	84.36 ± 15.12	82.68 ± 14.10	83.02 ± 13.89	83.76 ± 15.21
VE-VA	-18.41 ± 23.98	-16.38 ± 24.68	-16.53 ± 25.96	-10.25 ± 23.32*

*$p<0.05$; **$p<0.01$ study group compared on before and after training; #$p<0.05$ study group compared with control group after six months training.

Table 1. Cardiac function before and after training [22].

3.1.3. Qigong and serological data

There is always doubt whether Qigong would affect endocrine functions which could be revealed from serological markers like cytokines and blood sugar. A study done at Beijing Guang-on-Mun Hospital on patients suffering from diabetes showed that after four months' practice not only was the blood sugar level better controlled but the quality of life also improved [23].

Another study done at Talien on patients with high serum triglycerides showed that 60 minutes of Qigong per day for six months, resulted in improvements in all the relevant biological markers [24, 25].

Positive results after Qigong training were also demonstrated among patients with osteoporosis, reflected in the parameters of bone metabolism, viz. serum alkaline phosphatase and bone mineral density.

3.1.4. Qigong and mental activities

Psychologists are interested to know the effects of Qigong exercises on mental activities like cognitive abilities, calculation speed, memory, imitations, making sketches and motor reactions. Experts in Jiangxi have directed studies on elderly people and found that the trained group did better than the untrained group [26, 27].

3.2. Effects of *Tai Chi* on physiological functions

3.2.1. Tai Chi and musculoskeletal problems

Tai Chi is the most popular training exercise in the Chinese Communities, particularly among the elderly people. *Tai Chi* may appear to be gentle, dancing, purely relaxing activities. In fact

Tai Chi demands the same practice of stretching, controlled breathing and meditation. Training and practices give general physiological supports, very much similar to Qigong. *Tai Chi* is particularly indicated for the rehabilitation of back injuries. One impressive study done in Shanxi for 64 patients suffering from work-related spinal degenerations and back pain showed that *Tai Chi* gave very positive benefits at different stages of training [28] (Table 2).

Group	No.	Male / Female	Recovered	Improved	No Improvement	Cure rate	Effectiveness (%)
4 weeks							
Control	32	20/12	2	27	3	6.3	90.6
Tai Chi	32	22/10	4	28	1	9.4	96.9
8 weeks							
Control	32	20/12	40	21	1	31.3	96.9
Tai Chi	32	22/10	18	14	0	56.3*a	100
12 weeks							
Control	32	20/12	22	10	0	68.8	100
Tai Chi	32	22/10	27	5	0	84.4*b	100

*a $p < 0.01$; *b $p < 0.05$.

Table 2. Treatment results in 4, 8, 12 weeks [28]

3.2.2. *Tai Chi and balancing*

The dynamic dancing movements of *Tai Chi* would naturally be excellent for the training of people who find difficulties maintaining a normal balance. A large scale study covering 421 people practicing *Tai Chi* regularly, comparing with another group not doing exercise showed marked differences in the single leg stance durability.

3.2.3. *Tai Chi and cardio-pulmonary function*

Many scientific reports on the benefits given by *Tai Chi* to cardio-pulmonary function are available. A study conducted in Fujian on middle age and elderly people before and after *Tai Chi* training showed that, after one year, cardiac function, stroke volume, stroke index, cardiac output, pulse rate, cardiac oxygen consumption volume and index, all improved [16] (Table 3).

Although the general mediating effects of exercises on hypertension are well recognized, whether aerobic or otherwise, *Tai Chi* might provide the most remarkable results, when practiced together with regular therapeutic treatment [31]. Some studies have also shown that those suffering from milder hypertension are responding better than the severe ones [32, 33].

Indice	1996	1997	Rate
PR (min)	76.18 ± 11.73	72.08 ± 9.18**	5.38
SV (ml)	81.14 ± 1.72	84.05 ± 16.86*	3.59
CO (L/min)	6.10 ± 1.05	6.42 ± 1.20*	5.29
SI (ml/m2)	53.15 ± 9.51	55.41 ± 7.52*	4.24
HOI	2629.74 ± 616.08	2517.58 ± 593.45*	4.27
HOV (ml/min)	43.82 ± 10.27	40.23 ± 6.94*	8.19

*$p < 0.05$, ** $p < 0.01$.

Table 3. Changes in cardiac function [16].

Effects of *Tai Chi* are also shown in anti-oxidant studies. *Tai Chi* practices have been demonstrated to bring down tissue and serum anti-oxidants, viz. superoxide dismutase (SOD), glutathione peroxide (GSHPx), catalase (CAT) and malondialdehype (MDA). It was also apparent that the longer the duration of *Tai Chi* practice, the more active were the anti-oxidant effects (Table 4) [34].

	1-5 years		5-10 years		Over 10 years	
Markers	n	x ± s	n	x ± s	n	x ± s
SOD (NU/m l)	37	78.28 ± 15.27	21	99.66 ± 13.16	13	104.1 ± 12.48
GSH-Px (U/m l)	36	58.08 ± 2.88	22	72.21 ± 11.52	13	77.79 ± 8.75
CA T (U/m l)	37	1.78 ± 0.20	21	2.02 ± 0.19	13	2.05 ± 0.14
MDA (nmol/m l)	29	4.54 ± 0.19	10	4.03 ± 0.39	8	3.62 ± 0.17

Differences all reaching $p < 0.05$.

Table 4. Relationship between different duration of *Tai Chi* practice [34].

3.2.4. Tai Chi and endocrine function

Gross deficiencies of endocrine function lead to well-known pathologies and disease entities. Mild subclinical deficiencies are the causes of declining physical strength and deteriorating health status, particularly affecting the elderlies.The declining tendency with aging has been demonstrated in the evaluation of different hormonal levels in the blood, e.g. testosterone, estrogen, luteohormure, follicular stimulating hormone, thyroxine and thyroid stimulating hormone [Table 5]. *Tai Chi* exercises have been shown to alleviate some of the deficiencies [19].

Serum Homone				P		
Level	Tai Chi Group (A)	Elderly Group (B)	Young Group (C)	A:B	B:C	A:C
F (ng/dl)	14.74 ± 4.73	15.23 ± 7.67	14.20 ± 3.92	> 0.05	> 0.05	> 0.05
TSH (μU/ml)	4.80 ± 3.05	3.80 ± 1.55	3.10 ± 1.15	< 0.05	> 0.05	< 0.05
T3 (ng/ml)	0.93 ± 0.20	0.84 ± 0.21	1.51 ± 0.31	< 0.05	< 0.01	< 0.05
T4 (ng/ml)	69.97 ± 23.87	73.60 ± 31.96	104.97 ± 38.60	> 0.05	< 0.05	< 0.01
rT3 (ng/ml)	30.26 ± 7.77	28.79 ± 4.96	37.22 ± 7.64	> 0.05	< 0.01	< 0.01
FSH (mIU/ml)	16.54 ± 15.16	11.05 ± 6.08	4.85 ± 1.58	< 0.05	< 0.01	< 0.01
LH (mIU/ml)	11.74 ± 13.19	8.03 ± 5.95	4.41 ± 1.31	> 0.05	< 0.01	< 0.05
T (ng/dl)	680.00 ± 430.00*	510.00 ± 151.00	679.00 ± 173.00**	< 0.05	< 0.01	> 0.05
E2 (pg/ml)	63.91 ± 17.14	54.74 ± 18.62Δ	50.70 ± 7.14ΔΔ	< 0.05	> 0.05	< 0.05
PRL (ng/ml)	7.06 ± 3.46	6.34 ± 2.75	8.25 ± 3.21	> 0.05	> 0.05	> 0.05

*n = 50; **n = 12; $^{\Delta}$ n= 46; $^{\Delta\Delta}$ n = 10.

Table 5. Differences in serum hormone level [19].

3.2.5. *Tai Chi and general health*

General health could be reflected from the proneness to ailments of infective origin like common cold and/or influenza. Not only elderlies could be the victims but those suspected of being "low-resistant" against infections could be screened for immunologically related markers: the interleukins (IL's) of which IL2 is probably the most important member which controls the survival of T cells, NK cells and B cells. It has been found that six months of *Tai Chi* exercises among a group of women, aged between 55 and 65, boost up the IL2 level significantly [35, 36].

3.2.6. *Tai Chi and mental health*

Like Qigong, *Tai Chi* tends to bring up the psychosocial adaptation ability of the practitioner. Using standard mental assessment Indices, tendencies of depression, anxiety and tension questionaires, the effects of *Tai Chi* have been explored. Compared with non *Tai Chi* groups, advantages are well observed on the *Tai Chi* group [37].

3.3. Outlook of Yoga and Qigong practice on mental health

In the first place, both systems of physical training aim at the attainment of meditation i.e. mental serenity as the terminal stage of the self-disciplined exercises. Reaching the meditation level requires repeated practices and is subjectively felt by the individual. In the past decade Magnetic Resonance Studies carried out in different institutes have demonstrated that functional activities in different regions of the brain could be affected by sustained postures, musculoskeletal stretches and controlled breathings. These observations are early objective indications of the neurological outcome of Yoga and Qigong [38].

With the complexity of Neuroanatomy and Neuro-Physiology, it might take decades to get nearer to the scientific depths of how Yoga or Qigong influences brain functions. At this stage, we only have clinical evidences from different parts of the world, about the clinical values of Yoga and Qigong on the maintenance of mental health, from prevention to treatment of anxiety disorders and depression.

3.4. Yoga

In 2005 a systematic review on the effects of Yoga on anxiety was completed in the University of West-minister, United Kingdom. Eight studies were reviewed. In spite of many inadequacies in the methodologies, it appeared that many cases of anxiety state benefited from Yoga, although specific recommendations could not be made [38].

The same group reviewed the effects of Yoga for depression in 2005. They analyzed five randomized controlled trials which all reported positive results although the study methodologies were not perfect [39].

A systematic review done in Australia in 2008 on the effectiveness of Yoga and self-help for anxiety disorders found that Yoga was superior to medications like diazepam [40].

Looking through many other reviews of different academic levels, one realizes the general trend of encouraging results, which may be summarized in the Table 6.

Many other solitary reports on the effects of Yoga on the Mental State of people suffering from different degrees of anxiety disorders are available. Exercise training alone has been proven clinically effective in major depression and panic disorders [46]. Yoga should also provide enhancing effects on standard treatments. Since those maintained on anti psychotic medications are more vulnerable to obesity, diabetes and heart diseases, Yoga would be particularly indicated [47, 48], especially for those who are not suitable for aerobic exercises.

Since the 1970's, meditation and other stress-reduction techniques are more and more frequently practised and studied as possible means of treatments for depression and anxiety. The practice of Yoga, which combines exercises with meditation, unfortunately has been underlooked. The Harvard Medical School Health Review reported that in the recent decades an increasing number of Yoga practices revealed that Yoga reduced the unfavourable influences of exaggerated stress responses, hence should be helpful for anxiety and depression, equivalent to other self-soothing techniques like therapeutic relaxation, meditation and socialization. Yoga also helped through easing respiration and reducing heart rate which were considered indicators of the bodily ability to response to stress [49]. The tolerability to pain was also increased. Another study at Harvard found that after practicing Yoga for three months, the women involved felt improvements in mental states related to stress, depression, anxiety and fatigue feeling. They also felt stronger and better. Quantitatively, there was a 50% improve-

http://dx.doi.org/10.5772/60568

Source of Study	Summary of Results
Arias 2006 [41] Systematic review USA	82 studies, 20 RCTs. The strongest evidence for efficacy was found for epilepsy, symptoms of premenstrual syndrome and menopausal symptoms. Benefit was also demonstrated for nonpsychotic mood and anxiety disorders, autoimmune illness, and emotional disturbance in neoplastic disease.
Krisanaprakorn kit 2006 [42] Systematic review Thailand	Only two studies eligible for inclusion. Anti-anxiety drugs were continued in both. The duration of trials ranged from 12 to 18 weeks. Transcendental Meditation showed a reduction in anxiety symptoms.
Lafferty 2006 [43] Systematic review USA	27 clinical trials investigating massage or mind-body interventions, 26 showed significant improvements in symptoms such an anxiety, emotional distress, comfort, nausea and pain, difficult to judge the clinical significance of the results.
Kirkwood 2005 [38] Systematic review UK	Eight studies all reported positive results, quality of studies was poor and no firm conclusions can be drawn.
Pilkington 2005 [39] Systematic review UK	Five RCTs found that overall, yoga interventions for depressive disorders were potentially beneficial; however, methodological limitations prevented drawing firm conclusions.
Astin 2003 [44] Systematic review USA	There were moderate evidence of efficacy for mind-body therapies in the areas of hypertension and arthritis.
Jorm 2004 [45] Review Australia	Review for anxiety disorders found the treatments with the best evidence of effectiveness were kava, exercise, relaxation training and bibliotherapy.

Table 6. Yoga and meditation for stress, anxiety, anxiety disorders mood disorders, sleep disorders and depression.

ment in depression score, 30% improvement in anxiety score and 65% overall well-being. Other psychosomatic complaints of headache, back pain and sleep disorders also resolved better [50].

A review on Yoga would not be qualified without screening reports from India herself. Indeed the majority of research publications on Yoga has been conducted by Indian investigators and published in Indian journals, although there are increasing contributors from US and England, and increasing applications of Yoga are included in the new specialty of mind-body medicine [46]. A study done in Bangalore India in 2000, comparing the antidepressant effects between Yoga, meditation with imipramine, and electro-convulsive therapy for melancholia, showed that significant reductions in the total score rating of depression occurred in all three groups. At week 3, the Yoga group scored higher than the electro-convulsive group but was not different from the medication group. Remission rates at the end of the trial were 93, 73 and 67% in the electro-convulsive, medication and Yoga groups respectively [50].

3.5. Qigong

As stated earlier, Qigong is composed mainly of three essential self-attained activities, viz., stretching across joints, controlled breathing and meditation. Which mechanisms are most important towards the accomplishments of a physiological harmony presenting as both physical and mental well-being? Many theories have been postulated. One theory emphasizes on muscle relaxation, claiming that relaxation brings about improved blood circulation, better oxygen provision and removal of metabolic wastes. Another theory and limited experiments have shown the enhancement of the immunological defense. It is observed that relaxation, and controlled breathing could be giving the mind an effective training to relieve stress and pain. Other scientists have demonstrated changing hormonal levels in the blood during Qigong practice, while at the same time suppressing sympathetic output [51, 52].

With regard to research publications on Qigong, plentiful are available in Chinese language journals but the methodologies of studies are largely of low quality. The reports are mostly from sports related studies and analyses tend to be superficial.

A report from Wuhan, China, on the elderlies practicing Qigong showed that 6 weeks' practice reduced anxiety and depression primarily felt by the individuals while cardiac and pulmonary functions also improved [51]. Another study completed in Shanxi in 2005 approached from the ancient Chinese philosophers' context, but whether Confucian or Taoist philosophical views are suitable for the interpretation of harmonizing observations remain controversial [52].

A controlled study was done in 2006 on 600 people practicing and not practicing Qigong. Those who had long experience were found to have more stable mental health [53].

A group of hospital workers in USA were given Qigong training for six weeks after which they were assessed using the Perceived Stress Scale together with the quality of life, questionnaire, using the SF36 questionnaire. The outcome was compared with another group of hospital workers not trained. The Qigong group demonstrated statistically significant reduction of perceived stress compared to the control group ($p=0.02$) Greater improvement on the quality of life was also found in the Qigong group [54].

Medical Students who practiced Qigong for 12 weeks were studied on their mental adaptability: including depression, anxiety, aggressiveness, threat, stubbornness and social behaviors. 100 of them were compared with 50 others who did not practice Qigong. The practicing group showed significantly higher scores ($p<0.01$) [55].

A detailed case study done in Sweden on the mood recovery of a woman who lost her job and became dreadfully distressed was most interesting. After practicing Qigong, the woman was found to continuously benefit from the exercises. Exercise behaviour was recorded daily, stress-energy and wellness were followed up weekly and mindfulness after 4, 9 and 12 weeks. The woman felt that her mental state was enjoying progressive stabilisation to high levels: she could better adapt to stressful situations and was less worried about unexpected mishappenings in life [56]. She believed firmly that Qigong was the main cause of her achievements.

Reports about mental health after Yoga and Qigong training on the whole, are giving rather vague ideas of the state of the mind. "Stable mental health" is often stated. To the experts on mental health, it means little because specific psychiatric symptoms are not described.

http://dx.doi.org/10.5772/60568

4. Conclusion

Exercises have long been known to be good and effective means of self-administered treatment, not only for physical strengthening but also in attempts to sooth the mind. Indeed, many past and current studies have given good evidences to the objective reasoning and physiological changes behind the simple practice. Practicing meditations under various artificial initiations, have attracted a lot of attention as an effective means of promoting mental health.

When Yoga and Qigong both require sustained stretching and controlled breathing, leading gradually into a state of meditation, the self-initiating activities could be triggering off combined or synergistic effects derived from different levels of neurological activities. Harvard University has conducted a survey on Yoga practitioners in 2008, and found that they were mainly people (woman more than men) who were suffering from musculoskeletal or mental disturbances. The survey indicated that 5.1% of US populations have used Yoga for health in the last 12 months, representing 10.4 million individuals. The data gives sufficient support for further recommendation on the popular use of the simple safe practice, so easily learned and adopted by all [57]. When Mayo Clinic staff made wide papaganda on exercises, using this slogan: "Depression and Anxiety: Exercises ease Symptoms" and giving clear explanations and instruction on Yoga, they were well accepted [58].

Given the great similarities between Yoga and Qigong, there might be a great justification for exploring the two systems of therapies together, when they are recommended as alternative treatments for a holistic body-mind resolution against health deterioration, declining physique, stress, anxiety and depression. Yoga or Qigong is a safe prescription for healthy living and provides a rich ground for harmonized human existence basing on the mind's self-regulatory processes against mental stresses. The two alternative therapies may control mental health disruptions like anxiety and depression, helping to maintain an ideal quality of life [59].

The author is neither an expert on Yoga nor Qigong. He is a clinician researching on Alternative Medicine as a supplementary support to mainline scientific allopathic medicine. He does practice Qigong and has studied Yoga superficially. He realizes Yoga and Qigong could both be excellent additional support for physical and mental health. While searching for literal evidences to illustrate the value of Yoga and Qigong for mental health, he found many convincing conceptual literature, superficial in the scientific sense, but well covers the breadth that is required for those interested to know more about Yoga and Qigong. Readers need not be disappointed with the lack of specific evidences on specific mental diseases, because Yoga and Qigong are meant to be supplementary, not replacing the conventional specialist treatment. Likewise, strict scientific data like hormones and transmitters might have been included in some of the reports, but however, for the general proof of concept, being too specific might lead to a different direction of treatment specific application which should not be encouraged.

For those interested to develop alternative medicine, some prefers moving towards specific focci of their major concern. As far as the author is concerned, he is more capable of simply taking a general approach with the sincere wish of bringing more medical workers to the awareness of the importances of supplementary role of alternative medicine.

The World Health Organization, in its deliberations on Traditional Medicine Strategy, is emphasizing the importance of "Self-care Health" as a most practical way of improving global health [60]. Yoga and Qigong are effective traditional means of self-practice, not only for the musculo-skeletal aspects, as could be readily seen, but also for the mind.

Author details

Ping-chung Leung[1,2]

1 Professor Emeritus, Orthopaedics & Traumatology, The Chinese University of Hong Kong, Shatin, Hong Kong, China

2 State Key Laboratory of Phytochemistry and Plant Resources in West China, The Chinese University of Hong Kong, Shatin, Hong Kong, China

References

[1] World Health Organization. The world health report 2001 - Mental health: new understanding, new hope [Internet]. 2001 [cited 2014 Oct 31]. Available from: http://www.who.int/whr/2001/en/

[2] Pozuelo L, Ross J, Sussman N. The anxiety spectrum: which disorder is it? Patient Care. 1999 Aug; 33(13): 73-93.

[3] Scheweitzer E. Generalized anxiety disorder. Longitudinal course and pharmacologic treatment. Psychiatr Clin North Am. 1995 Dec; 18(4): 843-57.

[4] Stewart SH, Taylor S, Jang, KL, Cox BJ, Watt MC, Fedoroff IC, et al. Causal modeling of relations among learning history, anxiety sensitivity and panic attacks. Behav Res Ther. 2001 Apr; 39(4): 443-56.

[5] Paluska SA, Schwenk TL. Physical activity and mental health: current concepts. Sports Med. 2000 Mar; 29 (3): 167-80.

[6] Moses J, Steptoe A, Mathews A, Edwards S. The effects of exercise training on mental well-being in the normal population: a controlled trial. J Psychosom Res. 1989; 33(1): 47-61.

[7] Birdee GS, Legedza AT, Saper RB, Bertisch SM, Eisenberg DM, Phillips RS. Characteristics of Yoga users: results of a national survey. J Gen Intern Med. 2008 Oct; 23(10): 1653-8.

[8] Sancier KM. Medical application of Qigong. Altern Ther. Health Med. 1996 Jan; 2(1): 40-6.

[9] Leung PC. Natural Healing in Chinese Medicine: Qigong and Tai Chi. In: Leung PC, editor. Healthy Aging. Singapore: World Scientific Publishing; 2011.

[10] Melzack R, Wall PD. Peripheral nerve and spinal mechanisms. In: The Challenge of Pain. 2nd ed. London: Penguin Group; 1996.

[11] Kato T, Numata T, Shirayama M. Physiological and psychological study of Qigong. Japanese Mind-Body Science. 1992; 1(1): 29-38.

[12] Machi Y. Various measurements of Qigong masters for analyzing Qigong mechanism. Japanese Mind-Body Science. 1994; 3(1): 65-87.

[13] Spicuzza L, Gabutti A, Porta C, Montano N, Bernardi L. Yoga and chemoreflex response to hypoxia and hypercapnia. Lancet. 2000 Oct; 356(9240): 1495-6.

[14] Zeng YG, Zhou XQ, Wang AL, Yang BL, Wang ST. Research on the impacts of fitness Qigong Baduanjin on figure and physical function among the middle-aged and aged people. J Beijing Sport Univ. 2005 Sep; 28(9): 1207-9.

[15] Peng CK, Mietus JE, Liu Y, Khalsa G, Douglas PS, Benson H, et al. Exaggerated heart rate oscillations during two meditation techniques. Int J Cardiol. 1999 Jul; 70(2): 101-7.

[16] Lei XS, Ni HY, Chen QY. Effect of 42-form Taijiquan exercise on Cardiovascular function and respiratory endurance in middle-age and aged Intellectuals. Modern Rehabilitation. 2001 Jun; 5(11):64-65.

[17] Patel C, North WR. Randomized controlled trial of Yoga and bio-feedback in management of hypertension. Lancet 1975 Jul; 2(7925): 93-5.

[18] Schmidt T, Wijga A, Von Zur Muhlen A, Brabant G, Wagner TO. Changes in cardiovascular risk factors and hormones during a comprehensive residential three month kriya yoga training and vegetarian nutrition. Acta Physiol Scand Suppl. 1997; 640:158-62.

[19] Xu SW, Wang WJ. A study of the effects of Tai Ji Quan on endocrinology. Chinese Journal of Sports Medicine. 1986; 3:150-3.

[20] Sherman KJ, Cherkin DC, Erro J, Miglioretti DL, Deyo RA. Comparing Yoga, exercise and self-care book for chronic low back pain: a randomized controlled trial. Ann Intern Med. 2005 Dec; 143(12): 849-56.

[21] Peng PW. Tai Chi and chronic pain. Reg Anesth Pain Med. 2012 Jul-Aug; 37(4): 372-82.

[22] Du, SW, Chang, CL and Wang, S. A research on Health Qigong-Yi Jin Jing for strengthen cardiac function of the aged. Chinese Journal of Sports Medicine. 2006; 25(6): 721–2.

[23] Lin YN, Wang WD, Hang RR. Influence of different health cultivation methods on life quality and carbonhydrate metabolism among patients of diabetes Type II. Beijing Journal of Traditional Chinese Medicine. 2009; 28(1), 9–12.

[24] Yan, Y. Patient's cell blood disease to the high ester of the qigong five-animal exercises sticks the influence of molecules and level of fat of blood to build up body. Journal of Liaoning Normal University (Natural Science Edition). 2009; 32(3), 356–8.

[25] Brevetti, G, Schiano, V, Chiariello M. Cellular adhesion molecules and peripheral arterial disease. Vasc Med. 2006 Feb; 11(1), 39–47.

[26] Zhang WC, Zhong, ZB, Wu QH, Chen XF Wang SY, Zhang Y, et al. A research on Health Qigong-Yi Jin Jing for slowing down intelligence decline of aged. Chinese Journal of Behavioral Medical Science. 2006; 15(9), 827–8.

[27] Sun FL, Lei SP. Clinical method of evaluation of declining liquid intelligence with aging and its application in TCM research. Chinese Journal of Integrated Traditional and Western Medicine, 1989; 4: 203–6.

[28] Xiao L, Zhou Y. Recovered mechanism of the waist muscle injury by Taijiquan exercise. Journal of Shaanxi Normal University (Natural Science Edition). 2008 Sep; 36(5): 101–3.

[29] Taggart HM, Arslanian CL, Bae S, Singh K. Effects of Tai Chi exercise on fibromyalgia symptoms and health-related quality of life. Orthop. Nurs. 2003 Sep-Oct; 22(5), 353–60.

[30] Maki BE, Holliday PJ, Fernie GR. Aging and postural control. A comparison of spontaneous and indufced-sway balance tests. J Am Geriatr Soc. 1990Jan; 38(1), 1–9.

[31] Mao J, Li YJ, Zhong HS. Effect of exercise on blood pressure in aged patients with borderline hypertension. Chinese Journal of Clinical Rehabilitation. 2002 Jun; 6(11): 1673.

[32] Whelton SP, Chin A, Xin X, He J. Effects of aerobic exercise on blood pressure: A meta-analysis of randomized controlled trials. Ann Intern Med. 2002 Apr; 136(7), 493–503.

[33] Wang Y. Experimental study on treating hypertension of the aged by using Taijiquan and Artsport physical exercises. WuShu Science. 2007; 4(1), 44–46.

[34] Huang YX, Long YF, Zhan CL. Effects of Taijiquan exercise on activities of antioxidases and quantity of lipid peroxide in sera of middle aged people. Journal of Occupational Health and Damage. 2001; 16(3): 139–141.

[35] Wang XJ. Effect of Taijiquan on IL2 of aged people. Journal of Shangdong Physical Education Institute. 2003; 19(2): 48-50.

[36] Lewicki R, Tchorzewski H, Majewska E, Nowak Z, Baj Z. Effects of maximal physical exercise on T-lymphocyte subpopulations and on interleukin 1 (IL 1) and interleukin 2 (IL 2) production in vitro. Int J Sports Med. 1988 Apr; 9(2), 114–7.

[37] Luan LA. Healthy meaning of participating in Taijiquan activitaty among elderly people. China Journal of Health Psychology. 2008; 16(4), 477–478.

[38] Kirkwood G, Rampes H, Tuffrey V, Richardson J, Pikington K, Ramaratnam S. Yoga for anxiety: a systematic review of the research evidence. Br J Sports Med. 2005 Dec; 39(12): 884-91.

[39] Pilkington K, Kirkwood G, Rampes H, Richardson J. Yoga for depression: the research evidence. J Affect Disord. 2005Dec; 89(1-3): 13-24.

[40] Penman S, Cohen M, Stevens P, Jackson S. Yoga in Australia: Results of a national survey. Int J Yoga. 2012 Jel-Dec; 5(2): 92-101.

[41] Arias AJ, Steinberg K, Banga A, Trestman RL. Systematic review of the efficacy of meditation techniques as treatments for medical illness. J Altern Complement Med. 2006 Oct; 12(8): 817-32.

[42] Krisanaprakornkit T, Krisanaprakornkit W, Piyavhatkul N, Laopaiboon M. Meditation therapy for anxiety disorders. Cochrane Database Syst Rev [Internet]. 2006 [cited 2014 Oct 31]. Available from: http://onlinelibrary.wiley.com/doi/10.1002/14651858.CD004998.pub2/abstract;jsessionid=62EC69BCCF0B059D15D901CA2BD1668C.f03t04

[43] Lafferty WE, Downey L, McCarty RL, Standish LJ, Standish LJ, Patrick DL. Evaluating CAM treatment at the end of life: a review of clinical trials for massage and meditation. Complement Ther Med. 2006 Jun; 14(2): 100-12.

[44] Astin JA, Shapiro SL, Eisenberg DM, Forys KL. Mind-body medicine: state of the science, implications for practice. J Am Board Fam Pract. 2003 Mar-Apr; 16(2):131-47.

[45] Jorm AF, Christensen H, Griffiths KM, Parslow RA, Rodgers B, Blewitt KA. Effectiveness of complementary and self-help treatments for anxiety disorders. Med J Aust. 2004 Oct; 181(7 Suppl): S29-46.

[46] Khalsa SB. Yoga as a Therapeutic Intervention: a bibliometric analysis of published research studies. Indian J Physiol Pharmacol. 2004 Jul; 48(3): 269-85.

[47] Harvard Mental Health Letter. Yoga for anxiety and depression. [Internet]. 2009 Apr [cited 2014 Oct 31]. Available from: https://www.health.harvard.edu/newsletters/Harvard_Mental_Health_Letter/2009/April/Yoga-for-anxiety-and-depression

[48] Brown RP, Gerbarg PL. Sudarshan Kriya Yogic breathing in the treatment of stress, anxiety, and depression: part 1 – neurophysiologic model. J Altern Complement Med. 2005 Feb; 11(1): 189-201.

[49] Brown RP, Gerbarg PL. Sudarshan Kriya Yogic breathing in the treatment of stress, anxiety, and depression: part II – clinical application and guidelines. J Altern Complement Med. 2005 Aug; 11(4): 711-7.

[50] Janakiramaiah N, Gangadhar BN, Naga Venkatesha Murthy PJ, Harish MG, Subbakrishna DK, Vedamurthachar A. Antidepressant efficacy of Sudarshan Kriya Yoga (SKY) in melancholia: a randomized comparison with electroconvulsive therapy (ECT) and imipramine. J Affect Disord. 2000 Jan-Mar; 57(1-.): 255-9.

[51] Shi AQ, Li AM, Wang GL, Xiang HP, Lei B. Influence of Older's Psychology and Physiology by Practicing Yijinjing (Fitness Qigong). Journal of Chengdu Sport University. 2005; 31(3): 95-7.

[52] Shi J. Qigong and Mental Health. J. Xianning College. 2005; 25(6): 110-3.

[53] Zhai XY. Investigation on cultivating mental hygiene with gymnastic Qigong practice. Journal of Henan University of Chinese Medicine. 2006, 21(3): 47-8.

[54] Griffith JM, Hasley JP, Liu H, Severn DG, Conner LH, Adler LE. Qigong Stress reduction in hospital staff. J Altern Complement Med. 2008 Oct; 14(8): 939-45.

[55] Liu HF, An HY, Mung FY. Research on impact of health Qigong (Baduanjin) on mental health of medical college students. Medicine and Society. 2008 21(8):63-4.

[56] Jouper J, Johansson M. Qigong and mindfulness-based mood recovery: exercise experiences from a single case. J Bodyw Mov Ther. 2013 Jan; 17(1): 69-76.

[57] Saper RB, Eisenberg DM, Davis RB, Culpepper L, Phillip RS. Prevalence and patterns of adult Yoga use in United States: results of a natural survey. Altern Ther Health Med. 2004 Mar-Apr; 10(2): 44-9.

[58] Mayo Clinic. Depression and anxiety: exercise eases symptoms [Internet]. Mayo Clinic ;2014 [cited 2014 Oct 31]. Available from: http://www.mayoclinic.org/diseases-conditions/depression/in-depth/depression-and-exercise/art-20046495

[59] Rime J, Dwan K, Lawlor DA, Greig CA, McMurdo M, Morley W, et al. Exercise for depression. Cochrane Database Syst Rev [Internet]. 2012 [cited 2014 Oct 31]. Available from:http://onlinelibrary.wiley.com/doi/10.1002/14651858.CD004366.pub6/abstract

[60] WHO Traditional Medicine Strategy 2014-2023. WHO Geneva, 2013 [Internet]. 2013 [cited 2014 Oct 31]. Available from : http://apps.who.int/medicinedocs/documents/s21201en/s21201en.pdf

Chapter 9

Role of Acupuncture in the Treatment of Drug Addiction

Anfeng Xiang, Boyuan Zhang and Sheng Liu

Additional information is available at the end of the chapter

http://dx.doi.org/10.5772/60655

Abstract

This review systematically assessed the clinical evidence for and against acupuncture as a treatment for drug addiction. The existing scientific rationale and possible mechanisms for the effectiveness of acupuncture on drug addiction were also evaluated. We used computerized literature searches in English and Chinese and examined texts written before these computerized databases existed. We also used search terms of treatment and neurobiology for drug abuse and dependence. Acupuncture showed evidence for relevant neurobiological mechanisms in the treatment of drug addiction. Although positive findings regarding the use of acupuncture to treat drug dependence have been reported by many clinical studies, the data do not allow us to make conclusions that acupuncture was an effective treatment for drug addiction, given that many studies reviewed here were hampered by small numbers of patients, insufficient reporting of randomization and allocation concealment methods, and strength of the inference. However, considering the potential of acupuncture demonstrated in the included studies, further rigorous randomized controlled trials with long follow-up are warranted.

Keywords: acupuncture, addiction, heroin, cocaine, treatment

1. Introduction

Acupuncture originated in ancient China and has been used to manage various clinical disorders for thousands of years in China. Acupuncture needles insert into acupuncture points of the body to treat many different disorders. Acupuncture needles are manipulated manually. One of the recent technical developments was to use peripheral electrical stimulation applied via the acupuncture needles inserted into the acupoints, that is, "electroacupuncture" (EA). Currently, new methods for stimulating the acupuncture points include applying electric current to skin electrodes over the points, directing a laser light onto the points, or using finger pressure to massage selected points (acupressure). In addition, many new points and entire "microsystems" of points have been described for specific body parts, for example, scalp acupuncture and ear acupuncture (auricular acupuncture). In Western countries, acupuncture began to be known in the middle of the 1970s, yet its acceptance has increased rapidly. Many Western patients turn to acupuncture along with conventional medical therapy to make sure they are utilizing all possible medical options. A recent survey of acupuncture released by an NIH Consensus Development Panel indicated that although there are inherent problems of design, sample amount, and appropriate controls in the acupuncture literature, extensive work has shown that acupuncture is beneficial in treating various pain syndromes, postoperative and chemotherapy- induced nausea and vomiting, some forms of bronchial asthma, headache, migraine, and female infertility. For the past 40 years, a number of studies of acupuncture applied, as a medical technique, to the treatment of heroin, alcohol, nicotine, and cocaine addictions have been reported. In light of an increasing trend in the use of acupuncture and utilization of such approaches by patients suffering from drug addiction, we intend to review the existing scientific rationale and clinical data, which indicate that acupuncture may influence the prognosis of drug addicts.

2. Acupuncture: Theory and mechanisms

It has long been a dream to cure diseases by nonpharmacological measures that activate self-healing mechanisms, without using drugs. Recent efforts along these lines were the use of vagal nerve stimulation, repetitive transcranial magnetic stimulation (rTMS), deep brain stimulation, and acupuncture to stimulate certain brain areas. Evidence presented in the present review demonstrates that it is possible to facilitate the release of certain neuropeptides in the central nervous system (CNS) by means of peripheral acupuncture point's stimulation. In contrast to magnetic stimulation that stimulates the superficial areas of the brain (i.e., the cortex) [1], acupuncture activates various brain structures and/or the spinal cord via specific neural pathways. Any predictions made at this stage should not be overly optimistic. But the clinical efficacy demonstrated using acupuncture to ease postoperative pain [2,3], lower-back pain [4,5], and diabetic neuropathic pain [6], and the successful application of 100 Hz (but not 2 Hz) electroacupuncture for treating muscle spastic pain of spinal origin [7]E certainly hold exciting promise for the future. Gaining knowledge of therapeutic mechanisms is essential to validating therapies such as acupuncture that are difficult to test under double-blind, placebo-controlled conditions. If we try to answer the question "how the acupuncture works or what physical changes occur", it is appropriate first to give some theoretical background for acupuncture. Clinical treatment with acupuncture is done in light of symptom differentiation and therapeutic methods, by means of needling and moxibustion (lighted punks of *artemis vulgaris*) with certain manipulating methods to stimulate the selected acupuncture points for prevention and treatment of diseases. The theory of meridians and acupuncture points is the basic theory of therapy. In fact, traditional Chinese medicine is based on the concept of the flow of energy or Qi through meridian pathways in the body. Qi is postulated to flow through the body in precisely located pathways or channels called meridians. These meridians are thought to be connected to various body organs as well as to each other. According to the principles of traditional Chinese medicine, illness results from an imbalance of energy flow within these meridians. Acupuncture was developed according to the principle that human bodily functions are controlled by the "meridian" and "Qi" systems. There are 365 designated acupuncture points located along these meridians. Acupuncture stimulates the points located on "meridians" along which Qi flows, breaking the blockage, and subsequently restoring the flow of energy and healthy body functioning [8].

Acupuncture points on the body have both local and systemic influences. Pain, for example, is treated not only locally but distally as well, via acupuncture points further along the meridian, drawing energy away from the pain. Conditions caused by organ dysfunction such as asthma or drug addiction are differentiated according to the specific symptoms present. Acupuncture points are then selected appropriate to both the symptoms reported and the cause of that individual's problems.

Although different direction, angle and depth for inserting needles, stimulation intensity, such as rolling, raising, and thrusting, and Deqi may have an effect through different actions, the condition of the patient is the most important factor that influences the effectiveness of acupuncture. Numerous examples reveal that the regulatory effect of acupuncture has the characteristics of holism and bidirectional regulation. In acupuncture theory, bidirectional regulation is referred to a balancing effect of acupuncture interventions when the human body is experiencing a hyperactivity or hypoactivity due to abnormal intrinsic or external factors. The same acupuncture points' stimulation with different manipulating techniques or stimulation parameters can regulate different functional activities of the body bidirectionally, which means to balance the functions of the body when they become hyperactive with the inhibiting effect and to restore the normal functions of the body when they become hypoactive with the exciting effect. For example, when blood pressure is too high, needling Neiguan (PC.6) can reduce high blood pressure; when blood pressure is too low, needling PC.6 can elevate blood pressure. Acupuncture-induced correction of abnormal blood pressure is observed to be dependent on the nervous, endocrinal, humoral, and dielectric regulation. Take Zusanli (ST. 36) for another example, EA at Zusanli (ST.36) can biregulate gastric activity. For gastric hypermotility, EA at ST.36 can inhibit gastric movement; but for bradygastria, EA at ST.36 can promote the peristalsis of the stomach. In addition, it is notable that some of the acupuncture points can bear special or specific curative effect on certain diseases. For example, Dazhui (GV. 14) abates fever and Zhiyin (BL.67) rectifies the position of fetus [9].

The guidance of the theory of traditional Chinese medicine is traditionally believed to be essential in achieving acupuncture's therapeutic effect, but the metaphysical explanations may be hard to understand by modern science. In recent years, increasing research publications gave strong evidence that acupuncture could be explained on a physiological and neurobiological rather than a metaphysical basis [10, 11]. For example, in traditional Chinese medicine, the vision-related acupuncture point (VA1) (known as urinary bladder channel of BL67) is believed to be an effective acupuncture point that directly treats eye-related disorders. Various acupoints are related to corresponding specific organs rather than via the central nervous system. Based on the knowledge of Western medicine, it is difficult to believe that acupuncture treats disorders and diseases by direct control of organs or organ-related disorders and diseases. It is known that many disorders are either controlled or affected by the brain, i.e., specific corresponding brain functional areas. Recently, Cho et al. [12] demonstrated that when acupuncture stimulation is performed at VA1 (vision-related acupuncture point), activation of occipital lobes is seen by functional magnetic resonance imaging (fMRI). Stimulation of the eye by directly using light evokes similar activation in the occipital lobes. It may represent an important step toward understanding oriental acupuncture in relationship to brain function. In addition, the findings by Bruce Rosen of Harvard Medical School at the American Psychosomatic Society Meeting in Orlando showed that acupuncture on pain-relief points cut blood flow to key areas of the brain related with pain within seconds. Researchers applied acupuncture needles to acupuncture points on the hand linked to pain relief in traditional Chinese medicine. Blood flow decreased in certain areas of the brain, which was detected by fMRI within seconds of volunteers reporting a sense of heaviness in their hands, a sign that the acupuncture is working. The needling technique is not supposed to hurt if done correctly. When a few subjects reported pain, the fMRI scannings showed an increase of blood to the same brain areas. It may provide a clear explanation to date for how the ancient acupuncture might relieve pain.

Recently, the neurophysiology of acupuncture has been investigated extensively and reviewed in detail. The principal suggestion is that acupuncture operates largely through neurotransmitters, particularly endorphin-related mechanisms. These studies demonstrate conclusively that acupuncture's effects are related to the release of a variety of neurotransmitters including natural opiates and, furthermore, that this effect is naloxone-reversible. Basic research work carried out has demonstrated that any noxious stimulus will result in endorphin release through the neurophysiological mechanism described as diffuse noxious inhibitory control (DNIC). Therefore, DNIC represents a nonspecific physiological mechanism which triggers the natural opiate system in both man and experimental animal. It has been suggested that DNIC plays a relatively minor role in acupuncture analgesia and that other systems, mediated by serotonin and noradrenaline, may be important. The mechanism of acupuncture in internal diseases, such as asthma, irritable bowel, and the treatment of symptoms such as nausea is completely unknown. Acupuncturists have hypothesized that the autonomic nervous system plays an important, but not as yet ill-defined, part in the underlying mechanisms that are involved in the treatment of such internal problems.

3. Effects of acupuncture on drug dependence

Conventional detoxification methods such as methadone and buprenorphine are effective in reducing illicit opioid use, but problems associated with their use, such as social resistance to the idea of "replacing one drug of abuse with another"and difficulties in tapering patients off the medication due to long-lasting withdrawal effects, make the search for alternative therapies important [13].

Acupuncture's utility for treating drug abuse and dependence is best shown in opioid-dependent patients experiencing withdrawal [14, 15]. Over the past 40 years, acupuncture and

EA have been applied with great success to attenuate behavioral signs of opioid withdrawal in addicts [16-18]. Using acupuncture to treat drug withdrawal symptoms began in 1972. H. L. Wen, a neurosurgeon from Hong Kong, visited China to learn acupuncture anesthesia. Upon returning to his Hong Kong practice, he used electrical stimulation via acupuncture needles to reduce or eliminate the need for anesthetic drugs during surgery. Acupuncture treatment was given over several weeks prior to surgery, as well as during operational procedures. Dr. Wen was unaware that some patients were also heroin, opium, morphine, alcohol, and/or nicotine dependent. The addict patients later volunteered this information, and reported that they also lost their drug cravings after receiving acupuncture. Wen and his colleagues followed up 40 patients for opium and heroin addiction. They confirmed that 39 of 40 patients were considered improved in that they had gained basal weight and reported they did not crave drugs [19-21]. In the United States, Smith and coworkers [22-25] modified Wen's original protocol by eliminating electrical stimulation and by using an abbreviated prescription of five-point auricular acupuncture. This prescription was not designed for withdrawal from any class of drug or any single abused substance. Instead, it effectively reduced cravings, anxiety, and dysphoria of withdrawal in addict patients during withdrawal from a variety of drugs and alcohol. Patients consistently reported the dramatic relief during the early weeks of withdrawal, when the incidence of relapse is highest. By 1974, Smith had used this five-point auricular protocol as the sole detoxification method used in the outpatient clinic at Lincoln Hospital in the Bronx, NY. Over the past 40 years, this acupuncture protocol has grown in popularity. It is currently used to treat alcohol and other drug withdrawal in more than 800 substance abuse treatment centers across the United States and Europe.

Clinical studies and related research on acupuncture have been undertaken by independent groups. Some randomized trials have been done to compare the effects of auricular acupuncture at specific points for the treatment of substance abuse and at sham points [26-28]. Washburn et al. [29] conducted the first controlled study of acupuncture heroin detoxification. One hundred addicted persons were randomly assigned, in a single-blind design, to the standard auricular acupuncture treatment used for addiction or to a "sham" treatment that used points that were geographically close to the standard points. They observed that subjects assigned to the standard treatment attended the acupuncture clinic more days and stayed in treatment longer than those assigned to the sham condition. Zhang et al. [26] also found that acupuncture and electrical stimulation were more effective than clonidine in treating withdrawal syndromes such as insomnia, pain, and anxiety following acute withdrawal symptoms. Clinical studies have also demonstrated that this treatment has fewer side effects. In addition, Meade et al. [30] tested the effectiveness of transcutaneous electric acupoint stimulation (TEAS) as an adjunctive treatment for inpatients receiving opioid detoxification with buprenorphine–naloxone at a private psychiatric hospital. It is shown that TEAS is an acceptable, inexpensive adjunctive treatment that is feasible to implement on an inpatient unit and may be a beneficial adjunct to pharmacological treatments for opioid detoxification. Acupuncture also appears to be a useful adjunct to methadone maintenance therapy (MMT) in heroin addiction. Recently, one study examined the effectiveness of acupuncture for heroin addicts on methadone maintenance by measuring the daily consumption of methadone, variations in the 36-item Short Form Health Survey-36 (SF-36) and Pittsburgh Sleep Quality Index (PSQI) scores. It is shown that acupuncture was also associated with a greater improvement in sleep latency at follow-up. All adverse events were mild in severity [31].

A number of studies have examined the effects of acupuncture on cocaine and alcohol dependence. For example, severe recidivist alcoholic patients treated with acupuncture specifically for the treatment of substance abuse reported less craving for alcohol, fewer drinking episodes, and required fewer admissions to the county detoxification center than did control patients who received acupuncture at nonspecific points [27]. Lipton et al. [32] also reported that patients receiving acupuncture treatment had significantly lower levels of cocaine metabolites than the control subjects. Recently, researchers, headed by S. Kelly Avants, from the division of substance abuse in the Department of Psychiatry at Yale University, divided 82 cocaine addicts into three groups. One third received acupuncture at four specific points around the outer ear, another third received "sham" acupuncture at sites on the ear that would be ineffective, and the remaining third received relaxation therapy consisting of viewing a relaxing video. Treatment sessions were five times a week and lasted eight weeks. The subjects' urine was tested three times a week for traces of cocaine. They found that patients assigned to receive true acupuncture had less cocaine use compared to the two other groups, and there were a higher percentage of patients in the acupuncture group who were clean from cocaine use by the last week of the study than in the two other groups [6].

The effects of acupuncture on drug addiction have also been verified by animal experiments. It has been well shown that acupuncture suppressed morphine withdrawal syndrome and alcohol-drinking behaviors in rats [33-35]. Furthermore, morphine-induced conditioned place preference can be successfully suppressed by 2 or 100 Hz electroacupuncture, a substitute for classic acupuncture [36, 37]. A recent study by Chae et al. [38] found that acupuncture at ST36, but not the other acupuncture points, significantly attenuated the expected increase in nicotine-induced locomotor sensitization to subsequent nicotine challenge. Behavioral response to nicotine challenge in the repeated nicotine treated group (control) was significantly intenser. Stimulation of acupuncture at ST36 just before nicotine challenge as well as during 3 days of withdrawal period completely blocked the effects of nicotine on locomotor activity during the 60 min testing period. In our laboratory, we also found that acupuncture applied at the BL.23 acupuncture point, a novel acupuncture point, could effectively suppress withdrawal syndrome [39,40].

However, some large clinical trials have questioned the effectiveness of acupuncture for drug dependence. In these studies, the acupuncture treatment groups failed to show significant differences from the control group in the treatment of drug dependence [41]. One study has found that acupuncture offered no significant reduction of nicotine withdrawal symptoms or long-term improvement over placebo [42]. Bullock et al. performed a single-blind, randomized, placebo-controlled study to evaluate auricular acupuncture in the treatment of cocaine addiction. Their study had 236 residential and 202 day treatment clients. They did not find any significant treatment differences between true and sham acupuncture. They also found no differences among the three dose levels of true acupuncture [43].The Cocaine Alternative Treatment Study (CATS) [44] was a large-scale, multi-site study. In this study, 620 patients addicted to cocaine were enrolled from six treatment sites; 412 of the patients were "primary" cocaine-dependent, and 208 were opiate-dependent and maintained on methadone. Patients were randomized to the three treatment conditions: auricular acupuncture, a needle-insertion control condition, and a relaxation control condition. Treatments were offered five times weekly for 8 weeks. The patients maintained on methadone received standard care as offered in their methadone program. Concurrent drug counseling was also offered to patients in all conditions. The primary outcome measure was cocaine use during treatment and at the 3- and 6-month postrandomization follow-up based on urine toxicology screens and retention in treatment. Results of urine samples showed a significant overall reduction in cocaine use, but no differences by treatment condition. There were also no differences between the conditions in treatment retention (44%–46% for the full 8 weeks). In the last week of treatment, 24, 31, and 29% of patients in auricular acupuncture, needle-insertion control, and relaxation control conditions, respectively, were abstinent from cocaine. This large study does not support the use of acupuncture as a stand-alone treatment for cocaine addiction.

4. Effects of acupuncture on psychological symptoms associated with drug addiction

Easing psychological symptoms associated with heroin use and heroin relapse is an important goal in the treatment of heroin dependence. Notably, as the course of withdrawal followed its natural history and acute symptoms abated, acupuncture continued to reduce anxiety and cravings associated with protracted withdrawal. In fact, patients who had completed addiction programs often continued to enjoy stress reduction induced by occasional "booster" acupuncture treatments. There are many ancient and contemporary papers reporting the successful use of acupuncture for the treatment of patients with depression and anxiety disorders [45-50]. Given that the prevalence of depression and anxiety is very high in cocaine and other drug addicts, and depression and anxiety after prolonged abstinence become the main factors contributing to drug relapse and craving, it is very meaningful to pay close attention to the effects of acupuncture on depression treatment among addicts. In addition, acupuncture has been used to improve psychological status and lessen fatigue [51]. Chang et al. conducted a three-arm randomized controlled trial (RCT) on residents of a homeless veteran rehabilitation program. Sixty-seven enrolled participants were randomly assigned to acupuncture, the relaxation response, or usual care. They found that craving and anxiety levels decreased significantly following one session of acupuncture [52]. In another small, randomized controlled trial, Allen et al. [53] compared symptoms of depression in an acupuncture group, placebo group, and a waitlist control group. The acupuncture group showed greater improvements in depressive scores than the placebo group and the waitlist control group. Roschke et al. [54] studied the effects of adding acupuncture to antidepressant treatment and found that the acupuncture in combination with antidepressant treatment improved the alleviation of depression course compared with pharmaceutical treatment alone. In a clinical trial using TAES for the suppression of opiate craving in humans, a total of 117 heroin addicts who had completed the process of detoxification for more than 1 month were recruited [55]. They were randomly and evenly assigned into four groups. Three groups received TAES treatment of different frequencies (2, 100, or 2/100 Hz). Self-sticking skin electrodes were placed on four acupoints: Hegu and Laogong (palmar side of the Hegu point) in the left (or right) hand to complete a circuit, and Neiguan and Weiguan in the opposite arm to complete a circuit. The control group was processed as in the previous groups except that the intensity was minimal (15 Hz, threshold stimulation for 3 min, and then switched to 1 mA thereafter) to serve as a mock TAES control. Visual analog scale (VAS) was used to assess the degree of craving. There was a very slow decline of the VAS in the mock TAES control group in a period of 1 month. A dramatic decline of the degree of craving was observed in the groups receiving 2 and 2/100 Hz electric stimulation, but not in the group receiving 100 Hz stimulation. These results observed in humans were in line with the findings obtained in the rat: low-frequency TAES is more effective than high-frequency TAES in suppressing the morphine-induced CPP [56].

However, some studies [6, 30, 57, 58] did not show favorable effects of acupuncture on psychological symptoms associated with opioid addiction (anxiety, depression, and craving). For example, Black et al. [59] conducted a randomized controlled study to test the effect of auricular acupuncture in the treatment of anxiety associated with withdrawal from psychoactive drugs. They found that auricular acupuncture was not more effective than sham or treatment setting control in reducing anxiety. We reviewed the clinical studies that have investigated the clinical effectiveness of acupuncture and focused on psychological symptoms associated with opioid addiction. The clinical studies published in Chinese language journals were assessed carefully and included in our systematical reviews. We found that eight studies [26, 29, 41, 44, 60-62,64] included heroin/opioid craving. Seven studies [27, 28, 32, 60-63] included anxiety. Two studies included depression [60, 65]. All of the four studies [44, 66-68] published in English language journals did not show favorable effects of acupuncture on psychological symptoms associated with opioid addiction (anxiety, depression, and craving). Many studies published in Chinese language journals supported the use of acupuncture for controlling psychological symptoms associated with opioid addiction: craving [26, 41, 63, 69,], anxiety [29, 32, 60, 62, 63, 70], and depression [60, 68].

Treatment retention and abstinence are more important goals for the treatment of drug dependence. Effectiveness of the treatment of psychological symptoms associated with drug addiction should be assessed by including longer-term follow-up data. In fact, to determine whether initial improvements from the treatment persist for a reasonable period of time, participant observation should last for at least 3 months. However, most of the studies we reviewed did not provide follow-up data. In these studies, the duration of acupuncture interventions was also shorter than 1 month. In fact, it is unclear whether the extent to which acupuncture has therapeutic effects depends on the duration and frequency of acupuncture. Arguably, longer treatment periods are required for acupuncture to have any chance of showing clinical effects. These variable factors should be taken into account when assessing the effects of acupuncture. Future studies should therefore have sufficiently large samples, extended treatment, and follow-up periods.

5. Possible mechanisms for the effectiveness of acupuncture on drug addiction

It would be reasonable to suggest that an opioidergic mechanism is, at least partially, involved in mediating acupuncture antiwithdrawal. Han and his colleagues from Peking University China have made a detailed survey on the analgesic effect of EA. They found that analgesia induced by 100-Hz EA resulted from accelerating the release of dynorphin from the spinal cord of the rats [11, 71, 72]. In accord with this was the finding that the analgesic effect of 100-Hz EA observed in morphine-dependent rats could be blocked by a high dose of naloxone only [73]. On the other hand, dynorphin has been shown to be the endogenous ligand of the n-opioid receptor. Indeed, the withdrawal syndrome observed in rats dependent on morphine can be suppressed by high-frequency electroacupuncture, which accelerates the release of dynorphin in the spinal cord and brain [33, 70, 74]. Morphine-induced conditioned-place preference, an experimental model simulating the craving of heroin addicts, can be effectively suppressed by low-frequency electroacupuncture. This effect can be blocked by a small dose of naloxone, indicating the involvement of endogenous opioid peptides [36, 69]. Meanwhile, the clinical study by V. Clement-Jones et al. also showed that EA was associated with a rise in cerebrospinal fluid met-enkephalin levels in all addicts studied [67]. Recently, Wang et al. [75] found that a downregulation of preprodynorphin (PPD) mRNA level was observed in spinal cord, PAG, and hypothalamus 60 hours after the last morphine injection, which could be reversed by multiple sessions, but not a single session of EA. Accompanied with the decrease of PPD mRNA level, there was an upregulation of p-CREB in the three CNS regions, which was abolished by 100 Hz EA treatment. These findings suggest that downregulation of p-CREB and acceleration of dynorphin synthesis in spinal cord, PAG, and hypothalamus may be implicated in the cumulative effect of multiple 100Hz EA treatment for opioid detoxification.

The mesolimbic dopamine system originates in the ventral tegmental area (VTA) and projects to regions that include the nucleus accumbens and prefrontal cortex, which are believed to play a pivotal role in the development of opiate addiction [20]. Opiate abuse-induced changes in the levels of dopamine in the brain are associated with feelings of well-being and pleasure, providing positive reinforcement of continued opiate abuse [76, 39]. Conversely, withdrawal from chronic opiate administration reduces dopamine outflow in the nucleus accumbens [40, 77]. Furthermore, in the treatment of drug craving and relapse to drug use, the core symptoms of addiction, a non-endorphin-mediated mechanism is probably involved. Lu et al. [78] examined alterations in the firing rate of dopaminergic neurons by means of extracellular recording following chronic morphine exposure and applied 100 Hz electroacupuncture treatment to reverse the reduced firing rate of these neurons. They found that the electrophysiological response of VTA DA neurons to morphine was markedly reduced in chronic morphine-treated rats compared to saline-treated controls. A substantial recovery of the reactivity of VTA DA neurons to morphine was observed in rats that received 100 Hz EA for 10 days. Evidence also indicates that acupuncture acts on the nucleus accumbens to inhibit the elevation in dopamine [79, 80]. Yoon et al. demonstrated the acupuncture-mediated inhibition of ethanol-induced dopamine released in the rat nucleus accumbens through the $GABA_B$ receptor [80]. Chae et al. showed that acupuncture treatment at ST.36 attenuated the expected increase in nicotine-induced locomotor activity by reducing postsynaptic neuronal activity in the nucleus and striatum [38].

ΔFosB and FosB are members of the Fos family of transcription factors implicated in neural plasticity in drug addiction. Li et al. [81] found that the intake of and preference for ethanol in rats under 100 Hz, but not 2 Hz electroacupuncture, regiment were sharply reduced. The reduction was maintained for at least 72 hours after the termination of electroacupuncture treatment. Conversely, 100 Hz electroacupuncture did not alter the intake of and preference for the natural rewarding agent sucrose. Additionally, FosB/ΔFosB levels in the prefrontal cortex, striatal region, and the posterior region of ventral tegmental area were increased following excessive ethanol consumption, but were reduced after 6-day 100 Hz electroacupuncture. Interestingly, EA can inhibit CB1 receptor upregulation in the prefrontal cortex, striatum, hippocampus, amygdala, and ventral tegmental area in ethanol-withdrawn mice [82]. Furthermore, extracellular signal-regulated kinase (ERK) plays a role in neuronal changes induced by repeated drug exposure. EA can reverse ethanol-induced locomotor sensitization and subsequent ERK expression in mice [83]. These results suggest that acupuncture could play an important role in suppressing the potentiating effects of ethanol and other drugs.

Our recent study [41] showed that acupuncture attenuated elevated c-fos expression in the central nucleus of the amygdala (CeA) during morphine withdrawal in rats. Some studies emphasize that the motivational components of opiate withdrawal appear to be centrally mediated by limbic structures such as the nucleus accumbens and amygdale [2-4]. Therefore, elevated c-fos expression in the CeA might be associated with the motivational components of opiate withdrawal. Our observation that acupuncture suppressed elevated c-fos expression in the CeA indicated that acupuncture might have some therapeutic effects in the treatment of the negative motivations of opiate withdrawal. Of course, further studies must be performed to clarify this issue. In addition, the CeA and the basolateral amygdala have been extensively and differentially involved in associative learning and memory processes, attributing affective salience to environmental stimuli paired with drug effects [5]. One theory of the neural mechanisms of drug abuse focuses on various learning and memory systems in which the normal functions of these complex neural circuits become subverted leading to compulsive drug-seeking behaviors [84, 85]. In this model, drugs of abuse initiate plasticity mechanisms in different learning and memory systems that come to control behaviors of the individual over other preexisting memories. Experience with addictive drugs are encoded and stored like other experiences, except that drugs of abuse only mimic a subset of the actions of natural reinforcers in the brain. Acupuncture can affect learning and memorizing ability [1, 7, 86, 87]. Further work is needed to emphasize whether acupuncture can re-encode experience with addictive drug via affecting learning and memory systems, and modify the addictive behaviors. The amygdala acquires information that promotes approach and interaction with drug-associated stimuli. We also need to know which role the amygdale plays when acupuncture stimulation affects drug-associated learning and memory.

6. Discussion

In terms of lives and productivity, drug addiction remains one of the most serious threats to our public health. Addiction can be defined as the loss of control over drug use, or the compulsive seeking and taking of a drug regardless of the consequences. Available treatments for addiction remain inadequately effective for most individuals. Incorporating acupuncture into existing therapies offers a promising approach. Acupuncture has been widely recognized as a valuable, readily available, and safe means of health care. It is effective, inexpensive, and requires only simple equipment. In this review, we identify and summarize the evidence about the possible clinical effectiveness of acupuncture on drug addiction, including withdrawal symptoms, drug craving, depression, and anxiety. We also discuss the theory and possible mechanisms for the effectiveness of acupuncture. Some animal and clinical studies have provided supporting evidence for the promising effects of acupuncture. Unfortunately, the data do not allow us to make conclusions that acupuncture was an effective treatment for drug addiction. The evidence for its effectiveness has been inconclusive and difficult to interpret [63]. Some of the clinical studies were unable to detect statistically significant differences in treatment efficacy between their acupuncture treatment and control groups [66-68]. In addition, there are few randomized controlled clinical trials of acupuncture treatment for drug addiction, and the methodological methods used in several clinical trials of acupuncture treatment for drug dependence can be criticized for their poor quality. The quality issues include the following: small numbers of patients, no control subjects, lack of randomized assignment, lack of details regarding specific point locations for needle insertion, and no specification regarding the degree of blinding among research subjects.

In fact, there are some variable factors that need to be taken into account when assessing the effects of acupuncture on drug addiction. (1) The study protocol may influence the assessment of effectiveness of acupuncture. Methods and research designs have been issues of debate among acupuncture clinicians and researchers [88]. For a methodological perspective, randomized controlled trails are considered the gold standard in terms of identifying differences in treatment efficacy [89]. However, unlike the evaluation of a new drug, randomized controlled trials of acupuncture are extremely difficult to conduct, particularly if they have to be blind in design and acupuncture has to be compared with a placebo [90]. The efficacy of acupuncture is difficult to study empirically because of the fundamental divergence between the two schools of thought. The gold standard in Western science is randomized, double-blind, and controlled trails, utilizing one specific protocol for each condition. Randomized controlled trails can be used to answer questions about most clinical problems. However, this approach is not always a practical and cost-effective solution. Sometimes randomized controlled trails are open to error; for instance, patient preference may have an effect on the results as may certain cultural environments. In addition, in some Asian countries such as China where acupuncture is widely used, most patients know a great deal about acupuncture, including the special sensation that should be felt after insertion or during manipulation of the needle. Although various "sham" or "placebo" acupuncture procedures have been designed, they are not easy to perform in these countries. Moreover, acupuncturists consider these procedures unethical because they are already convinced that acupuncture is effective. In fact, most of the placebo-controlled clinical trials have been undertaken in countries where there is skepticism about acupuncture, as well as considerable interest. (2) Another difficulty in evaluating acupuncture practice is that the therapeutic effect depends greatly on the proficiency of the acupuncturists. Their ability and skill in selecting and locating the acupuncture points and in manipulating the needles are different. Needling techniques of inserting, retaining, stimulating, and withdrawing are difficult to standardize. This may partly explain the disparities or inconsistencies in the results reported by different authors, even when their studies were carried out on equally sound methodological bases. (3)In traditional Chinese medical system, such as acupuncture, where each individual is treated according to specific conditions and symptoms, it may be invalid to use the same protocol for every condition. Individualized protocols are critical to the success of the acupuncture treatment. For example, acupuncture stimulation typically elicits a composite of sensations termed deqi, manifesting as soreness, numbness, heaviness, and distention [91]. A body of clinical and experimental evidence indicates that the presence of the deqi sensation is a prerequisite for, and often an indicator of, a clinical acupuncture effect. Traditionally, patients are asked to remain aware of the sensation during acupuncture treatment. Deqi may be an important variable in studies of the efficacy and mechanism of the action of acupuncture treatment. Our previous study showed that the deqi sensations of heroin addicts were significantly higher than those of healthy subjects during acupuncture stimulation, indicating that heroin addicts are "good" responders to acupuncture stimulation [92]. (4) Acupuncture was developed as a branch of traditional Chinese medicine on the basis of oriental philosophy, which takes a holistic approach to regulating the balance of the human body. (Several different schools of acupuncture exist, each with its own principles.) These principles may vary with the types of acupuncture being investigated. The inconsistency in treatment protocols between studies, or the use of combined therapies, makes it impossible to draw a strong causal relationship between therapy and its treatment effect, thus making replication of studies difficult. To this end, traditional knowledge and experience of acupuncture should be duly represented by the investigation team when research is proposed, prepared, and conducted. A good clinical study on acupuncture may be conducted with the understanding and integration of both traditional and modern knowledge of medicine; (5) Most of the clinical research on acupuncture in the United States focused on auricular acupuncture, which is simply the insertion of acupuncture needles into prespecified locations in the ear, whereas studies from China used body acupuncture to treat opiate addiction. These findings are intriguing considering that acupuncture on body and auricular points exhibited different efficacies. According to our clinical experience and the theory of traditional Chinese medicine, body acupuncture may need more attention. Some acupuncture points represent discrete locations in the body, where manual or electrical stimulation can exhibit therapeutic effects on cocaine and other drug addiction [26, 28, 60, 61, 93]. Table 1 provides the summary of main acupoints/sites selected in the reviewed studies. In China, body acupuncture, rather than ear acupuncture, was commonly used for the treatment of drug addiction [26, 28, 60]. The acupuncture points most frequently selected are Zusanli (ST.36), Sanyinjiao (SP.6), Neiguan (PC.6), Shenmen (HT.7), Laogong (PC.8), Waiguan (TE.5), and Hegu (LI.15), located on the four limbs. In our recent work, we showed for the first time that acupuncture applied at the BL.23 acupuncture point, located on the back and commonly used for analgesia and sedation in our clinic, could effectively suppress withdrawal syndrome [40, 41]. Clinically, BL.23 could provide us with a new selection of effective acupuncture points for successful treatment of drug addiction. Further studies on the synergistic combination of BL. 23 and other effective acupuncture points, such as Zusanli (ST.36) and Sanyinjiao (SP.6), could assist acupuncturists to use a balanced and appropriate choice for combining points in the treatment of addicts.

Acupoints/sites	Frequency of appearance (N)	Percentage (N/26x %)	Acupoints appearing in the literature
Neiguan (PC6)	12	11.11	6,26, 27, 28, 29, 41,44, 62, 63, 64,65and68
Zusanli (ST36)	10	9.26	6,26, 63, 29, 68, 28, 27, 41, 44, and 62
Sanyinjiao (SP6)	8	741	6,26, 27,28,44,62,63,and 68
Shenmen (HT7)	7	6.48	26, 28, 41, 62,63,65, and 68
Hegu (LI4)	6	5.56	6, 26, 27,44, 64, and 68
Shenmen (ear)	4	3.70	3,5, 60, and 68
Kidney (ear)	4	3.70	3,5, 60, and 68
Liver (ear)	4	3.70	3,5, 60, and 68
Lung (ear)	4	3.70	3,5, 60, and 68
Sympathetic (ear)	4	3.70	3,5, 60, and 68
Laogong (PC8)	4	3.70	6,44,65, and 68
Sishencong (EX-HN1)	3	2.78	6, 27, and 65
Jiaji (EX-B2)	3	1.85	28, 62, and 63
Shenshu	3	1.85	28, 62, and 63
Taichong	2	1.85	29 and 63
Baihui (GV20/DU20)	2	1.85	41 and 61
Waiguan (SJ5)	2	1.85	26 and 44
Zhiyang (GV9)	2	1.85	29 and 61
Fengchi	1	0.93	29
Anmian	1	0.93	29
Dazhui (GV14/DU14)	1	0.93	61
Mingmen (GV4)	1	1.85	61
Shendao (GV11)	1	0.93	61
Lingtai (GV10)	1	0.93	61
Shenting	1	0.93	65
Naokong	1	0.93	65
Yintang	1	0.93	65
Yangbai	1	0.93	65
Yongquan	1	0.93	65
Quanzhong	1	0.93	65
Naohu	1	0.93	65
Ben Shen	1	0.93	65

Table 1. Summary of main acupoints/sites selected in the reviewed studies

In summary, acupuncture offer some advantages over existing pharmacological interventions: they are safer, have fewer side effects, and are less expensive. Since deteriorating health often accompanies long-term use of addictive drugs, pharmaceutical interventions with harsh side effects can be detrimental to the general health of long-term drug users. In contrast, acupuncture can enhance immune function and increase metabolism in organs necessary to fight infections and various acute and chronic illnesses. Although the definitive role of acupuncture in the treatment of drug addiction has yet to be established, its basic research and clinical data reviewed here justify further clinical trials to systematically examine the efficacy of acupuncture in treating various conditions related to drug addiction such as withdrawal symptoms, drug craving, anxiety, and depression. The next important step in acupuncture research is to get a better understanding of the neurochemical mechanism of acupuncture in order that the therapeutic effects of acupuncture can be further improved. Also scientifically conducted clinical research is needed to examine the effectiveness of acupuncture treatment of drug addicts. As we mentioned in this review, it has proved difficult to apply and integrate the basic principles and methodology of modern science that ensure the reliability of research subjects to clinical studies on acupuncture. However, researchers should be encouraged to ensure the highest possible standards of study design and reporting in future research in order to improve the evidence base in this field.

Acknowledgements

This work was supported by NSFC (81373753), Shanghai Natural Science Foundation (13ZR1441900), and Innovation Program of Shanghai Municipal Education Commission (11YZ68). We thank F.Q. Zhang for helpful comments on the manuscript.

Author details

Anfeng Xiang, Boyuan Zhang and Sheng Liu*

*Address all correspondence to: lskingcn@hotmail.com

Shanghai University of Traditional Chinese Medicine, Shanghai, China

References

[1] Wang L, Tang C, Lai X. Effects of electroacupuncture on learning, memory and formation system of free radicals in brain tissues of vascular dementia model rats. J Tradit Chin Med 2004;24:140-3. DOI:10.3969/j.issn.0255-2922.2004.02.021

[2] Heinrichs SC, Menzaghi F, Schulteis G, et al. Suppression of corticotrophin-releasing factor in the amygdala attenuates aversive consequences of morphine withdrawal. Behav Pharmacol 1995;6:74-80.DOI:10.1097/00008877-199501000-00011

[3] Stinus L, Le Moal M, Koob GF. Nucleus accumbens and amygdala are possible substrates for the aversive stimulus effects of opiate withdrawal. Neuroscience 1990;37:767-73.DOI:10.1016/0306-4522(90)90106-E

[4] Frenois F, Cador M, Caillé S, et al. Neural correlates of the motivational and somatic components of naloxone-precipitate morphine withdrawal. Eur J Neurosci 2002;16:1377-89.DOI:10.1046/j.1460-9568.2002.02187.x

[5] Everitt BJ, Parkinson JA, Olmstead MC, et al. Associative processes in addiction and reward. The role of amygdala-ventral striatal subsystems. Ann NY Acad Sci 1999;877:412-38.DOI:10.1111/j.1749-6632.1999.tb09280.x

[6] Avants SK, Margolin A, Holford TR, et al. A randomized controlled trial of auricular acupuncture for cocaine dependence. Archives of Internal Medicine 2000;160:2305-12.DOI:1 0.10 01/archinte.160.15.2305

[7] Deng QS, Fang ZC, Yin Y. Ionic mechanism of acupuncture on improvement of learning and memory in aged mammals. Am J Chin 1995;23:1-9.DOI:10.1142/S0192415X9500002X

[8] Maciocia G. The foundation of Chinese medicine. New York:Churchill Livingstone; 1989.

[9] Zhang XP. Researches on the mechanism of acupuncture and moxibustion. Anhui:Anhui Science and Technology Press;1983 [in Chinese].

[10] Ulett GA, Han S, Han J. Electroacupuncture: mechanisms and clinical application. Biol Psychiatry 1998;44:129-38.DOI:10.1016/S0006-3223(97)00394-6

[11] Han JS. Acupuncture: neuropeptide release produced by electrical stimulation of different frequencies. Trends Neurosci 2003;26:17-22.DOI:10.1016/S0166-2236(02)00006-1

[12] Cho ZH, Chung SC, Jones JP, et al. New findings of the correlation between acupoints and corresponding brain cortices using functional MRI. Proc Natl Acad Sci 1998;95:2670-3.DOI:10.1073/pnas.0602520103

[13] Comer SD, Sullivan MA, Yu E, et al. Injectable, sustained release naltrexone for the treatment of opioid dependence: a randomized, placebo-controlled trial. Arch Gen Psychiatry 2006;63:210-8.DOI:10.1001/archpsyc.63.2.210

[14] Cui CL, Wu LZ, Li YJ. Acupuncture for the treatment of drug addiction. Int Rev Neuro Biol 2013;111:235-56.DOI:10.1007/s11064-008-9784-8

[15] Jordan JB. Acupuncture treatment for opiate addiction: a systematic review. J Subst Abuse Treat 2006;30:309-14.DOI:10.1016/j.jsat.2006.02.005

[16] Clement JV, Mcloughlin L, Lowry PJ, et al. Acupuncture in heroin addicts: changes in metenkephalin and beta-endorphin in blood and cerebrospinal fluid. Lancet 1979;2:380-3.DOI:10.1016/S0140-6736(79)90401-X

[17] Montazeri K, Farahnakian M, Saghaei M. The effect of acupuncture on the acute withdrawal symptoms from rapid opiate detoxification. Acta Anaesthesiol Sin 2002;40:173-7.

[18] Shwartz M, Saitz R, Mulvey K, et al. The value of acupuncture detoxification programs in a substance abuse treatment system. J Subst Abuse Treat 1999;17:305-12.DOI:10.1016/S0740-5472(99)00010-0

[19] Wen HL. Acupuncture and electrical stimulation (AES) outpatient detoxification. Mod Med Asia 1979;15:39-43.

[20] Wen HL, Cheung SYC. Treatment of drug addiction by acupuncture and electrical stimulation. Asian J Med 1973;9:138-41.

[21] Wen HL, Teo SW. Experience in the treatment of drug addiction by electroacupuncture. Mod Med Asia 1975;11:23-4.

[22] Smith MO. Acupuncture and natural healing in drug detoxification. Am J Acupuncture 1979;7:97-107.

[23] Smith MO, Aponte J. Acupuncture detoxification in a drug and alcohol abuse treatment setting. Am J Acupunct 1984;12:251-5.

[24] Smith MO, Khan I. An acupuncture program for the treatment of drug-addicted persons. Bull Narc 1988;60:35-41.

[25] Smith MO, Squires R, Aponte J, et al. Acupuncture treatment of drug addiction and alcohol abuse. Am J Acupunct 1982;10:161-6.

[26] Zhang XF, Li X, Feng CX. Clinical study on electro-acupuncture treatment for protracted withdrawal syndromes of opiate dependence. Chin J Drug Depend 1998;7:152-5.

[27] Bullock ML, Culliton PD, Olander RT. Controlled trial of acupuncture for severe recidivist alcoholism. Lancet 1989;8659:1435-9.DOI:10.1016/S0140-6736(89)90135-9

[28] Shu R, Wen XY, Ru L. Advances in studies on acupuncture abstinence at home and abroad. Chin Acup Moxi 2003;23:121-5.

[29] Washburn AM, Fullilove RE, Fullilove MT, et al. Acupuncture heroin detoxification: a single-blind clinical trial. J Subst Abuse Treat 1993;10:345-51.DOI: 10.1016/0740-5472(93)90019-X

[30] Meade CS, Lukas SE, McDonald LJ, et al. A randomized trial of transcutaneous electric acupoint stimulation as adjunctive treatment for opioid detoxification. J Subst Abuse Treat 2010;38(1):12-21.DOI:10.1016/j.jsat.2009.05.010

[31] Chan YY, Lo WY, Li TC, et al. Clinical efficacy of acupuncture as an adjunct to methadone treatment services for heroin addicts: a randomized controlled trial. Am J Chin Med 2014;42(3):569-86.DOI:10.1142/S0192415X14500372

[32] Lipton DS, Brewington V, Smith M. Acupuncture for crack-cocaine detoxification: Experimental evaluation of efficacy. J Subst Abuse Treat 1994;11:205-15.DOI: 10.1016/0740- 5472(94)90077-9

[33] Wu LZ, Cui CL, Tian JB, et al. Suppression of morphine withdrawal by electroacupuncture in rats: dynorphin and kopioid receptor implicated. Brain Res 1999;851:290-6.DOI:10.1016/S0006-8993(99)02069-7

[34] Han JS, Zhang RL. Suppression of morphine abstinence syndrome by body electroacupuncture of different frequencies in rats. Drug Alcohol Depend 1993;31:169-75.DOI:10.1016/0376-8716(93)90069-3

[35] Yoshimoto K, Kato B, Sakai K, et al. Electroacupuncture stimulation suppresses the increase in alcohol-drinking behavior in restricted rats. Alcohol Clin Exp Res 2001;25:63S-68S.DOI: 10.1097/00000374-200106001-00015

[36] Wang B, Luo F, Xia YQ, et al. Peripheral electric stimulation inhibits morphine-induced place preference in rats. Neuroreport 2000;11:1017-20.DOI: 10.1097/00001756-200004070-00024

[37] Shi XD, Ren W, Wang GB, et al. Brain opioid-receptors are involved in mediating peripheral electric stimulation-induced inhibition of morphine conditioned place preference in rats. Brain Res 2003; 981:23-9.DOI:10.1016/S0006-8993(03)02798-7

[38] Chae Y, Yang CH, Kwon YK, et al. Acupuncture attenuates repeated nicotine-induced behavioral sensitization and c-Fos expression in the nucleus accumbens and striatum of rat. Neurosci Lett 2004;358:87-90.DOI:10.1016/j.neulet.2003.12.121

[39] Liu S, Zhou W, Liu H, et al. Electroacupuncture attenuates morphine withdrawal signs and c-Fos expression in the central nucleus of the amygdala in freely moving rats. Brain Res 2005;1044:155-63.DOI:10.1016/j.brainres.2005.02.075

[40] Liu S, Zhou W, Liu H, et al. Effects of acupuncture at Shenshu (BL.23) on morphine withdrawal syndrome and c-fos expression in addiction-relative brain regions. J Acupunct Tuina Sci 2005;3:16.DOI:10.1007/BF02845486

[41] Avants SK, Margolin A, Chang P, et al. Acupuncture for the treatment of cocaine addic tion. Investigation of a needle puncture control. J Subst Abuse Treat 1995;12:195-205.DOI:10.1016/0740-5472(95)00014-V

[42] Clavel-Chapelon F, Paoletti C, Benhamou S. Smoking cessation rates 4 years after treatment by nicotine gum and acupuncture. Prev Med 1997;26:25-8.DOI:10.1006/pmed.1996.9997

[43] Bullock ML, Kiresuk TJ, Pheley AM, et al. Auricular acupuncture in the treatment of cocaine abuse: a study of efficacy and dosing. J Subst Abuse Treat 1991;16:318.DOI: 10.1016/S0740-5472(98)00002-6

[44] Margolin A, Kleber HD, Avants SK, et al. Acupuncture for the treatment of cocaine addiction: a randomized controlled trial. JAMA 2002;287:55-63.DOI:10.1001/jama. 287.1.55

[45] Bresler DE, Cohen JS, Kroening R, et al. The potential of acupuncture for the behavioral sciences. Am Psychol 1975;30:411-4.DOI:10.1037/0003-066X.30.3.411

[46] Maciocia G. The treatment of mental and emotional problems with acupuncture and Chinese herbs: Part II. Am J Acupunct 1994; 22:305-34.

[47] Peterson JR. Acupuncture in the 1990s: a review for the primary care physician. Arch Fam Med 1996;5:237-40.DOI:10.1001/archfami.5.4.237

[48] Allen JJ, Schnyer RN, Hitt SK. The efficacy of acupuncture in the treatment of major depression in women. Psychol Sci 1998;9:397-401.DOI:10.1111/1467-9280.00074

[49] Röschke J, Wolf C, Müller MJ, et al. The benefit from whole body acupuncture in major depression. J Affect Disord 2000; 57:73-81.DOI:10.1016/S0165-0327(99)00061-0

[50] Luo HC, Jia YK, Li Z. Electroacupuncture vs. amitriptyline in the treatment of depressive states. J Tradit Chin Med. 1985;5:3-8.

[51] Stux G, Pomeranz B. Basics of acupuncture, 3rd edn. Berlin: Springer-Verlag; 1995,4-60,230-236.DOI:10.1007/978-3-642-18988-3

[52] Chang BH, Sommers E. Acupuncture and relaxation response for craving and anxiety reduction among military veterans in recovery from substance use disorder. Am J Addict 2014;23:129-36.DOI:10.1111/j.1521-0391.2013.12079.x

[53] Allen JJ, Schnyer RN, Chambers AS, et al. Acupuncture for depression: a randomized controlled trial. J Clin Psychiatry 2006;67(11):1665-73.DOI:10.4088/JCP.v67n1101

[54] Roschke J, Wolf C, Muller MJ, et al. The benefit from whole body acupuncture in major depression. J Affect Disord 2000;57(1-3):73-81.DOI:10.1016/S0165-0327(99)00061-0

[55] Wang B, Zhang BG, Ge XC, et al. Inhibition by peripheral electric stimulation of the reinstatement of morphine induced place preference in rats and drug-craving in heroin addicts. J Peking Univ Health Sci 2003;85(3):241-7.

[56] Chan JH, Liang J, Wang GB, et al. Repeated 2 Hz peripheral electrical stimulations suppress morphine induced CPP and improve spatial memory ability in rats. Exp Neurol 2005;194(2):550-6.DOI:10.1016/j.expneurol.2005.04.001

[57] Lua PL, Talib NS. Auricular acupuncture for drug dependence: an open-label randomized investigation on clinical outcomes, health-related quality of life, and patient acceptability. Alt Therap Health Med 2013;19:28-42.

[58] Bearn J, Swami A, Stewart D, et al. Auricular acupuncture as an adjunct to opiate detoxification treatment: effects on withdrawal symptoms. J Subst Abuse Treat 2009;36:345-9.DOI:10.1016/j.jsat.2008.08.002

[59] Black S, Carey E, Webber A, et al. Determining the efficacy of auricular acupuncture for reducing anxiety in patients withdrawing from psychoactive drugs. J Subst Abuse Treat 2011;41(3):279-87.DOI:10.1016/j.jsat.2011.04.001

[60] Wang ZT, Yuan YQ, Wang J, et al. Treatment of heroin dependence by acupuncture combined with traditional Chinese herb. Chin Acup Moxi 1999;11:657-8.

[61] Li F, He XP, Chen YL, et al. The effect of acupuncture on heroin withdrawal symptoms. Fujian Trad Chin Med 1998;29:30-1.

[62] Clement-Jones V, McLoughlin L, Lowry PJ, et al. Acupuncture in heroin addicts; changes in met-enkephalin and beta-endorphin in blood and cerebrospinal fluid. Lancet 1979;2:380-3.DOI:10.1016/S0140-6736(79)90401-X

[63] Wells EA, Jackson R, Diaz RO, et al. Acupuncture as an adjunct to methadone treatment services. Am J Addict1995;4:198-214.DOI:10.3109/10550499509038105

[64] Margolin A, Avants SK, Chang P, et al. Acupuncture for the treatment of cocaine dependence in methadone maintained patients. Am J Addict1993;2:194-201.DOI: 10.1111/j.1521-0391.1993.tb00419.x

[65] Konefal J, Duncan R, Clemence C. The impact of the addition of an acupuncture treatment program to an existing metro-Dade County outpatient substance abuse treatment facility. J Addict Dis 1994;13:71-99.DOI:10.1300/J069v13n03_07

[66] Ter Riet G, Kleijnen J, Knipschild P. A meta-analysis of studies into the effect of acupuncture on addiction. Br J Gen Pract 1990;40:379-82.DOI:10/1990; 40(338):379-82

[67] Bullock ML,Kiresuk TJ,Pheley AM, et al. Auricular acupuncture in the treatment of cocaine abuse. A study of efficacy and dosing. J Subst Abuse Treat 1999;16:31-8.DOI: 10.1016/S0740-5472(98)00002-6

[68] A R White, K L Resch, E Ernst. A meta-analysis of acupuncture techniques for smoking cessation. Tob Control 1999; 8:393-7.DOI:10.1136/tc.8.4.393

[69] Wang B, Luo F, Zhang WT, et al. Stress or drug-priming induces reinstatement of extinguished conditioned place preference. Neurosci Lett 2000;11:1017-1020.DOI: 10.1097/00001756-200008210-00034

[70] Cui CL, Wu LZ, Han JS. Spinal k-opioid system plays an important role in suppressing morphine withdrawal syndrome in the rat. Neurosc Lett 2000;295:45-8.DOI: 10.1016/S0304-3940(00)01593-7

[71] Chen XH, Han JS. Analgesia induced by electroacupuncture of different frequencies is mediated by different types of opioid receptors: another cross-tolerance study. Behav Brain Res 1992;47:143-9.DOI:10.1016/S0166-4328(05)80120-2

[72] Fei H, Xie GX, Han JS. Low and high frequency electroacupuncture stimulations release (Met5) enkephalin and dynorphin A in rat spinal cord. Chin Sci Bull 1987;32:1496-509.

[73] Wu LZ, Cui CL, Tian JB, et al. Suppression of morphine withdrawal by electroacupuncture in rats: dynorphin and kopioid receptor implicated. Brain Res 1999;851:290-6.DOI:10.1016/S0006-8993(99)02069-7

[74] Shi XD, Wang GB, Ma Y, et al. Repeated peripheral electrical stimulations suppress both morphine-induced CPP and reinstatement of extinguished CPP in rats: accelerated expression of PPE and PPD mRNA in NAc implicated. Mol Brain Res 2004;130:124-33.DOI:0.1016/j.molbrainres.2004.07.016

[75] Wang GB, Wu LZ, Yu P, et al. Multiple 100 Hz electroacupuncture treatments produced cumulative effect on the suppression of morphine withdrawal syndrome: Central preprodynorphin mRNA and p-CREB implicated. Peptides 2011;32(4): 713-21.DOI:10.1016/j.peptides.2010.12.006

[76] Gerhard I, Postneek F. Auricular acupuncture in the treatment of female infertility. Gynecol Endocrinol 1992;6:171-81.DOI:10.3109/09513599209015552

[77] Eisenberg DM, Davis RG, Ettner SL, et al. Trends in alternative medicine use in the United States, 1990-1997: results of a follow-up national survey. JAMA 1998;280:1569-75.DOI:10.1001/jama.280.18.1569

[78] Hu L, Chu NN, Sun LL, et al. Electroacupuncture treatment reverses morphine-induced physiological changes in dopaminergic neurons within the ventral tegmental area. Addict Biol 2009 14(4):431-7.DOI:10.1111/j.1369-1600.2009.00163.x

[79] Watkins SS, Koob GF, Markou A. Neural mechanisms underlying nicotine addiction: acute positive reinforcement and withdrawal. Nicotine Tob Res 2000;2:19-37.DOI: 10.1080/14622200050011277

[80] Yoon SS, Kwon YK, Kim MR, et al. Acupuncture-mediated inhibition of ethanol induced dopamine release in the rat nucleus accumbens through the GABA (B) receptor. Neurosci Lett 2004;369:234-8.DOI:10.1016/j.neulet.2004.07.095

[81] Li J, Sun Y, Ye JH. Electroacupuncture decreases excessive alcohol consumption involving reduction of FosB/ΔFosB levels in reward-related brain regions. PLoS One 2012;7(7):e403 47.DOI:10.1371/journal.pone.0040347

[82] Escosteguy-Neto JC, Fallopa P, Varela P, et al. Electroacupuncture inhibits CB1 upregulation induced by ethanol withdrawal in mice. Neurochem Int 2012;61(2): 277-85.DOI:10.1016/j.neuint.2012.05.014

[83] Fallopa P, Escosteguy-Neto JC, Varela P, et al. Electroacupuncture reverses ethanol-induced locomotor sensitization and subsequent pERK expression in mice. Int J Neuropsychopharmacol. 2012;15(8):1121-33.DOI:10.1017/S1461145711001325

[84] Everitt BJ, Dickinson A, Robbins TW. The neuropsychological basis of addictive behavior. Brain Res Rev 2001;36:129-38.DOI:10.1016/S0165-0173(01)00088-1

[85] White NM. Addictive drugs as reinforcers: multiple partial actions on memory systems. Addiction 1996;91:921-49.DOI:10.1046/j.1360-0443.1996.9179212.x

[86] Sher L. The role of the endogenous opioid system in the effects of acupuncture on mood, behavior, learning, and memory. Med Hypotheses 1998;50:475-8.DOI: 10.1016/S0306-9877(98)90265-1

[87] Chang YH, Hiseh MT, Wu CR. Effects of acupuncture at pai-hui on the deficit of memory storage in rats. Am J Chin Med 1999;27:289-98.DOI:10.1142/S0192415X99000331

[88] Margolin A, Avants SK, Kleber HD. Investigating alternative medicine therapies in randomized controlled trials. J Am Med Assoc 1988;280(18)1626-8.DOI:10.1001/jama.280.18.1626

[89] Marlatt GA. Relapse prevention: theoretical rationale and overview of the model. In Relapse Prevention1985;3-70.

[90] Jadad AR, Moore RA, Carroll D, et al. Assessing the quality of reports of randomized clinical trials: is blinding necessary. Control Clin Trials 1996;17:1-12.DOI: 10.1016/0197-2456(95)00134-4

[91] Kong J, Fufa DT, Gerber AJ, et al. Psychophysical outcomes from a randomized pilot study of manual, electro, and sham acupuncture treatment on experimentally induced thermal pain. J Pain 2005;6:55-64.DOI:10.1016/j.jpain.2004.10.005

[92] Liu S, Zhou W, Ruan X, et al. Activation of the hypothalamus characterizes the response to acupuncture stimulation in heroin addicts: a functional MR imaging study. Neurosci Lett 2007;421:203-8.DOI:10.1016/j.neulet.2007.04.078

[93] Wu LZ, Cui CL, Han JS, et al. Effect of 2/100 HZ transcutaneous electrical stimulation on the sexual dysfunction of 33 heroine addicts as revealed by behavioral questionale and serum testosterone and leutinizing hormone examination. J Chin Tradit West Med 2000;20:15-8.

Section 3

Soul

Distant Healing Techniques and Distant Intercessory Prayer – A Tentative Scientific Conciliation

Marcelo Saad and Roberta de Medeiros

Additional information is available at the end of the chapter

http://dx.doi.org/10.5772/60722

Abstract

Currently there is a lack of a universally accepted theory that would constitute the base for the DH paradigm, and some fundamental issues about the mechanisms of DH remain non-responded. Even so, there is sparse documentation that intentions of one person can remotely influence mental and body functions of another person. With the available data, it becomes difficult to formulate an opinion about the validity of such techniques in healthcare. The question of DH may be put under the frame "Is the glass half empty or half full?". People who look at the issue of DH and see a half empty glass usually raise these points: Scientific evidence of benefit is poor, from scarce studies, many of them with methodological limitations; There is a lack of a coherent theory aligned to the ordinary reality based upon Newtonian science; Practical obstacles for healthcare include high variability of outcomes and low relevance of clinical effects. People who look at the issue of DH and see a half full glass usually raise these points: the positive results from some serious and well designed researches may indicate a possible hidden reality; emerging understanding of the mind and its non-local properties may explain the gap of distance; commitment to the patients' claims for a humanistic, comprehensive and integrative healthcare. We may cite two poles of ignorance and the balanced position related to the discussion of DH. The first pole is the obstinate skepticism (arrogant and prejudiced attachment to materialism), that denies the full half. The opposite pole is the naive mysticism (unrealistic trust on paranormal potentialities), that denies the empty half. The balanced position is called here the option for the open-minded scientificism. Some opportunities of advancement in this field would arise from these points: new and adequate research designs complying with limitations of the phenomenon; the progressive consolidation of a new, post-materialist scientific paradigm; optimizing the efficacy of the phenomenon knowing better its interfering factors.

Keywords: Complementary Therapies, Mental Healing, Prayer Healing, Spiritual Therapies, Faith Healing, Metaphysical Mind-Body Relations, Holistic Health, Mind-Body Therapies

1. Introduction

"The day science begins to study non-physical phenomena, it will make more progress in one decade than in all the previous centuries of its existence. To understand the true nature of the universe, one must think it terms of energy, frequency and vibration" (Nikola Tesla, 1856–1943).

1.1. Motivation of authors

For a long time, the authors have had an interest in broader healing concepts than those of conventional biology and medicine. What has inspired the authors is the occasional observation of some health outcomes that do not follow an expected pattern. On the one hand, there are people with chronic health problems that suddenly, following some simple intervention, have an unexpected improvement. On the other hand, there are people with simple health problems who do not improve even after getting every conventional care available. The easiest path would be to put these events in the account of the placebo effect or unknown genetic variations. But the authors are attracted to the more difficult path, in which unknown potentialities of the human being collaborate to determine its state of equilibrium.

Four years ago, the authors began to be interested in the phenomenon of healing from a distance. This is an intriguing phenomenon, because the components of the easy route described above are not in play. Distant healing could only be explained by elements not yet described by science. Saint Augustine said that miracles do not happen in contradiction to nature but only in contradiction to what we know of nature. In the same spirit, the authors have searched in the scientific literature for extraordinary phenomena reports, as well as data to support theories to explain them. This work has been a bit frustrating because the information available form a puzzle in which many pieces are missing.

The authors decided that an ultimate model that is fully understood scientifically cannot still be mounted. At the same time, they have the conviction that the gaps of an imperfect model can be overcome with goodwill and the benefit of doubt. The authors engaged in gathering information found in a logical and orderly way so that readers can draw their own conclusions. There are arguments against and in favor of the existence of unexplored human potential, consistent with the events of healing from a distance. In particular, the authors think that in the near future, medicine will recognize that its progress will involve going through these fields.

http://dx.doi.org/10.5772/60722

Each one of us, at some point in life, may have experienced the situation of a beloved person in difficulty, maybe affected by a severe disease. In such moments, we feel helpless and feel the need to share with this person our deepest resources. Our cultural background may determine whether this attitude will assume the format of a prayer or a secular engagement in sending to this person our best intentions. But despite these exceptional situations of personal desperation, there are descriptions of techniques for health purposes based on the supposed power of compassive intentionality.

1.2. What is known and gaps of knowledge

Distant healing (DH) techniques are defined as acts of conscious intent, wish, or focus, dedicated to improve the health or well-being of another person who is far away [1]. Such approaches for health purposes, described for thousands of years and called by different names, are maybe the oldest ancestral curative practice, present in virtually all cultures worldwide throughout recorded history [2]. Examples include techniques from structured systems (such as distant Reiki) to nonstructured actions (such as informal healers); from ancient shamanistic traditions to modern civilized developments; from laic visions to religion-rooted rituals; from familiar initiatives to professional consultancy.

Perhaps the most widely used DH intervention is intercessory prayer (IP). This is a form of prayer characterized by petitions on behalf of others for their health and well-being [3]. Intercessory prayer is advocated by many religions and philosophies and involves an effort on behalf of someone who is with a special need, aiming to alleviate disease and promote health. Especially in the monotheistic traditions, a prayer is a dialog between man and God (or His messengers). But the term "prayer" used in the current text is broader than the one from main Western religions. Here, it means any concentrated mental effort to conduct the reality to a wished outcome, by appealing to a force which may not be religious. Sometimes, this action is done far from the target beneficiary, when it may be called distant intercessory prayer.

Regarding self-prayer or healing techniques before the presence of a practitioner, the changes in health parameters are explainable by mind–body pathways. Plausible mechanisms by which such techniques deliver health benefits include relaxation response, placebo effect, expression of positive emotions, improved coping strategies from certain spiritual beliefs, and feeling of psychosocial support [4]. All these mechanisms may be related to better physical and mental balance. But a problem arises when considering DH techniques. For the present text, the word "distant" means that the two parts are shielded from any kind of ordinary physical and psychological influence, including those from sensory, informational, and electromagnetic natures [5]. Even thousands of miles of separation do not appear to limit the beneficial effects of healing or prayer [6]. Obviously, such a situation excludes the placebo effect.

For the issue of DH to be properly analyzed, it is necessary to separate the study of the CAUSES (the mechanisms involved in the DH phenomenon) and the EFFECTS (what can be observed in the recipient's body). The first item is the most obscure. Currently, there is a lack of a universally accepted theory that would constitute the base for the DH paradigm. DH appears to contradict our ordinary sense of reality and the laws defined by Newtonian science. The observations point to the existence of a subtle interconnection between living beings, a phenomenon not constricted to the known laws of cause and effect, in ways that go beyond ordinary sense perception. Some fundamental issues about the mechanisms of DH remain non-responded: What is the source of healing and the pathway by which it is transmitted to the client? What is it that is precisely being transmitted or channeled or worked with? What do exactly practitioners do when they perform healing? and What is required of the client in order to receive healing [7]?

The second element regarding DH and its effects may receive another consideration. Although many of the studies about distant influence are not well designed, there are also some serious and well-controlled researches. In such cases, the results cannot be explained by chance or coincidence, natural internal rhythms, uncontrollable external stimuli, errors on recording or reading the registries, placebo effect, or systematic changes in the studied phenomenon [8]. Many researchers studying distant IP used methodologies designed to rule out the possible influence of psychological variables or placebo effects, including double-blinding procedures and control group (prayer vs. no prayer) [9]. Under such conditions, there is documentation that intentions of one person can remotely influence mental and body functions of another person, interacting with his/her physiological, psychological and/or behavioral status. But the effects are not restricted to person-to-person interactions, and distant intention has also influence in other biological systems.

Remote interference of human intention over living systems has been documented over gene functions, such as cell division (which reflects DNA synthesis), cell differentiation, mutagenesis, and apoptosis [10]. Significant effects of mind intentionality are demonstrated through randomized-controlled trials in the germination of seeds, and the growth of plants has also been described [11, 12, 13], as well as over simple life forms such as cells, bacteria, yeast, and the kinetics of biochemical reactions [14, 15, 16]. Considering complex beings interactions, a study [17] examined the effects of IP over wound healing in bush babies, primates with chronic self-injurious behavior. All animals were treated with dietary L-tryptophan, and some also received IP (daily for 4 weeks). Prayer-group animals showed significant differences from the standard group: (a) greater reduction in wound size; (b) better physiological parameters associated with wound healing: red blood cells, hemoglobin, hematocrit, mean corpuscular hemoglobin, and corpuscular volume; (c) better behavioral parameters associated with wound healing: a reduction in wound grooming and total grooming behaviors.

In humans, a variety of physiological effects can be modulated in transpersonal transmissions, known as telesomatic interactions [18]: they consist of physiological changes triggered in a targeted person by the mental processes of another. The effects are detected, especially in both the central and peripheral nervous system. Upon the brain, many studies showed that the status of a subject "A" (either sending intentions or being stimulated) produces changes over the electroencephalogram or the functional magnetic resonance activity of an isolated and distant subject "B" [19, 20, 21, 22, 23, 24, 25]. Upon the autonomic nervous system, there is an observed effect of distant intentions on the electrodermal activity of another subject, in a small but significant effect size [26]. Besides these physiologic modulations, there is also a documented positive effect in performance capabilities, such as the effect of benevolent intentions over the mind focus of a remote person during a specific task [27].

1.3. Is the glass half full or half empty?

The above citations, though exciting, are a minority among many other studies with negative results. Research to investigate the health benefits of receiving prayers from distant intercessors produced conflicting results [28]. A major problem is that positive results in these studies are very unpredictable, probably due to unknown and uncontrollable variables, either related to the practitioner and the beneficiary. With the available data, it becomes difficult to formulate a unique opinion about the validity of such techniques in healthcare. The body of knowledge about DH is a collection of information, each one with defects and qualities, strengths and weaknesses. Given these contradictory possibilities, someone could focus more on one or other side, and yet he would be right. If one prefers to work only with what is concrete and guaranteed, this person will say that there is no evidence enough on DH even for it to be taken seriously. If someone else believes that the advance of knowledge goes through unexplored areas, this person will say that this matter should be thoroughly discussed.

The question "Is the glass half empty or half full?" is a common expression, generally used rhetorically as a challenge for an individual's worldview. This idiom is used to explore how people perceive events and objects. The purpose of the question is to demonstrate that one situation may be seen in very different ways depending on personal background. In any situation, there may be opportunity as well as trouble. Perception is subjective to each individual and it is simply his/her interpretation of reality. Thus, the preference to see a half full or a half empty glass illustrates one's psychological and philosophical worldview regarding pessimism or optimism. The question of DH may be put under the frame of the "half full/ half empty" perspective. Based upon previous personal values, anyone may choose to see the problem in a positivist or a negativist optic. Figure 1 shows the arguments for both interpretations, which will be discussed as follows.

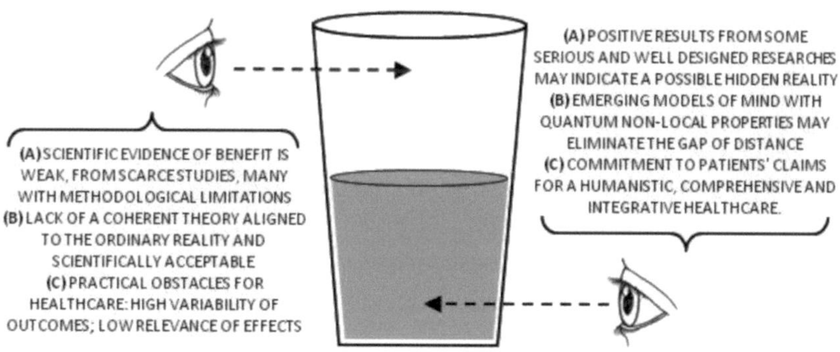

Figure 1. The question of DH under the frame of the "half full / half empty glass" and the main arguments for both interpretations

People who look at the issue of DH and see a "half empty glass" usually raise the following points: (A) the scientific evidence of benefit is weak, from scarce studies, many of them with methodological limitations; (B) there is a lack of a coherent theory aligned to the ordinary reality and scientifically acceptable; and (C) practical obstacles for healthcare include high variability of outcomes and low relevance of clinical effects. On the other hand, people who see a "half full glass" usually raise the following points: (A) the positive results from some serious and well-designed researches may indicate a possible hidden reality; (B) emergent models of the mind with quantum non-local properties may eliminate the gap of distance; and (C) the commitment to the patients' claims for a humanistic, comprehensive, and integrative healthcare. All these points will be discussed below.

2. The empty part of the glass

2.1. Poor evidence of benefit

Evidence-Based Medicine, at its introduction in 1992, was defined as "the conscientious, explicit, and judicious use of current best evidence in making decisions about the care of individual patients" [29]. A main impediment to the acceptance of DH techniques as established forms of therapies has been its seeming irregular reproducibility on empirical research. In fact, clinical trials on DH therapies produce variable results. At least for distant intercessory prayer, the most studied modality, there is no scientifically discernible effect over health. The omnibus effect size across studies, at best, has borderline statistical significance [9]. Roberts et al. [30] reviewed thoroughly the effects of intercessory prayer as an additional intervention to healthcare. Overall, they found no significant difference in recovery from illness or death between those prayed for and those not prayed for. They concluded that, although some of the results of individual studies suggest a positive effect of IP, the majority does not, and the evidence does not support a recommendation either in favor or against the use of IP.

Ideally, any health intervention should be tested by randomized-controlled trials. Science is the backbone of our medical practice. Evidence-based medicine places systematic reviews and meta-analyses at the pinnacle and excludes numerous sources of research information, such as basic research and epidemiology [31]. However, for most CT, there will never be adequate studies following this research model. Investigating CT following rigorous clinical research can be methodologically challenging. This approach is radically different from the experientially rich healing practices found throughout the world that presumably date to the beginning of humanity [32]. Some characteristics of complementary therapies make them less prone to be studied by randomized trials [33].

2.2. Lack of a coherent theory

The most sensitive point of any argument about DH is to explain how any interaction may occur between two separated organisms. No model provides an ultimate explanation for the mechanism of action of DH. This gap reinforces the skepticism among scientists. Generally, most theories about DH systems are comprised of [34]: (a) a source which generates an emanation and modulates it in some manner such that it conveys information; (b) the transfer of a modulation factor or signal at a distance; (c) a transfer medium through which the curative element flows; (d) a terminal sink which includes a mechanism for the perception of information; (e) the ability of the beneficiary to tune in to this frequency and decode this modulation.

http://dx.doi.org/10.5772/60722

DH is the hypothesized form of healing intentionality occurring beyond the reach of the physical senses and that appears to be unmediated by any demonstrable form of physical signal [35]. Traditional DH theories were born in the past and reflect the worldview of that time. Even if they do not fit the current biomedical model, old theories have considerable value, although they may have some structural errors. In the past, conclusions were drawn from the intensive observation of nature, and they have insights we could not draw today. A way to recover this ancestral wisdom is to adapt their concepts to the contemporary knowledge, as a simple matter of language.

The traditional concepts of DH technique are often elaborate, transcending biophysical models and employing metaphysical terms, which don't correlate to conventional biologic concepts. Ancient traditions have explanations that involve manipulation of a supposed subtle vital elements, or intervention of invisible entities, such as spirits, saints, Christ, and even God. But all these interpretations have no correspondence to current scientific constructs. Many practitioners claim for the manipulation of some kind of subtle "energy". Virtually all ancient medical systems pose the existence of some form of vital principle, which determines life and health state. The nature of this supposed principle cannot be described in scientific field. Many DH techniques propose the activation or unblocking of patients' energies, projection of the practitioners' own energies, channeling of energies by the practitioner from nature (the earth, or cosmic energies).

Biofield is the name used for the supposed endogenous energy fields of the living biological bodies [36-37]. It is hypothesized to involve information for regulating homeodynamics. The biofield may act as a resonance target for external forms of energy used as treatment modalities in DH. The biofield would have functional role in the body's innate self-healing mechanisms, based on the concept of bioinformation which, mediated by consciousness, functions globally at the quantum level to regulate and heal physiologic processes. This model [36] is used to explain anomalies reported in the scientific literature, which cannot be explained by traditional biophysics and bioelectromagnetics. However, the analogies between these technical terms of physics and the concepts from DH models are inexact approximations. In physics, the term ''energy'' refers to ''the capacity to do work and overcome resistance'', and the term ''field'' refers to ''a force which can cause action at a distance'' [38].

Thus, this solution brings some embarrassment between defenders and opponents of DH. Firstly, because this "energy" is not currently detectable, albeit most current instruments of measurement are based on detection of electromagnetic signals. Secondly, the DH effects occur even in conditions of isolation between organisms by a Faraday cage [22], ruling out the participation of ordinary electromagnetic waves in the phenomena. We are limited to propose that, somehow, by an unknown mechanism, the intention of the practitioner reaches the beneficiary by a subtle connection medium.

2.3. Practical clinical obstacles

When testing healthcare interventions, it is necessary to explore the concepts of efficacy and effectiveness [39]: Efficacy is the extent to which an intervention brings results under ideal circumstances, and its exploratory question is: "can it work?". Effectiveness refers to whether an intervention brings results under usual healthcare practice, and its exploratory question is: "does it work in practice?". The lack of uniformity on the patients' responses to DH is responsible for many reports of bad results on researches. DH may work well for some patients while it doesn't work at all for others. There may be factors determining these differences, which remain still unknown because they must be beyond the data obtained from randomized, double-blind clinical trials. So, the attempt to predict the benefit of DH for a specific person becomes a lottery.

In addition to the obvious limitation of DH due to the unpredictability of the results, there is another main obstacle: the effects of DH do not appear to be clinically relevant. In both healthy people and patients, there are promising results of DH modalities mainly over mild subjective symptoms such as anxiety, muscle relaxation, stress reduction, and well-being. Over pain, DH techniques may modestly help to decrease it, roughly 1 point on the 10-point scale [40]. In a randomized, blinded study [41], patients with cancer who received IP had small but significant improvements in spiritual dimension of well-being. For the small magnitude of its clinical effect, the feasibility of DH as a clinical treatment may be limited to collaborate with conventional treatment.

In fact, many negative results in clinical trials appear when the focus of the study is the rate of morbidity or mortality in patients with serious illnesses. A study [42] about effects of IP over status health of patients in an intensive care unit received many commentaries for its negative results. It was a multicenter, randomized controlled trial, seemingly very well designed. However, the premise was perhaps flawed, assuming that the intervention is so powerful that it would support clinical success in frail patients who underwent coronary artery bypass graft. The health outcomes in seriously debilitated patients may be determined by more concrete clinical elements than the subtle interference of DH. Thus, the term "cure at distance" may be a little ambitious. As DIP is not intended to treat a disease, but rather to improve general well-being, perhaps it would be more adequate to call it "*complementary health practice*", instead of complementary therapy.

3. The full part of the glass

3.1. A possible hidden reality

As Dossey [14] posed, the key question is not how large the effects are, but whether they exist at all. In other words, what matters is whether human consciousness can act non-locally to affect the material world, beyond the reach of the senses. Events that cannot be explained by existing science are regularly reported in high-quality scientific literature [44]. The inability of existing paradigms to explain these observations elucidates a need for more research [44]. Such findings invite us to consider a nonphysical aspect of reality. These phenomena are a calling for the emergence of a new paradigm [45]. Science advancement begins with observations which cannot be explained, in such manner that what is paranormal in one era can become mainstream science in another [44].

On the biologic field, the available data point to the existence of several levels of distant communication [46]: neuron-to-neuron (in vitro, isolated cells responding collectively to a stimulus), brain-to-brain (stimulus in one subject leading to physiologic changes in other one), and person-to-person (intention from one person leading to well-being in other one). Furthermore, on this astonishing field, there are also some studies about mind–matter interaction besides the biological interest. Such experiments about consciousness-related physical anomalies brought the verification that the mind exchanges information with the environment. Mind interference over machines generating random effects has been studied [47, 48, 49]. In such research, an operator tries to exert some mental influence on an external system to achieve a specific desired outcome. They concluded that human intention is able to elicit anomalous variations on random event output in a very small size but statistically significant effect. The replicability of results is irregular in ordinary trials, but statistically robust over large databases.

Although the positive data are not unanimous in studies of DH, these outcomes cannot be viewed as anomalous or as exceptions to natural laws. Instead, they call our attention to a dimension of reality yet to be explored, which need a broader explanatory framework. The increasing knowledge on this subject will dictate what role these phenomena can play in our lives. Anyway, the academic medical centers should seek new knowledge concerning therapeutics, irrespective of the source of the original hypotheses. Scientific research centers exist for the purpose of the generation, conservation, and dissemination of new knowledge concerning the causes, prevention, and treatment of human disease. Thus, they should go on rigorously investigating such a widely used treatment modality, the IP [50].

3.2. Emergent nonlocal mind model

Quantum mechanics, the physics of subatomic particles, is commonly said to be a theory applicable for submicroscopic level. Nearly all physicists, though, think it applies to everything, no matter what the size [51]. Quantum effects may be not limited to subatomic particles. These effects are perhaps more pervasive, and some evidence points toward quantum physics applicable to the macro world. Many experimentalists have seen quantum effects in a growing number of macroscopic systems. The quintessential quantum effect, entanglement, can occur in experiments with large systems, and it may even operate in the cells of living systems [51]. Physicists thought the bustle of living cells would blot out quantum phenomena. Now they find that cells can nurture these phenomena—and exploit them [51]. Nonlocal consciousness, in which the intention of the practitioner may connect to the mind of the beneficiary, is an alternative explanation for some of the effects [52].

The quantum mind hypothesis proposes that quantum mechanical phenomena, such as quantum entanglement and superposition, can explain nonlocal consciousness. In quantum mechanics, the term non-locality describes effects of spatially separated particles. Non-locality [35] is the state of being unconfined and unrestricted to a particular place. In modern physics, it is a property in which entities once in contact demonstrate correlated behaviors, instantly and to the same degree, regardless of the extent of spatial separation. Entanglement is the concept in which separated particles can still remain connected, with the state of one particle affecting the state of another. By analogy, the term "biological non-locality" would refer to correlations between spatially separated living beings. In fact, telesomatic interactions mean to have the characteristics of quantum non-locality [53]: they are unmediated (not propagated by any known form of force, energy, or signal); unmitigated (strength of the effect doesn't diminish with increasing spatial separation); and immediate (correlations take place with no time delay).

An approach in this direction [54] proposes quantum computations in microtubule networks embedded within gap junction-linked cortical dendrites. According to this theory, consciousness depends on biologically orchestrated coherent quantum processes in microtubules within brain neurons, and these quantum processes correlate with, and regulate, neuronal synaptic and membrane activity. This theory suggests that there is a connection between the brain's biomolecular processes and the basic structure of the universe.

Mind could operate in a nonlocal fashion, being unconfined to specific points in space, such as brains and bodies [55]. Thus, we could receive information without the use of ordinary senses, in ways that transcend the habitual space and time constraints. Instead of energy exchange, there may be an exchange of information of biological interest, in a subliminal way. Information, in the present context, means any array of stimuli to which consciousness or its environment is capable of sensing and reacting 35]. A form of information transfer is due to resonance, which is the inducing of a synchronizing effect in a beneficiary. It is conjectured that the information content transferred by the practitioner may create a resonance phenomena within the beneficiary [34]. It is also possible that the healing potential is not emitted. Maybe the only element that travels from the practitioner to the beneficiary is the pure intention. Healing potential may already be present in the beneficiary, and it is then only awakened [56].

3.3. Humanistic healthcare

Paradoxically, modern medicine understands more the serious diseases than the minor functional deviations. Current conventional model best explains mechanical (material) problems, but has gaps to explain functional disorders (which are actually related to most of the medical appointments). If we imagine the human being as a computer, the current biomedical model would better take care of the hardware, whereas it has few resources to fix the software. Somatic pathology, in many cases, is due to subtle imbalances, since the ideal health results from an integrated state. DH techniques may serve to strengthen or reinforce the client's resources to enable one to withstand pathogenic exposures or threats, thus ameliorating susceptibility to disease and/or facilitating recovery, to correct a slight pathological deviation and to restore balance and wellness. DH may empower one's innate salutogenic resources, complementing the treatment of the disease process made by conventional medicine [57].

The World Health Organization defined health as a state of complete physical, mental and social well-being, not merely the absence of disease or infirmity [58]. By this definition, conventional medical treatment, in its strict sense, would not encompass everything the patient needs to balance his/her health. As a result, many patients currently show dissatisfaction with characteristics of conventional medicine. In this scenario, complementary therapies have become an attractive option for some people, play a role in filling this gap by correcting the deviated pathway [59]. DH techniques are part of the so-called holistic therapies, as such activities consider the whole person, including physical, mental, emotional, and spiritual aspects.

Although clinical studies of DH have yielded equivocal results, this is one of the most frequently practiced healing modalities. Prayer is probably the best-known and widely practiced form of DH in the western world [60]. Even small clinical effects derived from DH are noteworthy for many people. Patients with debilitating symptoms will not wait until unquestionable evidence is available; they tend to try CT regardless of the uncertainties associated with it. DH modalities may be chosen by patients, challenging the physician to conciliate the expectations of patients with the lack of solid evidence, in an ethical counseling. So, medical community has the ethical and moral obligation to accompany the patient in his search for relief. The "north" cardinal reference must always be the "*primum non nocere*" (first, do no harm) principle. But the "south" must be the principle of "put yourself in someone else's shoes", remaining sympathetic and respectful to the aspirations and desires of the patients [61].

Harding [62] asks whether there is no place in medicine for a multiple approach to healing, and, further, if reported studies of efficacious prayer therapies are meaningful, are physicians not using these additional treatments withholding something curative from their patients? The IP findings are strong enough to accept them and incorporate them into medical practice. DH would be used even without solid evidence of efficacy if the condition causes a heavy burden of suffering. Adequate physician characteristics include partnership on a real patient-centered care, respecting the values of the patient. We would use more IP studies even if we don't understand the underlying mechanisms. This situation is similar to the case of scurvy and its treatment by consumption of citrus fruit long before we understood the role of vitamin C [63].

4. Two poles of ignorance and a balanced position

Attitudes to medical literature can create belief systems which are analogous to those of religious traditions [64]. In science as in religion, there are fundamentalist, conservative, or liberal people. Such variations reflect the different ways of reading the data and the disparity in the value placed on the evidence. Whether a scientist takes a fundamental or liberal view of available evidence will affect how he/she interprets it [64]. In both the religious and medical context, debate difficulties (either on scriptures or evidence) arise when attitudes become polarized in an atmosphere of intolerance, denying the validity of alternative world views.

According to this analogy [64], fundamentalist scientists take a strict and literal view of the literature. They give little allowance for individualization, ignore the limitations of the literature, and tend to undervalue nonrandomized papers. The fundamentalist approach sees the literature as sacred texts to be applied literally, and any deviation is seen as heresy. On the other hand, a liberal approach sees the literature as a guide to establish principles to be adapted to specific situations. However, an excessive liberal perspective would result in important deviations from the evidence. Summing up these erroneous positions, we would say that acceptance without criterion is characteristic of blind mysticism, whereas rejection without criterion is characteristic of blind skepticism.

The famous British physicist and cosmologist Stephen Hawking stated: the greatest enemy of knowledge is not ignorance; it is the illusion of knowledge. A conservative scientific position employs observation, empirical investigation, and theoretical explanation of each phenomenon. Figure 2 represents what we call here the two poles of ignorance and the balanced position related to the discussion of DH. The first pole is the obstinate skepticism (arrogant and prejudiced attachment to materialism), that denies the full half. The opposite pole is the naive mysticism (unrealistic trust on paranormal potentialities), that denies the empty half. The balanced position is the option for the enlightened scientificism, a non-dogmatic, open-minded method of acquiring knowledge about nature.

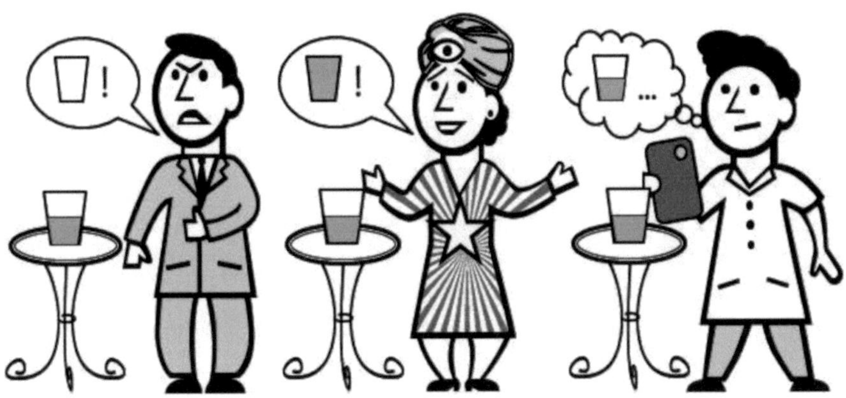

Figure 2. Representation of the two poles of ignorance (the obstinate skepticism and the naive mysticism), and the balanced position

4.1. The option for obstinate skepticism

Many people ridicule DH even before collecting all information for a critical analysis, in a position like "I didn't read it and I didn't like it". Prejudice and disinterest from some scientists are ingredients to creating a comfort zone of sloth. Skepticism may be healthy and constructive when it is a careful doubt until enough data have been collected to draw a conclusion. But the unhealthy and destructive form of skepticism is manifested by a dogmatic insistence in a particular conclusion in absence of data, and denial of findings that contradict that conclusion [65].

Some materialistically inclined scientists and philosophers refuse to acknowledge these phenomena because they are not consistent with their conception of the world. But science should not be committed to any particular beliefs, dogmas, or ideologies. The term "paradigm paralysis" [66] refers to the tendency to be unable to see beyond the current models of thinking. To justify their attachment to conventions, these scientists usually claim their commitment to evidence-based medicine, as if it is the pure expression of the true.

Evidence-Based Medicine is a useful tool, but has drawbacks when used in isolation in the practice of individual patient care. The authoritative aura given to the "best available evidence" may lead to inappropriate guidelines or doctrinaire dogmas for clinical practice. Many criticism to evidence-based medicine have been raised [67, 68, 69], and the main are: definition of "evidence" is narrow and excludes important information; limited usefulness of applying populational conclusions to individual patients; ignores the autonomy of the doctor/patient relationship and patient preferences; being a "cookbook" in medicine, giving an average overview; under-valued issues such as rare diseases, clinical circumstances, and surgeon expertise; discrepancies in health care systems worldwide.

4.2. The option for naïve mysticism

Acceptance of anything without checking the source, with free association of smithereens from scientific idiom, may generate "mumbo jumbo" stuff such as "quantic weight loss". This attitude, on the verge of charlatanism, may be motivated either by greed or by ignorance. Ideally, practitioners must be adequately informed, motivated, and expectant. An example of realistic purpose may be the pursuit for well-being; an unrealistic purpose may be the intention to stop all conventional remedies in a chronic disease; and an impossible purpose may be to cure advanced cancer. The challenge of the correct expectation may also include the user behavior. Patient may seek a practitioner for wrong motivations, as a shortcut to resolve problems.

Any harmless complementary therapy is welcome as a support for medical approach. But its nemesis, the concept of alternative therapy, may be very dangerous when it means a substitute for conventional treatment. This path may lead to consequences, ranging from disappointment to retardation of clinical investigation in serious diseases. This disaster may happen when some practitioners, making exaggerated claims about curing diseases, ask their clients to abandon the medical follow-up. Whereas direct harm to the patient is virtually impossible with DH, an indirect harm is possible to occur, which results in a delay of appropriate treatment. Also, unreasonable expectations may discourage patients and their families from accepting and dealing effectively with their medical conditions.

4.3. The option for enlightened scientificism

The word science derives from a Latin verb, *"scire"*, meaning to know or to understand; it could thus properly apply to any process of comprehension of any topic or form of experience. True science is characterized by thorough and respectful cognizance of relevant past and present work by others, humility in the face of empirical evidence, openness of mind to new topics, new approaches, new ideas, and new scholars; and a profound respect for demonstrable experimental and theoretical anomalies [70].

The dedicated scientist does not discard what is proposed by other theories, including ancient philosophical or religious doctrines. Supposed subtle fluid and/or invisible intelligent entities could naturally coexist with the physical nature. It would make sense to infer that both tangible and intangible realities could be supplemented by information from each other. We must respectfully consider any nonphysical and transpersonal aspect of reality that would contribute to a broader explanatory framework. Open-minded scientists may see comprehensively all the aspects of the glass in a naturalistic point of view. In such context, the answer of whether a glass is half full or half empty would be: the content of the vessel is 50% of its capacity; the glass is both half full and half empty. The enlightened scientificism comprises the acknowledgment of the potentials of DH as well as its limitations.

5. Further sources to fill up the glass

Some opportunities for advancement in this field would arise from the following points: (A) new and adequate research designs complying with limitations of the phenomenon; (B) the progressive consolidation of a new, Post-Materialist scientific paradigm; and (C) optimizing the efficacy of the phenomenon knowing better its interfering factors. Figure 3 illustrates such sources from which the question about DH will be reinforced. Each item will be discussed below.

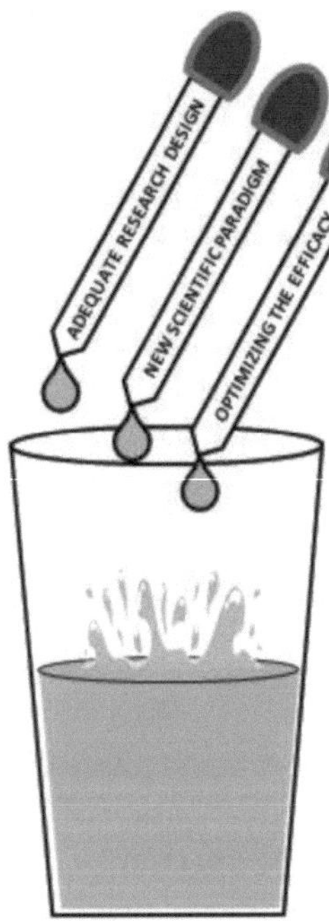

Figure 3. Sources from which the question about DH will be reinforced

5.1. Adequate research designs

Even in controlled and blinded experimental designs, many interfering factors would not be completely isolated. Main scientific biases have been cited [71, 72]. The most important is probably the difficulty for creation of a pure control group, without intervention. The relatives of the beneficiary may be praying for him/her, and there are anonymous benefactors who pray for the restoration of the sick people in general. Studies of IP fail to adequately measure and control exposure to prayer from others, which is likely to exceed IP and to vary widely from subject to subject, and whose magnitude is unknown [63]. This supplemental prayer greatly attenuates the differences between the treatment and control groups. Another important bias may be the quality assurance of the prayer offered. At least for prayer, it is said that its power is related to intention, motivation, focus capacity, compassion, empathy, sincerity, commitment, and trust [73]. In a study with many practitioners, the uniformity of the intervention may be compromised. A speculative bias would include the artificiality of the environment for the experiment and its possible interference with the subtle phenomena it would intend to capture.

Future scientific studies must comply with limitations of the technique, by the creation of suitable models to study this phenomenon. As a rule, studies in complementary therapies would follow a different dynamic from that of studies with drugs. It makes no sense to study remote IP as if it were just another drug [72]. Further research must be conducted in different molds. Research designs more adequate for complementary therapies include [74]: Pragmatic trials (intervention intended to represent the real world to enhance external validity); factorial designs (comparing single modalities to a combination of modalities); preference trials (respecting treatment preferences of participants); and "N-of-1" (a single patient trial with multiple crossovers between treatment and placebo).

The worship of a particular research method (such as the randomized controlled trial) and a dogged determination to employ it, in spite of its shortcomings, has been called "methodolatry" [46]. There is a need to critically reappraise core elements of the evidence-based medicine paradigm: the hierarchical ranking of evidence, RCTs or systematic reviews as the gold standard for all clinical questions or situations, the statistical tests that have become integral to the "measurements" for analyzing evidence, and reincorporating a role for evidence from basic sciences and pathophysiology [75]. To provide patients with best care at lowest cost, EBM must balance priorities by [76]: expanding to include new methods of study design and integration; adapting to the needs of both patients and the health care system; dealing with the need for individualized care, incorporating patient values.

Future research to accelerate the progress of understanding the source and the biological effects of DH must focus on [77]: (a) clarifying the scientific hypotheses and developing further theories to resolve questions of mechanism of action; (b) developing preclinical models (cell, tissue, animal) to validate their biological effects and mechanisms of action; (c) validating markers attesting to the biological effects, such as biomarkers associated with stress and relaxation response; (d) investigating at least as a shadow or a trace of bioelectric signaling, as the purported phenomenon cannot be directly measured; and (e) clarifying practical issues, such as characteristics of the practitioner and potential interfering factors (e.g., empathic resonance).

5.2. New scientific paradigm

Scientific ideas are subject to change, for the process for producing knowledge brings new observations, which may challenge prevailing theories. In science, improving and occasional discarding of theories, whether new or old, go on all the time [78]. The improvement of ideas, rather than their outright rejection, is the norm in science. For example, in formulating the theory of relativity, Albert Einstein did not discard the Newtonian laws of motion but rather showed them to be only an approximation of limited application within a more general concept [78]. A paradigm is a set of assumptions, concepts, and beliefs that define the way we frame our thoughts. Paradigms shape the way we see, and cause us to notice some things and ignore others and to anticipate what is likely to occur based on a particular set of assumptions. The development of a new paradigm demands a learning to "think outside the box" (i.e., outside the prevailing paradigm).

Studies already indicate that we can mentally influence living organisms at a distance, and that intention can influence the state of the physical world in a nonlocal fashion. So, many contemporary scholars and researchers believe a transition is currently required in science, because the materialistic focus that has dominated it in the modern era cannot account for an ever-increasing body of empirical findings in the domain of consciousness and spirituality. Some of these scientists signed the Manifesto for a Post-Materialist Science [55]. Their purpose was to discuss the impact of the materialist ideology on science and the emergence of a new paradigm for science, spirituality, and society.

As they argued [55], the nearly absolute dominance of materialism in the academic world has seriously constricted the sciences and hampered the development of the scientific study of mind and spirituality. In the view of these scholars and researchers, science methodology is not synonymous with materialism. The true spirit of scientific inquiry is that empirical data must always be adequately dealt with. Data which do not fit favored theories and beliefs cannot be dismissed a priori. Such dismissal is the realm of ideology, not science. According to these authors, it is time to free ourselves from the shackles and blinders of the old materialist ideology, to enlarge our concept of the natural world, and to embrace now a post-materialist paradigm.

5.3. Optimization of the efficacy

The more we know about the interfering factors involved in DH outcomes, the more we can set the conditions to induce the positive result. However, it is very difficult to investigate such factors, as they may be more subjective than the scientific methods could detect. Some factors are traditionally cited, and they will be described as follows. Practitioner-beneficiary emotional connection seems to be an important factor, since telesomatic interactions occur more clearly among emotionally close people, such as identical twins, couples, or relatives [56]. The studies in DH and IP reveal that nonlocal mind is intimately connected with love, compassion, and deep caring, just as healers throughout history have maintained [79]. Thus, the starting point for a favorable DH outcome would be a practitioner with appropriate empathy, focus, and motivation. The practitioner mentally focuses the receiver, establishing a figurative connection that will transfer his/her healing intention.

There are no clues about the role of the practitioner's background elements (such as the kind of graduation; amount of experience; etc.). Thus, we could infer this is not a decisive factor. Maybe the correct attitude of the practitioner is more important than his/her background. Some ethical posture items from healers have been suggested [60]: do not promise something (either relief or cure); not working in competition with medical treatments; not tempt a client to delay or omit a medical consultation or treatment, to interrupt or stop it; not recommend any drugs and give no advice to stop taking a drug; not giving any diagnosis; not enter into sexual relationships with my clients; not put pressure on clients to begin or continue the healing process; not using misleading titles; not charge money in advance for healing sessions.

These moral elements seem to be more important than the faith tradition of the intercessor or either the format of the prayer [7]. DH research did not show that prayers within any particular religious framework are more effective than any other, or than secular DH practitioners [6]. The experiments in nonlocal healing show that the prayers of all religions appear to be effective [15]. Even secular intentions that are not associated with any traditional religion, appears to result in healing [15]. These findings universalize healing intentions and nonlocal effects of prayer to all systems. The use of a formal technique or a religious routine may only serve as a support to fasten the practitioner thought, for the unbroken conduction of the task.

The level of wellness and health state of the practitioners may interfere with the process. Their physical and mental well-being, states of wholeness and balance that they seek to engender in their clients, can affect the outcomes. Rubik et al. [80] measured the effects of Reiki treatments on heat-shocked bacterial cultures and, secondarily, the role of the practitioner well-being. Reiki improved growth of bacteria in a healing context. Reiki-treated cultures overall exhibited significantly more bacteria than controls, but the level of well-being social, physical, and emotional of the practitioners correlated strongly with this outcome. For practitioners with a higher level of well-being, Reiki-treated bacterial counts were likely to be higher than control counts. The inverse result occurred for practitioners with diminished well-being.

Another concept, purely speculative, involves the receptiveness of the beneficiary on his/her healing process. DH techniques can produce effects even when the beneficiary is unaware that the effort is being made [15]. However, it is possible that the beneficiary could block the benefit, either consciously or unconsciously, for secondary gains of illness or due to personality types. At least to some degree, the beneficiary must desire or be motivated to be healed, keeping receptive openness, with minimal mismatch of impedance. As stated by Roman philosopher Seneca (4bC-65aD), it is part of the cure to wish to be cured. In a study [81], a prayer intervention reduced the subject's level of concern only for the subjects who initially believed that the problem could be resolved. Those in the intervention group who did not believe in a possible resolution to their problem were not different from controls. Among those with a higher belief in prayer in the intervention group, a better physical functioning was observed.

6. Conclusion

6.1. Summary of the main points

Currently, there is a lack of a universally accepted theory that would constitute the base for the DH paradigm, and some fundamental issues about the mechanisms of DH remain non-responded. Even so, there is sparse documentation that intentions of one person can remotely influence mental and body functions of another person. With the available data, it becomes difficult to formulate an opinion about the validity of such techniques in healthcare. The question of DH may be put under the frame "Is the glass half empty or half full?".

People who look to the issue of DH and see a half empty glass usually raises these points: Scientific evidence of benefit is poor, from scarce studies, many of them with methodological limitations; There is a lack of a coherent theory aligned to the ordinary reality based upon Newtonian science; Practical obstacles for healthcare include high variability of outcomes and low relevance of clinical effects. People who look to the issue of DH and see a half full glass usually raises these points: the positive results from some serious and well-designed researches may indicate a possible hidden reality; emerging understanding of the mind and its nonlocal properties may explain the gap of distance; commitment to the patients' claims for a humanistic, comprehensive, and integrative healthcare.

We may cite two poles of ignorance and the balanced position related to the discussion of DH. The first pole is the obstinate skepticism (arrogant and prejudiced attachment to materialism), that denies the full half. The opposite pole is the naive mysticism (unrealistic trust on paranormal potentialities), that denies the empty half. The balanced position is called here the option for the open-minded scientificism. Some opportunities of advancement in this field would arise from these points: new and adequate research designs complying with limitations of the phenomenon; the progressive consolidation of a new, post-materialist scientific paradigm; optimizing the efficacy of the phenomenon knowing better its interfering factors.

6.2. Closing considerations

The fragmentary reasoning of the present paper does not constitute an ultimate explanation. The affirmations posed here are contestable, if analyzed separately. However, taken as a whole, the sum indicates a possibility to conciliate the scattered data and at the same time overcome their apparent contradictions. The present text doesn't have the intention to deny or to confirm any interpretation. Nor does this paper have the presumption to present an ultimate dictate to close the discussion. The objective of this chapter is to expose different views that lead to the acceptance or refusal of assumptions regarding DH. The acceptance of DH is still a jump of faith. But it may be a rational faith.

http://dx.doi.org/10.5772/60722

Author details

Marcelo Saad[1,2*] and Roberta de Medeiros[3]

*Address all correspondence to: msaad@uol.com.br

1 Medical Spiritist Association of S. Paulo, S. Paulo, Brazil

2 Medical College of Acupuncture of S. Paulo, Brazil

3 Centro Universitário S. Camilo, Brazil

References

[1] Astin JA, Harkness E, Ernst E. The efficacy of "distant healing": a systematic review of randomized trials. Ann Intern Med. 2000;132(11):903-10.

[2] Jain S, Mills PJ. Biofield therapies: Helpful or full of hype? A best evidence synthesis Int. J Behav Med. 2010; 17:1-16.

[3] Jantos M, Kiat H. Prayer as medicine: how much have we learned? Med J Aust. 2007 May 21;186(10 Suppl):S51-3.

[4] Andrade C, Radhakrishnan R. Prayer and healing: A medical and scientific perspective on randomized controlled trials. Indian J Psychiatry. 2009 Oct-Dec; 51(4): 247-253. doi: 10.4103/0019-5545.58288.

[5] Schlitz M, Radin D, Malle BF, Schmidt S, Utts J, Yount GL. Distant healing intention: definitions and evolving guidelines for laboratory studies. Altern Ther Health Med. 2003;9(3 Suppl):A31-43.

[6] Benor DJ. Distant healing. Subtle Energies & Energy Medicine. 2000; 11(3):249-64.

[7] Levin J. Energy healers: Who they are and what they do. Explore. 2011; 7:13-26.

[8] Bonilla E. Distant mental influence on living organisms. Invest Clin. 2013; 54(4): 427-54.

[9] Masters KS, Spielmans GI. Prayer and Health: Review, Meta-Analysis, and Research Agenda. J Behav Med. 2007; 30:329–338. doi 10.1007/s10865-007-9106-7.

[10] Sidorov L, Chen K. Biophysical mechanisms of genetic regulation: Is there a link to mind-body healing? DNA Decipher Journal. 2012; 2(2):177-205.

[11] Shinde V, Sances F, Patil S, Spence A. Impact of biofield treatment on growth and yieldof lettuce and tomato. Australian Journal of Basic & Applied Sciences. 2012; 6(10):100.

[12] Sances F, Flora E, Patil S, Spence A, Shinde V. Impact of biofield treatment on ginseng and organic blueberry yield. Agrivita. 2013; 35(1):22-9.

[13] Patil SA, Nayak GB, Barve SS, Tembe RP, Khan RR. Impact of biofield treatment on growth and anatomical characteristics of pogostemon cablin (Benth.). Biotechnology. 2012; 11(3).

[14] Dossey L. Healing research: What we know and don't know. Explore (NY). 2008; 4(6): 341-52.

[15] Dossey L. PEAR lab and nonlocal mind: why they matter. Explore (NY). 2007; 3(3): 191-6.

[16] Benor DJ. Energy medicine for the internist. Med Clin North Amer 2002; 86(1): 105-25.

[17] Lesniak KT. The effect of intercessory prayer on wound healing in nonhuman primates. Altern Ther Health Med. 2006; 12(6): 42-8.

[18] Laszlo E. The convergence of science and spirituality. Syntropy. 2005; 3: 69-84.

[19] Wackermann J, Seiter C, Keibel H, Walach H. Correlations between brain electrical activities of two spatially separated human subjects. Neurosci Lett. 2003; 336(1): 60-4.

[20] Standish LJ, Kozak L, Johnson LC, Richards T. Electroencephalographic evidence of correlated event-related signals between the brains of spatially and sensory isolated human subjects. J Altern Complement Med. 2004; 10(2): 307-14.

[21] Radin DI. Event-related electroencephalographic correlations between isolated human subjects. J Altern Complement Med. 2004; 10(2): 315-23.

[22] Thaheld FH. A method to explore the possibility of nonlocal correlations between brain electrical activities of two spatially separated animal subjects. Biosystems. 2004; 73(3): 205-16.

[23] Richards TL, Kozak L, Johnson, C, Standish, LJ. Replicable functional magnetic resonance imaging evidence of correlated brain signals between physically and sensory isolated subjects. J Altern Complement Med. 2005; 11(6): 955-63.

[24] Achterberg J, Cooke K, Richards T, Standish LJ, Kozak L, Lake J. Evidence for correlations between distant intentionality and brain function in recipients: a functional magnetic imaging analysis. Journal of Alternative and Complementary Medicine. 2005; 11(6): 965-71.

[25] Charman RA. Has direct brain to brain communication been demonstrated by electroencephalographic monitoring of paired or group subjects? Journal Society for Psychical Research. 2006; 70(882): 1-24.

[26] Schmidt S, Schneider R, Utts J, Walach H. Distant intentionality and the feeling of being stared at: two meta-analyses. Br J Psychol. 2004; 95(Pt 2): 235-47.

[27] Schmidt S. Can we help just by good intentions? A meta-analysis of experiments on distant intention effects. J Altern Complement Med. 2012; 18(6): 529-33. doi: 10.1089/acm.2011.0321.

[28] Yang FY. Intercessory prayer: Issues in investigating medicinal faith. meducator. Mcmaster's Undergraduate Health Sciences Journal. 2008; 12:6.

[29] Sackett DL, Rosenberg WM, Gray JA, Haynes RB, Richardson WS. Evidence based medicine: what it is and what it isn't. BMJ. 1996 Jan 13; 312(7023): 71-2.

[30] Roberts L, Ahmed I, Hall S, Davison A. Intercessory prayer for the alleviation of ill health. Cochrane Database Syst Rev. 2009; 15(2): CD000368. doi: 10.1002/14651858.CD000368.pub3.

[31] Rosner AL. Evidence-based medicine: Revisiting the pyramid of priorities. J Bodyw Mov Ther. 2012; 16(1): 42-9.

[32] Wilson KH. Medicine's missing dimension. Trans Am Clin Climatol Assoc. 2010; 121: 309-17.

[33] Kienle GS, Albonico HU, Fischer L, Frei-Erb M, Hamre HJ, Heusser P, Matthiessen PF, Renfer A, Kiene H. Complementary therapy systems and their integrative evaluation. Explore (NY). 2011 May-Jun.

[34] Hintz KJ, Yount GL, Kadar I, Schwartz G, Hammerschlag R, Lin S. BioEnergy definitions and research guidelines. Altern Ther Health Med. 2003; 9: 13-30

[35] Jonas WB, Chez RA. Recommendations regarding definitions and standards in healing research. J Altern Complement Med. 2004; 10(1): 171-81.

[36] Rein G. Bioinformation within the biofield: beyond bioelectromagnetics. J Altern Complement Med. 2004 Feb; 10(1): 59-68.

[37] Rubik B. The biofield hypothesis: Its biophysical basis and role in medicine. J Altern Complement Med. 2002; 8(6): 703–17.

[38] Movaffaghi Z, Farsi M. Biofield therapies: Biophysical basis and biological regulations? Complementary Therapies in Clinical Practice. 2009; 15: 35-37.

[39] Haynes B. Can it work? Does it work? Is it worth it? BMJ 1999.

[40] Rindfleisch JA. Biofield therapies: Energy medicine and primary care. Primary Care: Clinics in Office Practice. 2010; 37(1): 165-79.

[41] Olver IN, Dutney A. A randomized, blinded study of the impact of intercessory prayer on spiritual well-being in patients with cancer. Altern Ther Health Med. 2012; 18(5): 18-27.

[42] Benson H, Dusek JA, Sherwood JB, Lam P, Bethea CF, Carpenter W, et al. Study of the therapeutic effects of intercessory prayer (STEP) in cardiac bypass patients – A

multicenter randomized trial of uncertainty and certainty of receiving intercessory prayer. Am Heart J. 2006; 151(4): 934-42.

[43] Dossey L. Mind-Body medicine: Whose mind and whose body? Explore (NY). 2009; 5(3): 127-34. doi: 10.1016/j.explore.2009.03.002.

[44] Bobrow RS. Paranormal phenomena in the medical literature sufficient smoke to warrant a search for fire. Med Hypotheses. 2003 Jun; 60(6): 864-8.

[45] Bonilla E. Is the brain the creator of psychic phenomena or is a paradigm shift inevitable? Invest Clin. 2014 Jun; 55(2): 103-6.

[46] Dossey L. The next decade: How it might unfold. Explore (NY). 2012; 8(2): 73-80.

[47] Jahn RG, Dunne BJ. The PEAR proposition. Explore (NY). 2007; 3(3): 205-26.

[48] Bösch H, Steinkamp F, Boller E. Examining psychokinesis: the interaction of human intention with random number generators - a meta-analysis. Psychol Bull. 2006; 132(4): 497-523.

[49] Caswell JM. The potential role of consciousness in the collapse of random physical systems: a quantitative biophysical investigation of cognitive intention. A thesis submitted in partial fulfillment of the requirements for the degree of Master of Arts (MA) in Human Development. The School of Graduate Studies Laurentian University Sudbury, Ontario, Canada. May 2014.

[50] Halperin EC. Should academic medical centers conduct clinical trials of the efficacy of intercessory prayer? Acad. Med. 2001; 76: 791-7.

[51] Vedral V. Living in a quantum world. Scientific American. 2011; 304(June): 38-43. doi:10.1038/scientificamerican0611-38.

[52] Dossey L. The millennium of consciousness: Reflections on the one mind. Explore (NY). 2013; 9(2): 67-74. doi: 10.1016/j.explore.2012.12.007.

[53] Dossey L. How healing happens: Exploring the nonlocal gap. Altern Ther Health Med. 2002; 8(2): 103-10.

[54] Hameroff S, Penrose R. Consciousness in the universe - A review of the 'Orch OR' theory. Physics of Life Reviews. 2014; 11: 39–78.

[55] Beauregard M, Schwartz GE, Miller L, Dossey L, Moreira-Almeida A, Schlitz M, et al. Manifesto for a post-materialist science. Explore (NY). 2014; 10(5): 272-4.

[56] Dossey L. Unbroken wholeness: The emerging view of human interconnection. Explore (NY). 2013; 9(1): 1-8. doi: 10.1016/j.explore.2012.11.001.

[57] Levin J. Scientists and healers: toward collaborative research partnerships. Explore (NY). 2008; 4(5): 302-10.

[58] WHO. Constitution of the World Health Organization as adopted by the International Health Conference, New York, 19-22 June, 1946.

[59] De Medeiros R, Saad M. Complementary Therapies – Considerations Before Recommend, Tolerate or Proscribe Them. In: Saad M & De Medeiros R (book editors), Complementary Therapies for the Contemporary Healthcare. InTech Publisher, Rijeka, Croatia, 2012, ISBN: 978-953-51-0801-6, doi: 10.5772/50446.

[60] Walach H, Bösch H, Haraldsson E, Marx A, Tomasson H, Wiesendanger H, Lewith G. Efficacy of distant healing--a proposal for a four-armed randomized study (EU-HEALS). Forsch Komplementarmed Klass Naturheilkd. 2002 Jun; 9(3): 168-76.

[61] Saad M, De Medeiros R. Complementary therapies for fibromyalgia syndrome - a rational approach. Curr Pain Headache Rep. 2013 Aug; 17(8): 354.

[62] Harding OG. The healing power of intercessory prayer. West Indian Med J. 2001 Dec; 50(4): 269-72.

[63] Sloan RP, Ramakrishnan R. Science, medicine, and intercessory prayer. Perspect Biol Med. 2006; 49(4): 504–14. doi:10.1353/pbm.2006.0064.

[64] Links M. Analogies between reading of medical and religious texts. BMJ. 2006 Nov 18; 333(7577): 1068-70.

[65] Leary M. Why are some scientists so opposed to parapsychology? Explore 2011; 7(5): 275-7.

[66] Harrison JC. Redefining stuttering: What the struggle to speak is really all about. ISBN 1-929773-08-4.The National Stuttering Association, New York, USA. 2011 Edition. ISBN 1-929773-08-4.

[67] Cohen AM, Stavri PZ, Hersh WR. A categorization and analysis of the criticisms of evidence-based medicine. Int J Med Inform. 2004 Feb; 73(1): 35-43.

[68] Darlenski RB, Neykov NV, Vlahov VD, Tsankov NK. Evidence-based medicine: Facts and controversies. Clin Dermatol. 2010 Sep-Oct; 28(5): 553-7. doi: 10.1016/j.clindermatol.2010.03.015.

[69] Bhandari M, Giannoudis PV. Evidence-based medicine: What it is and what it is not. Injury. 2006; 37(4): 302-6. DOI: http://dx.doi.org/10.1016/j.injury.2006.01.034.

[70] Jahn RG, Dunne BJ. Science of the subjective. Explore (NY). 2007; 3(3): 295-305.

[71] Warber SL, Cornelio D, Straughn J, Kile G. Biofield energy healing from the inside. J Altern Complement Med. 2004; 10(6): 1107-13.

[72] Turner DD. Just another drug? A philosophical assessment of randomised controlled studies on intercessory prayer. J Med Ethics. Aug 2006; 32(8): 487-90.

[73] Levin J. How faith heals: a theoretical model. Explore (NY). 2009; 5(2): 77-96. doi: 10.1016/j.explore.2008.12.003.

[74] Verhoef MJ, Lewith G, Ritenbaugh C, Boon H, Fleishman S, Leis A. Complementary and alternative medicine whole systems research: beyond identification of inadequacies of the RCT. Complement Ther Med. 2005 Sep; 13(3): 206-12.

[75] Seshia SS, Young GB. The evidence-based medicine paradigm: Where are we 20 years later? Part 2. Can J Neurol Sci. 2013; 40(4): 475-81.

[76] Bluhm R, Borgerson K. Evidence-Based Medicine (Chapter). In: Gabbay D, Thagard P, Woods J (editors), Philosophy of Medicine. 2011, Elsevier. ISBN: 9780080930916.

[77] Anonymous (National Center for Complementary and Alternative Medicine). Expanding Horizons of Health Care - Strategic Plan 2005-2009. National Institutes of Health, USA. Publication number 04-5568, December 2004.

[78] Rutherford FJ, Ahlgren A. Science for All Americans: Education for a Changing Future. 2nd Edition.ISBN-13 978-0-19-506771-2. Oxford University Press, 1991. ISBN-13 978-0-19-506771-2.

[79] Saad M, De Medeiros R. Distant Healing by the Supposed Vital Energy. In: Saad M & De Medeiros R (book editors), Complementary Therapies for the Contemporary Healthcare. InTech Publisher, Rijeka, Croatia, 2012, ISBN: 978-953-51-0801-6, doi: 10.5772/50446.

[80] Rubik B, Brooks AJ, Schwartz GE. In vitro effect of Reiki treatment on bacterial cultures: Role of experimental context and practitioner well-being. J Altern Complement Med. 2006 Jan-Feb; 12(1): 7-13.

[81] Palmer RF, Katerndahl D, Morgan-Kidd J. A randomized trial of the effects of remote intercessory prayer: interactions with personal beliefs on problem-specific outcomes and functional status. J Altern Complement Med. 2004 Jun; 10(3): 438-48.

Chapter 11

Why is Qi-Invigorating Therapy in Chinese Medicine Suitable for Mitochondrial Diseases? A Bioenergetic Perspective

Xing-Tai Li, Hai-Xue Kuang and Jia Zhao

Additional information is available at the end of the chapter

http://dx.doi.org/10.5772/59418

Abstract

The central player in bioenergetics is the mitochondrion. Bioenergetic dysfunction is emerging as a cornerstone for understanding the pathophysiology of mitochondrial diseases. Accompanying the depth of mitochondrial research and the rapid development of mitochondrial medicine, however, is rapid amplification of the number of mitochondrial diseases; mitochondrial dysfunction would undermine the function of cells, tissues, and organs, thereby causing cancer, diabetes, obesity, strokes, cardiovascular diseases, neurodegenerative diseases, and ageing, etc. Currently, there are no effective treatments; Western medicine is in crisis when it comes to mitochondrial diseases.

According to traditional Chinese medicine (TCM) theory, all kinds of diseases are born from Qi: Qi refers to the most basic motive force and maintains life's functional activities. Both life and death of humans depends on Qi. Qi always underpins the basic theory of TCM and acts as its cornerstone. Qi has been used as a healing technique in China for 4000 years. The author proposes a scientific hypothesis that "Qi" is "bioenergy", that Qi-deficiency can lead to bioenergetic dysfunction, which can be improved by Qi-invigoration, and demonstrates that Qi-invigoration was achieved through improved mitochondrial bioenergetics. Qi-deficiency is the common cause of mitochondrial diseases and Qi-invigoration is the basic principle for treatment of Qi-deficiency; therefore, Qi-invigorating therapy for mitochondrial diseases is logical. This chapter will focus on the role of mitochondrial bioenergetics in the aetiology and progression of several mitochondrial diseases and explore the potential therapeutic benefits of improving mitochondrial bioenergetics in mitigating the disease processes by Qi-invigorating therapy. It will also provide a comprehensive overview of why Qi-invigorating therapy in TCM is suitable for mitochondrial diseases from a bioenergetics perspective, try to find its underlying mechanism, and to propose a novel way of thinking and provide scientific evidence in guiding Qi-invigorating therapy for the prevention and treatment of mitochondrial diseases.

The chapter will give an overview of some potential breakthroughs and the many challenges remaining in pursuit of the first effective treatment for mitochondrial disease by Qi-invigorating therapy. There seems to be light at the end of the tunnel; efforts to develop effective drugs should be devoted to the design of Qi-invigorating prescriptions that work in synergy to protect the mitochondria. It is hoped that the next few years will see a further convergence of Qi-invigorating therapy with mitochondrial bioenergetics, which will provide a comprehensive view of mechanisms on mitochondrial diseases. It seems likely that we are on the right track to acquiring this understanding, and that it will involve mechanisms rich with ideas from both the modern bioenergetics and the old Qi-invigorating therapy in TCM on mitochondrial diseases and how to counteract them.

Keywords: Qi-invigorating therapy, mitochondrial diseases, bioenergetics, mitochondria, energy metabolism

1. Introduction

As we all know, traditional Chinese medicine (TCM) is the summary of Chinese people's experiences in fighting diseases for thousands of years. Its theoretical system contains the essence of Chinese classical philosophy, embodies the Chinese people's own culture and profound speculative dialectical relationship between man and nature, and has made a great contribution to the healthcare of the Chinese people and the prosperity of the Chinese nation. TCM is also a unique treasure of the world's medical knowledge, and contributed to world civilization via the Silk Road and other external communication channels from very early on.

With the changes of the concept of people's health and the transformations of medical models in recent years, TCM pays more attention to the "preventive treatment of disease" and follows the "overall theory, system theory". It has ushered in a new development, not only having a significant effect on many common diseases but also plays an important role in the prevention and treatment of major incurable diseases and emerging infectious diseases, providing a source of knowledge and technology, and research and development ideas, for the development of a modern pharmaceutical industry and health services, and the evolution of medical science.

In the development of medical and health services with Chinese characteristics, the Chinese government has adhered to the policy of juxtaposing Chinese and Western medicines. The practice proves that the two medical systems have complementary advantages, promote each other. Both systems have salient features and advantages for China's medical and health

http://dx.doi.org/10.5772/59418

protection, and not only provide a unique impetus for the development of Chinese medical science, but also play an increasingly significant role for the realization of a healthy China. TCM is a treasure, this ancient wisdom should be respected and applied to the modern medical system; it will provide more choice and a wider field of vision for modern medicine at the two cognitive crossroads of East and West.

The mitochondria, whose main function is the production of the energy substance adenosine triphosphate (ATP), and are the hub and core of all life's activities, have been recognized as a cellular "Achilles heel". Interest in the roles that mitochondria play in human health and disease have grown markedly over the past two decades. Mitochondria lie at the heart of systemic metabolic regulation, they regulate the life and death of cells by manipulating several factors, including bioenergetics, mitochondrial permeability transition (MPT), and mitochondrial redox status. They are usually regarded as specialized organelles for cellular respiration and oxidative phosphorylation (OXPHOS). A lack of cellular energy, excessive free radical production, and dysregulated apoptosis are found alone or in combination in most human diseases, including neurodegenerative diseases, strokes, cardiovascular disorders, ischemia/ reperfusion, and cancer [1].

Mitochondrial dysfunction has severe cellular consequences and is linked to ageing and mitochondrial diseases in humans. Since the discovery of the first case of mitochondrial disease in 1962 [2], the depth and development of mitochondrial research and medicine has increased rapidly, as has the number of mitochondria-related diseases; mitochondrial dysfunction would undermine the function of cells, tissues, and organs, thereby causing cancer, diabetes, obesity, strokes, cardiovascular diseases, age-related diseases, neurodegenerative diseases, and ageing, etc. Mitochondria have become a new target for the treatment of diseases, and mitochondrial dysfunction was listed as one of the nine hallmarks of ageing in the journal *Cell* in 2013 [3]. Therefore, mitochondrial protection is an important mechanism for the treatment of mitochondrial diseases.

Currently there are no highly effective mitochondrial disease treatments. Though related symptoms, such as seizures or attention problems can be managed with various medications, the mitochondrial disease itself is unchanged. As scientists have learned more about mitochondria's role in health and in disease, research suggests that mitochondrial function may be the unifying theme — the Holy Grail of medicine, perhaps — of understanding a spectrum of diseases, conditions, and why we grow old. Mitochondrial research across different disease disciplines will help all of us access treatments, and ultimately cures, much faster.

Continually increasing resources are being expended to combat mitochondrial diseases. Yet the causes of these diseases remain a mystery, while their incidence and morbidity either remain constant or are increasing. Huge investments in biomedical research in recent years have resulted in some striking accomplishments, but have failed to reveal the anticipated causes for the diseases. Western medicine is in crisis [4].

1.1. Mendelian paradigm of genetics and mitochondrial diseases

Western biomedical science has stood on two philosophical pillars: the anatomical paradigm of medicine and the Mendelian paradigm of genetics. The Mendelian paradigm of genetics argues that genetic traits are transmitted across generations according to the laws of Gregor Mendel. However, Mendelian genetics is specific for nuclear DNA (nDNA) genes and have been powerful predictors of medical relationships for the past century, but fails to direct us toward answers for mitochondrial diseases. Since mitochondrial DNA (mtDNA) encodes genes for proteins of energy metabolism, human diseases affect many organs that could originate from systemic energy metabolism defects and could result from mutations in mtDNA [4]. The classical Mendelian genetic perspective has failed to explain the aetiology of mitochondrial diseases, because they are primarily systemic bioenergetic diseases, and the most important energy genes are located in mtDNA [5].

1.2. mtDNA and mitochondrial bioenergetics

In many animal species, mtDNA is a circular intron-free genome consisting of 14,000–17,000 base pairs (16,569 in humans), although in some species it is much larger, noncircular, and contains introns [6–7]. It is typically maternally inherited and present in multiple copies within each cell; the mtDNAs are grouped in DNA-protein complexes referred to as nucleoids [8–9] that are anchored to the inner mitochondrial membrane. Most somatic cells in mammals have 10^3–10^4 mtDNAs [10], but this number varies significantly by cell type and developmental stage [11].

Mitochondria are at the centre of bioenergetics and generate about 90% of cellular energy, regulate cellular redox status, and produce reactive oxygen species (ROS). The mitochondrial genome consists of thousands of copies of mtDNA, plus between 1,000 and 2,000 nDNA genes. mtDNA codes for 13 OXPHOS polypeptides, the 22 tRNAs, and the 12S and 16S rRNAs. mtDNA polypeptides encompass seven of OXPHOS complex I (ND1, ND2, ND3, ND4, ND4L, ND5, and ND6), one of complex III (cytochrome b), three of complex IV (COI, COII, and COIII), and two of complex V(ATPase6 and ATPase8). Consequently, mitochondrial biology and genetics become excellent candidates for expanding the anatomical and Mendelian paradigms to address the complexities of age-related diseases, ageing, and cancer [12], and life involves the interplay between structure and energy [4].

Both variation in the mtDNA and nDNA-coded mitochondrial genes sequences can perturb mitochondrial bioenergetics and result in disease. Since different tissues depend on mitochondrial energy to different extents, partial systemic energy deficiency can result in tissue-specific symptoms. Tissues with high energy demands include the brain, heart, muscles, kidneys, and the endocrine system: the organs commonly affected in metabolic and degenerative diseases [5]. A decline in energy is common in ageing, and the restoration of mitochondrial bioenergetics may offer a common approach for the treatment of numerous age-associated diseases [13].

The basic role of mitochondria in sustaining the normal cellular function has made dysfunction of this organelle a central feature of numerous diseases in any organ system at any stage of life [14–15]. "Mitochondrial medicine" has emerged as an active field of research. However, the mystery remains as to how tissue or cell type specificity occurs, and how a systemic disorder of one mitochondrial complex can cause a selective disease phenotype while leaving other tissues intact. It is believed that many of the mitochondrial diseases might actually be an expression of progressive organ system failure due to disruption of specific aspects of mitochondrial function. Even though dysfunctional mitochondria appear to be a common underlying problem for all these diseases, they each exhibit unique triggers and symptoms.

1.3. Mitochondrial dynamics and bioenergetics

Mitochondria are highly dynamic organelles that show constant movement, fusion, and fission [16–17]. The role of mitochondrial dynamics is enabling content mixing of mitochondrial matrix and membranous components between mitochondria [18]. Disruption of mitochondrial dynamics causes a series of diseases, including neurodegenerative disease, cardiovascular disease [19], and even cancer [20]. Benard et al. describe the fundamental mechanisms by which mammalian cells regulate energy production, and put emphasis on the importance of mitochondrial dynamics for the regulation of bioenergetics. In addition, most neurodegenerative diseases such as Alzheimer's disease (AD), Parkinson's disease (PD), Huntington's disease (HD), and Hereditary Spastic Paraplegia are associated with defects in mitochondrial dynamics and bioenergetics [21]. Therefore, to unravel the fundamental mechanisms by which mitochondrial form interacts with mitochondrial function could permit us to increase our basic knowledge on the regulation of energy metabolism and to decipher the pathophysiology of a group of rare neuronal diseases.

Pathogenic mutations in genes essentials for mitochondrial fusion and fission have complicated the mechanisms of these diseases [22]. Thus, the mitochondrial network organization is a new parameter for physiopathological analyses of mitochondrial diseases [21]. The possible interaction between mitochondrial dynamics and energy production could offer an opportunity for the discovery of drugs that target mitochondrial fusion or fission with a stimulatory effect on energy metabolism, to the benefit of patients suffering from mitochondrial diseases [23–24].

1.4. Qi-invigoration and mitochondrial bioenergetics improvement

In TCM, "Qi" is expressed as the basic material that constitutes the body, maintains human life activities, and is its basic driving force. Qi, as the master of the brain, regulates Yin-Yang and five elements, tonifies the five vital organs of the human body, and keep the six hollow viscera unobstructed, and is in charge of chemical and biological transformation and defences, Qi dominate the whole vital activities. Qi is the centre in TCM from basic theory to clinical practice. According to TCM, "Qi is the root of the human"; "All the diseases originate from Qi"; "Both life and death depend on Qi, if Qi gets together, it will result to the birth; if Qi is strong, then the human body is healthy; if Qi is waning, the body will be weak; if Qi is disordered, the human will be sick; if Qi is depleted, the human will die". This shows that Qi is closely related to health, disease, and life.

Qi can make the human body work in an orderly fashion by promoting a variety of physiological activities; "Qi-deficiency" will lead to a decline of physiological functions. As one part of a central medical classic *The Yellow Emperor's Inner Canon*, 'Plain Questions' pointed out that consumption of the vital essence Qi leads to deficiency, 'Miraculous Pivot' says that Qi-deficiency in the heart, liver, spleen, lung, or kidneys becomes worse with increasing age, and ultimately all five internal organs of the body become deficient, spirit and Qi leave the body, and eventually the human will die. The basic idea of TCM to prevent and cure diseases is strengthening vital Qi to eliminate pathogenic factors. Strengthening vital Qi can improve body's resistance to disease, in order to eliminate weakness syndromes, ward off illnesses, and be physically strong. On the understanding of the aetiology, TCM theory emphasizes the cause of disease — "vital Qi-deficiency", especially.

Due to the fact that both Qi and bioenergy are at the centre of life activity, the author suggests that Qi and bioenergy are closely related, and proposes a scientific hypothesis that "Qi" is "bioenergy" [25]; that Qi-deficiency can lead to mitochondrial energy metabolism obstacles, which can be improved by Qi-invigoration; and demonstrates that Qi-invigoration can be achieved through improved mitochondrial bioenergetics [26]. Qi-deficiency is the common cause of a variety of diseases (including mitochondrial diseases) and Qi-invigoration is the basic principle for the treatment of Qi-deficiency. Doctors of TCM usually compose prescriptions made up of Qi-invigorating herbal medicines (QIHM) for Qi-deficiency, and have accumulated abundant clinical experience for a long time. QIHM is a group of herbal medicines which can invigorate Qi and treat syndromes of Qi-deficiency.

1.5. The central premise of the chapter

This chapter will examine the role of mitochondrial bioenergetics in the aetiology and progression of several mitochondrial diseases and explore potential therapeutic benefits of improving mitochondrial bioenergetics in mitigating the disease processes by Qi-invigorating therapy. The chapter aims to provide a comprehensive overview of why Qi-invigorating therapy in TCM is suitable for mitochondrial diseases from a bioenergetic perspective, try to find its underlying mechanism, and provide a novel way of thinking and scientific evidence in guiding Qi-invigorating therapy for the prevention and treatment of mitochondrial diseases.

2. Mitochondrial bioenergetics dysfunction and diseases

2.1. A Primer on mitochondrial bioenergetics

The standard model of mammalian cellular bioenergetics is based on the pioneering work of Krebs and Mitchell over half a century ago [27]. In 1961, Peter Mitchell published a unique hypothesis regarding cellular bioenergetic conservation, to elucidate the role of mitochondria in energy generation — Mitchell theory, namely the chemiosmotic theory of OXPHOS, is one of the most fascinating discoveries in the history of science. ATP synthase was driven to produce ATP by the transmembrane proton gradient induced when electrons transfer along a series of respiratory enzyme complexes in the mitochondrial inner membrane, an insight for which Mitchell was awarded the Nobel Prize in Chemistry in 1978 [28]. Studies on bioenergetics have occupied an important position in the life sciences, the generation mechanism of ATP (the most important energy molecule in life activity) was elucidated by an academic of the National Academy of Sciences — Boyer — who proposed binding change and rotational catalysis mechanism of ATP synthase, and won the 1997 Nobel Prize in Chemistry. Products of the Krebs cycle, such as nicotinamide adenine dinucleotide (NADH) and succinate, are the obligatory factors that drive mitochondrial electron transport and maintain OXPHOS and ATP production (Figure 2) [27]. Mitochondrial bioenergetic processes are central to the production of cellular energy, and a decrease in the expression or activity of enzyme complexes responsible for these processes can result in an energy deficit that correlates with many metabolic diseases and ageing [29].

An increase in the slippage of complex I and III of the electron transport chain (ETC) [30–32] can lead to overproduction of ROS, which can further damage the mtDNA and create a vicious feed-forward loop of energetic decline. The consequence of such an energetic decline is potentially grave, which might be manifested as either the normal progression of ageing, or as the onset of major diseases such as diabetes, AD, PD, and cancer [33–34]. Interest in the roles that mitochondria play in health and disease has grown markedly over the past two decades [35]. Mitochondria are involved both in male and female germ-line formation, which may also be affected by sexual antagonism of mitochondrial-nuclear gene interaction. Mitochondrial energy metabolism is also involved in tissue and organism differentiation. The mitochondrial bioenergetics system should be recognized as a candidate key driver of speciation events, at least in animals [36].

Cardiolipin is a unique phospholipid which is almost exclusively located in the inner mitochondrial membrane, where it is biosynthesized. Cardiolipin plays the functional role in several reactions and processes involved in mitochondrial bioenergetics [37]. Cardiolipin contains unsaturated fatty acyl chains which are readily oxidizable targets. Peroxidation of cardiolipin is now considered an important event in mitochondrial dysfunction in cellular pathophysiology and also an early step in apoptotic cell death. Abnormalities in cardiolipin content, fatty acyl chain composition, and remodelling appear to be, at least in part, responsible for mitochondrial dysfunction associated with several pathophysiological situations, including hypo- and hyperthyroid states, heart ischemia/reperfusion, heart failure, diabetes, Barth syndrome, as well as ageing and age-related cardiovascular and neurodegenerative disorders. Pharmacological strategies designed to prevent cardiolipin oxidation may open new perspectives for treatment of these disorders [37].

High-fat feeding is associated with reduced whole body respiration and, over sufficient duration, results in reduced mitochondrial respiration and ATP production. High-fat feeding also results in more ROS per unit respiration and per unit ATP being produced. The impaired high-fat-induced bioenergetics is, in part, mitigated by partial substitution of n-3 fatty acids in the diet [38]. Most of the beneficial effects of melatonin in a number of physiopathological situations, which may depend on its effect on mitochondrial bioenergetics, involve mitochondrial dysfunction as a primary cause of disease [39].

2.2. Mitochondrial bioenergetic dysfunction

Bioenergetic dysfunction is emerging as a cornerstone for understanding the pathophysiology of cardiovascular disease, diabetes, cancer, and neurodegeneration. A substantial bioenergetic reserve capacity of cells is a prospective index of 'healthy' mitochondrial populations, which appears to be essential for cell survival under conditions of pathological stress [40].

It has long been known that mitochondria show a diminished functional activity when isolated from a broad range of tissues subjected to pathological stress. Well-established examples are alcohol-dependent hepatotoxicity, cardiac ischemia/reperfusion, and neurodegenerative diseases [41–43]. In all of these cases, a role for reactive oxygen or nitrogen species (ROS/RNS) in causing mitochondrial dysfunction has been proposed. Typically, mitochondrial damage is defined as a relative decrease in respiratory parameters, such as a change in oxygen consumption in the presence of substrates and ADP (state 3 respiration), in the presence of substrates alone (state 4), or the ratio of these parameters (i.e., respiratory control ratio (RCR)). Other parameters include decreased activity of specific enzymes, deletions in mtDNA, and increases in oxidative markers such as protein oxidation. The challenge with these data is in integrating them into an overall model of cellular and tissue bioenergetic function. It is becoming apparent that mitochondria under pathological stress exhibit multiple defects that overall can be viewed as a decrease in mitochondrial quality [43–44].

An existing mitochondrial population is examined that was subjected to pathological stress with the formation of reactive oxygen, nitrogen, and lipid species (ROS/RNS/RLS). This oxidative stress damages mtDNA, impairing the ability of the organelle to replace damaged electron transport proteins and decreasing bioenergetic reserve capacity; the resulting increased mitochondrial ROS then oxidatively damage previously unmodified mitochondria. The damaged mitochondria are turned over by a mitophagic mechanism that then suppresses this vicious cycle. The mitochondrial population is now renewed through mitochondrial biogenesis. The bioenergetic reserve capacity is essential for resistance to oxidative stress and supplying ATP demand. Once the bioenergetic reserve is depleted, bioenergetic failure occurs and the cell is programmed for cell death [40].

A unique feature of the molecular machinery controlling cellular bioenergetics is that the proteins necessary for electron transport and OXPHOS are encoded by both nuclear and mitochondrial genomes. An emerging concept in the energetics field is that the reserve capacity can be used as an index of mitochondrial health [45–47]. It appears that a higher bioenergetic reserve capacity results in a greater ability to withstand oxidative stress [40].

The mitochondrial genome encompasses in the order of one to two thousand nDNA genes and thousands of copies of the mtDNA. Hence, a large number of mitochondrial gene targets can mutate and have significant effects on cellular bioenergetics. Given that a human has in the order of 10^{17} mitochondrial capacitors, this is a great deal of potential energy, the vital force that animates our life. When breathing stops, the membrane potential collapses, energy transduction ceases, and death ensues [48–51]. However, there is a clear need to determine whether the contribution of mitochondrial dysfunction to different age-related diseases is explained by a cellular bioenergetic deficiency or by changes in mitochondrial ROS production affecting oxidative damage and signalling [52].

2.3. Bioenergetics and disease

2.3.1. mtDNA mutation and mitochondrial heteroplasmy

The mitochondrial genome encompasses both mtDNA and nDNA genes and the assembly and function of mitochondrial OXPHOS requires the cooperation of both genomes. Hence, the

http://dx.doi.org/10.5772/59418

interaction of the Mendelian and non-Mendelian mitochondrial genes generates a "complex genetics" that nicely explains many of the hereditary anomalies of many "common" clinical problems. Moreover, the central importance of energy metabolism for health provides a direct explanation of the pathophysiology of many diseases [53]. The frequency of mtDNA diseases is indeed high, currently estimated as having an incidence of 1.65/10,000 [54]. Moreover, mtDNA mutations have been linked to a broad spectrum of clinical problems affecting the central nervous system, the heart and cardiovascular system, the musculoskeletal system, and the renal and endocrine systems — many of the same systems that are affected by ageing and the age-related diseases. The appearance of a new mtDNA mutation in a cell results in an intracellular mosaic of mutant and normal mtDNAs, a state known as heteroplasmy. Identical twins derived from the same heteroplasmic egg can have different mtDNA genotypes and different clinical phenotypes and manifestations [4].

Rodell et al. present the contrasting view that the effects of mitochondrial heteroplasmy, in a broader sense, are not limited to a decline from a healthy norm, leading to unhealthy ageing and disease, but may also serve as the fabric of positive adaptive responses, at the genetic and epigenetic levels, to challenging bioenergetic events. The roles of mitochondrial biogenesis and dynamic fission and fusion mechanisms are vital to the maintenance of healthy mitochondrial populations, and impairment of the respective mechanisms is implicated in many age-related diseases [55]. Recently, Jose et al. reviewed the adaptive biology of mitoplasticity as a protective mechanism against ageing, diabetes, cancer, and neurodegenerative diseases, which Rodell et al. extend to the specific and directed promotion of healthy ageing [55–56].

Ageing is associated with decreasing bioenergetic capacity, as mitochondria increasingly become unable to meet the respiratory energy demands of cells [57]. Free radicals increasingly damage mtDNA with age, leading to an age-dependent state of variable heteroplasmy in individual cells, with detrimental effects on the bioenergetic capacity of the tissue [58]. Studies of mtDNA mutator mice show that increased accumulation of damaged mtDNA exacerbates the heteroplasmic conversion, with rapid onset of unstable health as the hallmark of ageing and the onset of age-related diseases. Such heteroplasmic variation can be described as the consequence of an age-dependent lack of selection [59].

2.3.2. Bioenergetic deficiency for mitochondrial diseases

The role of mitochondria in mitochondrial diseases aroused people's concern due to the central role of mitochondria in producing chemical energy (ATP) to meet cellular requirements. Old mitochondria appear morphologically altered and functionally produce more ROS and less ATP. Mitochondrial bioenergetic processes are central to the production of cellular energy, and energetic deficit correlates with many metabolic diseases and ageing. As the mutant mtDNAs accumulate, they progressively erode the individual cell's energetic capacity. Ultimately, cellular energetics drops below the threshold necessary for normal cellular and tissue function, and leads to a decline in organ function, tissue failure, and an ageing phenotype [12,60].

While mitochondrial defects are systemic, the clinical manifestations are often organ specific. This is because different organs and tissues have different needs and roles in energy homeostasis. Certain tissues require high levels of mitochondrial ATP, such as the central nervous system, the heart, and the muscles. These organs are preferentially affected as mitochondrial energy production declines. Other tissues store energy in fat. The liver is an energy homeostatic tissue, maintaining the serum glucose level within acceptable limits [49].

Mitochondrial disease or dysfunction (a cellular energy deficiency problem) is at the root of all these diseases. It is generally accepted that minimizing mitochondrial dysfunction is of central importance in maintaining cellular and body's fitness and also in counteracting mitochondrial diseases. The chapter may hold an important key to understanding mitochondrial disease (i.e., the body cannot make enough energy, or ATP). Mitochondrial diseases primarily affect the brain, heart, and muscle tissues at varying levels of severity. Almost all cells in the body have mitochondria, which are tiny "power plants" that produce the body's essential energy. When someone has mitochondrial disease, their power plants do not work properly and some functions in the body (e.g., muscles and neurological pathways) do not work normally. The body can have a power failure similar to a "brown out" or a "black out".

Mitochondria are highly dynamic organelles which play a central role in cellular homeostasis. Mitochondrial dysfunction leads to life-threatening disorders and accelerates the ageing process. A common denominator of these lifespan-modulating interventions seems to be defined by their ability to impact on cellular energy metabolism and stress response [61].

Alterations in mitochondrial structure and function, nDNA, and/or mtDNA mutations can impair OXPHOS, which in turn can reduce energy production, alter the cellular redox state, increase ROS production, deregulate Ca^{2+} homeostasis, and ultimately activate the mitochondrial permeability transition pore (MPTP), leading to apoptosis. The consequences of OXPHOS perturbation result in decline of mitochondrial function, and energy output declines, which accounts for ageing, degenerative diseases, metabolic deregulation, endocrine dysfunction, and symptoms such as diabetes, obesity, and cardiovascular disease. As inflammatory response initiates, this will contribute to autoimmune diseases. Finally, cancer cells must manage energy resources to permit rapid replication [5] (Figure 1).

The milder mtDNA variants can also affect caloric metabolism and result in metabolic diseases, such as diabetes and obesity, and degenerative diseases, such as psychiatric disorders, Parkinson's disease (PD), and Alzheimer's disease (AD). The more severe mtDNA mutations, like MERRF (myoclonus epilepsy with ragged red fibres) and MELAS (myopathy, encephalopathy, lactic acidosis, stroke-like episodes), cause progressive multisystem diseases, frequently resulting in premature death. The most severe mtDNA mutations can lead to lethal childhood diseases, such as Leigh syndrome [62].

While mtDNA mutations have permitted humans to adapt to stable regional environmental energetic differences, many energy resources and demands fluctuate cyclically, for example, seasonal changes in temperature and food supply. As these mitochondrial bioenergetic parameters fluctuate with the environment, they drive posttranslational modification of the proteins of the epigenome and the signal transduction pathways. In this way, the expression of nDNA-coded bioenergetic genes is coupled to environmental changes through mitochondrial energy flux [63–64]. This new bioenergetic perspective not only provides a framework

http://dx.doi.org/10.5772/59418

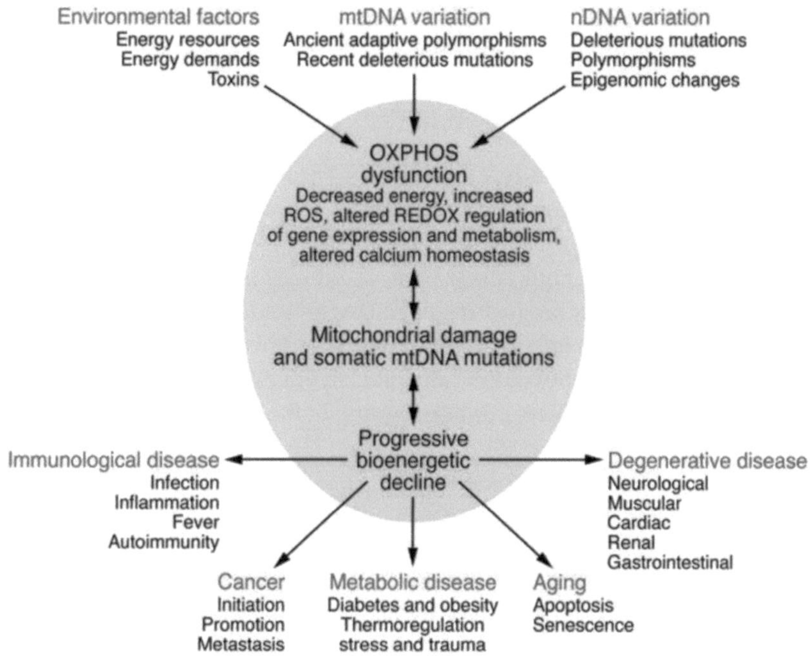

Figure 1. Bioenergetic paradigm for metabolic and degenerative diseases, cancer, and ageing. Figure adapted from reference [5].

within which the genetics and pathophysiology of "complex" diseases, such as PD, AD, autism spectrum disorders (ASDs), and psychiatric disorders [5] can be re-evaluated, it also provides a coherent theory for the aetiology of the "complex" metabolic and degenerative diseases, suggesting powerful new approaches for their presymptomatic diagnoses, reliable prognosis, and effective treatment and prevention.

3. Mitochondrial diseases

Enormous strides have recently been made in our understanding of the biology and pathobiology of mitochondria. Many diseases have been identified as having been caused by mitochondrial dysfunction, and many pharmaceuticals have been identified as previously unrecognized mitochondrial toxicants. Meyer et al. reviewed the importance of mitochondrial function and maintenance for health based on the genetics of mitochondrial diseases and the toxicities resulting from pharmaceutical exposure [11]. There are, however, currently no pharmaceutical cures for any mitochondrial disease [65].

The diseases described above are unambiguously caused by mitochondrial dysfunction. There are also many very common diseases for which there is strong correlative evidence suggesting that mitochondrial dysfunction is at least partially causative [50]. These are frequently diseases of old age or energy homeostasis and include neurodegenerative diseases such as PD and AD

[42], many cancers [34,66], diabetes, metabolic syndrome, cardiovascular disease [67], and others [68]. Considerable effort is currently devoted to investigate whether these relationships are causal. There is experimental evidence demonstrating that defective mtDNA replication and repair can accelerate organismal ageing [52].

The existence of so many mitochondrial diseases illustrates the critical importance of mitochondria for health. Why did it take us so long to realize that many diseases are in fact mitochondrial diseases? Part of the answer is surely that they are very complicated, although they often target tissues with high energy use, and there is significant variability in their presentation. Some mtDNA mutations result in single-tissue diseases, others affect a wide spectrum of tissues, and others affect different tissues in different patients, with varying ages of onset [69]. However, the absence of fundamental knowledge about the biology and genetics of the mitochondrion limited a deeper understanding of the inheritance and pathophysiology of mitochondrial diseases.

3.1. Classic mitochondrial disorders

Classic mitochondrial disorders result from mutations in mtDNA or nuclear genes that disrupt mitochondrial respiratory function. These diseases typically have brain and skeletal muscle manifestations, and therefore they are often referred to as mitochondrial encephalomyopathies. Based on the tissues typically affected in mtDNA diseases, it is generally thought that tissues such as brain, skeletal muscle, heart muscle, and endocrine glands are particularly dependent on respiratory function and have a lower bioenergetic threshold [70].

Leber's hereditary optical neuropathy (LHON) and mitochondrial myopathies were in 1988 the first diseases demonstrated to be caused by mtDNA mutations [71–72]. There are now more than 200 such diseases, including MELAS, MERRF, and many others [73]. Importantly, cellular dysfunction and clinical disease do not occur until a threshold proportion of mtDNAs carrying mutations (heteroplasmy) is reached [74–75]. Together, these diseases affect at least 1/10,000 people clinically [76], establishing mtDNA mutations as a major cause of disease.

Most patients with mtDNA diseases caused by deletions that cross two or more gene boundaries (intergenic mutation) generally do not reproduce. Therefore, most intergenic mutations arise *de novo*, resulting in sporadic disease [71]. Common presentations of this class of diseases include chronic progressive external ophthalmoplegia (CPEO) and the Kearns-Sayre syndrome (KSS) [77]. In contrast, most maternally inherited mtDNA diseases are the result of mutations confined within the gene commonly involving one or few base changes (intragenic mutations). Examples of this latter class of mtDNA mutations include LHON [72], MERRF syndrome [78–79], and neurogenic muscle weakness, ataxia, retinitis pigmentosum (NARP), and Leigh syndrome [80]. Over 200 pathogenic mtDNA base substitution mutations associated with a broad spectrum of clinical phenotypes have been identified, including encephalomyopathy, mitochondrial myopathy, exercise intolerance, gastrointestinal syndromes, dystonia, diabetes, deafness, cardiomyopathy, AD, and PD, etc [81].

In addition to recent deleterious mutations and ancient adaptive mtDNA variants, somatic mtDNA mutations play an important role in human health. Moreover, somatic mtDNA

http://dx.doi.org/10.5772/59418

intergenic and intragenic mutation levels are elevated in the organs of patients with degenerative diseases. The accumulation of somatic mtDNA mutations causes an age-related decline in mitochondrial function, thus exacerbating partial inborn defects in mitochondrial function leading to the delayed onset and progression course of age-related diseases [53]. Experimental results from mtDNA mutator mice suggest that mtDNA mutations in somatic stem cells may drive progeroid phenotypes without increasing oxidative stress, thus indicating that mtDNA mutations that lead to a bioenergetic deficiency may drive the ageing process [52]. Thus, somatic mtDNA mutations provide the ageing clock. Large-scale deletions in some cell types can attain a threshold to directly affect OXPHOS. Single-cell studies have shown that deletions can occur in ~32 to 80% of mtDNA molecules in *substantia nigra* neurons of brains from patients with PD [82].

Since most mitochondrial proteins are nuclear encoded, it is not surprising that mutations in many nuclear genes also cause mitochondrial diseases. For example, mutations in DNA polymerase γ — the only mtDNA polymerase and thus responsible for all mtDNA replication and repair — cause a wide range of mitochondrial diseases including progressive external ophthalmoplegia, and Leigh's syndrome, among others [83]. Friedreich's ataxia is caused by mutations in the gene encoding frataxin which is involved in iron-sulphur cluster assembly [84]. Diseases caused by mtDNA and nDNA mutations are estimated to collectively have an incidence of ~1/4000 individuals [85–86].

These and related studies will permit determination of exactly how important the mitochondrial and mtDNAs are in determining the complex physiology and inheritance of the common "complex" metabolic and degenerative diseases that demand much of the healthcare resources in both developing and developed countries.

3.2. Mitochondria and cardiovascular diseases

Cardiovascular disease remains the commonest form of mortality and morbidity in the Western world. There remains an urgency to identify and translate therapies to reduce the effects of this disease and its associated co-morbidities. Vascular smooth muscle cells are the primary source of extracellular matrix and collagen, and it has been suggested that loss of viability and vitality of these cells contributes to plaque vulnerability and rupture. It is the loss of ATP that may ultimately be more detrimental. Finding alternative sources of ATP synthesis by energetic reconfiguration may also provide a vital link in delaying the kinetics of plaque rupture [87].

Excitation–contraction coupling in cardiac myocytes consumes vast amounts of ATP that need to be replenished by OXPHOS. During a single heartbeat, ~2% of the cellular ATP is consumed, and the whole ATP pool of cardiac myocytes is turned over within one minute. To orchestrate OXPHOS in response to constantly changing workloads of the heart, constant availability of ATP must be secured [88].

A large body of work has shown that endothelial dysfunction contributes to the pathogenesis of cardiovascular disease, and considerable effort has been put into defining operative mechanisms. Recent work has emphasized the importance of mitochondria for endothelial function. Although they have long been recognized for their role in bioenergetics, mitochondria participate in a host of other cellular processes. It is now recognized that endothelial mitochondria play a prominent role in signalling cellular responses to environmental cues. An important mode of mitochondrial signalling is the regulated production of ROS. Blood markers of mitochondrial dysfunction, such as mtDNA damage and mitochondrial oxygen consumption in circulating leukocytes or platelets, may facilitate studies of systemic abnormalities of mitochondrial function and their relation to cardiovascular disease [89]. The presented studies suggest that mitochondria-directed therapies have potential for the prevention and management of cardiovascular disease, in part by improving mitochondrial function in the endothelium.

3.3. Mitochondria and metabolic diseases

Metabolic syndrome is a growing epidemic in the United States and worldwide. Currently, approximately 34% of the US population are living with this diagnosis [90–91] and it is expected that this number will continue to increase. One of the hallmarks of metabolic syndrome is central obesity, an increase in visceral white adipose tissue (WAT) around the midsection. Central obesity not only contributes to metabolic syndrome but also increases individual risk for type 2 diabetes mellitus (T2DM) and cardiovascular disease [92].

3.3.1. Obesity

An excess consumption of high-calorie foods appears to be one of the key factors in the epidemic of obesity [93], which increases the risk for developing diseases with a bioenergetic component [94]. As described above, these include cardiovascular disease [95], hepatotoxicity, and neurodegenerative diseases. While a high caloric intake can be offset by exercise (for example, the gold medallist Michael Phelps remains lean despite consuming up to ~12,000 calories per day), increasing evidence suggests that physical activity, on average, is declining [95]. This has led to heightened efforts to promote increased energy utilization and to better understand how altered intermediary metabolism, perturbations in cellular bioenergetics, and genetic differences contribute to the risk for becoming obese and insulin resistant [40].

Obesity is a primary risk factor for numerous metabolic diseases including metabolic syndrome, T2DM, cardiovascular disease, and cancer. Although classically viewed as a storage organ, the field of white adipose tissue biology is expanding to include the consideration of the tissue as an endocrine organ and major contributor to overall metabolism. Given its role in energy production, the mitochondrion has long been a focus of study in metabolic dysfunction, and a link between the organelle and white adipose tissue function is likely [90]. Physical exercise is a promising strategy to counteract liver mitochondrial damage [96–98]. Exercise is considered a non-pharmacological tool against several lifestyle disorders in which mitochondrial dysfunction is involved. Both exercise types (voluntary physical activity and endurance training) counteracted oxygen consumption (RCR, P/O ratio, and FCCP-uncoupling state) impairments and improved mitochondrial membrane potential ($\Delta\psi_m$) (lag-phase). In conclusion, exercise prevented or reversed the bioenergetic impairment induced by non-alcoholic steatohepatitis, and both prevents and mitigates non-alcoholic steatohepatitis-induced liver mitochondrial structural and bioenergetic impairments [96].

Mitochondria lie at the heart of systemic metabolic regulation. They act as end-point regulators of metabolic rate and affect thermogenesis primarily by increasing proton leak. In brown fat, the relatively high expression of uncoupling protein 1 (UCP1) allows re-entry of protons into the mitochondrial matrix without generating ATP. This uncoupling therefore generates an increase in substrate utilization and ETC turnover, as well as energy in the form of heat [99]. Despite the low amounts of brown fat in humans, as little as 50g of brown fat has been estimated to be capable of utilizing up to 20% of basal caloric needs [100]. This suggests that decreasing mitochondrial efficiency is an attractive therapeutic option for obesity [40].

3.3.2. *Diabetes Mellitus (DM)*

DM is a common degenerative disease and one of the leading causes of morbidity and mortality in developed countries. DM is a heterogeneous disease, affecting nearly every organ in the body. It has a common phenotype of impaired glucose tolerance and can be divided in type 1 (T1DM) and type 2 (T2DM). T1DM occurs mainly in childhood and puberty and is characterized by an absolute insulin deficiency, requiring daily insulin replacement therapy. T2DM usually develops in adults over the age of 40, accounts for 90–95% of all DM cases and is characterized by insulin resistance and/or inadequate compensatory insulin secretion response [101–102].

DM has become a worldwide epidemic with a substantial social and economic burden [103]. The prevalence of this disorder is rising dramatically; an estimated 370 million people worldwide will be suffering from diabetes in 2030 [104]. Among the wide range of chronic complications associated with diabetes, brain degenerative events, cognitive deterioration, and dementia have assumed pivotal importance in the last few decades [105]. In particular, diabetes is considered to be a major risk factor for the development of AD and PD [106–107]. Mitochondria take centre stage in the brain since neurons have a limited glycolytic capacity, making them highly dependent on aerobic OXPHOS to fulfil their energetic requirements [108].

Mitochondrial dysfunction is at the centre of many metabolic disorders, such as obesity and T2DM. It is widely believed that these disorders can be avoided by regular exercise and restricted food intake [109–110]. Imbalanced energy homeostasis is characteristic of obese and T2DM patients. Interestingly, metabolic inflexibility can already be observed in pre-diabetic individuals suffering from insulin resistance [111], limiting the ability to switch from fatty acid breakdown to fat storage after a meal, and vice versa [112]. Diverse mitochondrial parameters vary between insulin-resistant and insulin-sensitive subjects, such as mitochondrial number, structure, and function. This suggests that mitochondrial dysfunction might contribute to metabolic inflexibility and insulin resistance [113].

Chronic overnutrition and physical inactivity are major risk factors for insulin resistance and T2DM. Recent research indicates that overnutrition generates an increase in hydrogen peroxide (H_2O_2) emission from mitochondria, ultimately decreasing insulin sensitivity. Fisher-

Wellman et al. review the principles of mitochondrial bioenergetics and redox systems' biology, and offer new insight into how H_2O_2 emission may be linked via redox biology to the aetiology of insulin resistance [28]. This concept is consistent with the principles of cellular energetics and suggests that, in the absence of lifestyle (e.g., exercise) and/or dietary (e.g., caloric restriction) interventions designed to restore metabolic balance, pharmacological strategies must be devised [28].

More importantly, the dynamic behaviour was impaired in high-fat diet-induced (HFD) obese mice, accompanied with disturbed mitochondrial respiratory function and decreased ATP content in skeletal muscle. Altogether, mitochondria are dynamic organelles *in vivo* in skeletal muscle, and are essential in maintaining mitochondrial respiration and bioenergetics. It appears that mitochondrial dynamics and bioenergetics in diabetic skeletal muscle are impaired [16]. Dysfunctional mitochondrial bioenergetics and oxidative stress exist in T1DM [114].

Disruption of mitochondrial function is also implicated in the aetiology of the disease. For example, mitochondria of T2DM patients have reduced ETC capacities [115]. The ability of pancreatic β-cells to regulate blood glucose levels rely on mitochondrial ATP generation. Mitochondrial dysfunction or reduced mitochondrial number could impair the insulin-signalling cascade. Excess mitochondrial ROS in β-cells inhibits OXPHOS, leading to a decrease in ATP for glucokinase and the low ATP/ADP ratio will result in inactivated K_{ATP} channels and impaired insulin secretion [15]. A decline in ATP generation affects the glycolysis ratio, decreasing glucose, fructose, and several amino acids' utilization [116–117], leading to severe energetic impairment. Therefore, improving mitochondrial respiratory activity seems to be a metabolic adjustment to circumvent injury in hepatocytes. It seems plausible that similar decreases in ATP/ADP ratio occur in streptozotocin-treated rats, and the enhanced activity of the respiratory chain of diabetic rats can be a consequence of these decreased ratios [101].

Pre-diabetes, a risk factor for type 2 diabetes development, leads to metabolic changes at a testicular level. Every year, about 5–10% of the individuals with pre-diabetes become diabetic [118], and population habits may increase these rates. Adenylate energy charge was decreased in pre-diabetic rats, as were ATP and ADP levels. Conversely, AMP levels were increased, evidencing a decreased ATP/AMP ratio. Testicular mitochondrial function was compromised by inhibiting the PGC-1α/Sirt3 axis and the mtDNA copy number, decreasing respiratory capacity, and increasing oxidative stress in pre-diabetes [119].

3.4. OXPHOS disorders

OXPHOS disorders can be classified genetically according to whether the primary defect is in the nuclear or mitochondrial genome, as well as by the pathway primarily affected. There remains a considerable lack of understanding of the pathogenic mechanisms involved in clinical symptoms and the deterioration. The central role of OXPHOS in metabolism suggests that many features are related to abnormal metabolic consequences of the defects.

In addition, OXPHOS defects can be tissue specific, due to the variable metabolic thresholds for the different OXPHOS enzyme complexes in each tissue [120]. Tissue specificity may limit

http://dx.doi.org/10.5772/59418

the systemic effect of metabolic changes while still inducing marked abnormalities within the affected tissue. There are, however, likely to be many contributing factors including tissue-specific expression of nuclear OXPHOS genes, different metabolic needs of a tissue (for example, burst activity seen in some neurons versus cells with predominantly continuous biosynthetic functions), and tissue-dependent segregation of heteroplasmy [121].

The treatment of patients with OXPHOS disease remains very limited, but counteracting the most damaging metabolic changes may be beneficial in some patients, and is the mainstay of treatment at present. An inability of mitochondria to supply sufficient ATP to meet cellular needs is often assumed to be the primary effect of mitochondrial disease mutations [122].

3.5. Mitochondria and neurodegenerative diseases

The neurodegenerative diseases are a key health issue because they are profoundly debilitating [123]. In the past decade, the genetic causes underlying many familial neurodegenerative disorders, such as Huntington's disease (HD), Parkinson's disease (PD), Alzheimer's disease (AD), dominant optic atrophy, Friedreich ataxia, amyotrophic lateral sclerosis, and Leber's hereditary optic atrophy have been elucidated. However, the common pathogenic mechanisms of neuronal death are still largely unknown. Mitochondrial dysfunction has emerged as a potential 'lowest common denominator' linking these disorders [124]. Oxidative damage to mitochondrial membranes, enzymes, and the ETC components, culminate in impaired mitochondrial ATP production and facilitated MPTP opening [125]. Mitochondria play multiple roles in the maintenance of neuronal function under physiological and pathological conditions [126].

Brain function is almost totally dependent on a continuous supply of glucose and oxygen. Although the brain represents only 2% of the body weight, it receives 15% of the cardiac output, and consumes 20% of total body oxygen and 25% of total body glucose [127]. A high aerobic capacity of the brain is required for the mitochondria to generate sufficient ATP to maintain and restore ion gradients across the enormous area of plasma membrane, to maintain the compartmentation of neurotransmitters, and to drive exocytotic and endocytotic synaptic vesicle cycling [126]. Given the brain's high energy requirements, any decline in brain respiratory chain enzyme complexes' activity with ageing could have a significant impact on brain function, as well as on the aetiology and progression of age-associated neurodegenerative disorders [128–130].

An aged brain has a decreased capacity to produce ATP by OXPHOS and this becomes limiting under physiological conditions in aged individuals. The impairment of brain mitochondrial function in ageing is mainly due to decreased electron transfer rates in complex I and IV [131]. Previous results have shown an impairment of complex I activity in brain mitochondria of aged rats which was ascribed, in part, to oxidation of cardiolipin [132]. The age-associated alterations to brain mitochondrial cardiolipin were prevented by treatment of aged rats with melatonin [133]. It is reasonable to assume that melatonin's ability to prevent the age-related alterations of mitochondrial bioenergetic parameters in rat brains, could be ascribed (in addition to other factors) to its protective effect against cardiolipin peroxidation. Thus, the effect of long-term administration of melatonin against the age-dependent mitochondrial oxidative damage could be accompanied by an improvement of mitochondrial bioenergetics and brain function, and therefore to health in general [128].

Deficiency in complex IV activity may be a crucial factor in the aetiology, progression, and prevalence of several neurodegenerative diseases associated with ageing, in particular AD. The results may prove useful in elucidating the molecular mechanisms underlying mitochondrial dysfunction associated with the brain's ageing process, and may have implications in the aetiopathology of age-associated neurodegenerative disorders, and in the development of potential treatment strategies. Melatonin treatment may represent a valid therapeutic strategy for combating brain ageing process and age-related neurodegenerative disorders, in which complex IV deficiency and oxidation/depletion of cardiolipin could play a critical role [128].

In recent years, the field of neurometabolism has been greatly amplified by the recognition that bioenergetic dysregulation may be a critical pathophysiological factor in diseases of the nervous system [130]. Indeed, there is increasing appreciation for the concept of energy failure – principally from mitochondrial dysfunction – as a key mechanism resulting in neuronal death seen in neurodegenerative diseases [134].

Previous studies have suggested that mitochondrial dysfunction plays a central role in the pathogenesis of neurodegenerative disorders, including AD [135]. Alzheimer's pathology is accompanied by a decrease in expression and activity of enzymes involved in mitochondrial bioenergetics, which would be expected to lead to compromised ETC complex activity and reduced ATP synthesis [136]. Mitochondrial bioenergetic deficit precedes Alzheimer's pathology; in addition to the lowered mitochondrial bioenergetic capacity, impairment of OXPHOS is associated with increased free radical production and the resultant oxidative damage. Overproduction of ROS and higher oxidative stress is characteristic of brains from AD [137]. Mitochondria and brain bioenergetics are increasingly thought to play an important role in AD [138]. In summary, mitochondrial dysfunction and deficits in bioenergetics occur early in pathogenesis and precede the development of observable plaque formation of AD. Mitochondrial dysfunction provides a plausible mechanistic rationale for the hypometabolism in the brain that precedes AD diagnosis and suggests therapeutic targets for prevention of AD. Further, the age of reproductive senescence markedly exacerbated mitochondrial and bioenergetic dysfunction, which is coincident with marked increases in AD pathology. In addition, one consequence of oxidative damage to mtDNA may be impairment of mitochondrial respiratory capacity. Mitochondrial DNA damage is associated with reduced mitochondrial bioenergetics in Huntington's disease. HD cells may be more dependent on glycolysis than respiration to compensate for ATP production [139]. A number of studies have identified mitochondrial abnormalities within neuronal cell bodies in progressive multiple sclerosis, leading to a deficiency of mitochondrial respiratory chain complexes or enzymes [140].

3.6. Mitochondria and cancer

Cancer cells exhibit large varieties of metabolic changes which are associated with alterations in mitochondrial structure, dynamics, and function. Mitochondria can regulate tumour growth through modulation of the TCA cycle and OXPHOS, and are also crucial in controlling redox homeostasis in the cell, inducing them to be either resistant or sensitive to apoptosis. All these reasons locate mitochondria on centre stage in understanding the molecular basis of tumour growth [141]. A change in cellular bioenergetics is one of the key hallmarks of cancer. The Nobel prize-winning German physician and scientist, Otto Warburg, discovered that mitochondria in cancer cells do not efficiently generate energy; that almost all neoplastic cells demonstrate enhanced uptake and utilization of glucose for glycolysis to generate ATP. While increased glycolytic flux may provide some benefit to cancer cells by increasing ATP production, recent studies suggest that it is advantageous mainly because it generates chemical "building blocks" required for the anabolic processes that must occur prior to cell division [142]. The most glycolytic tumour cells were found to be most resistant to therapy, and most aggressive in metastasis [143–144].

Altered metabolism was among the first cancer biomarkers [145]. Nevertheless, the notion that glycolysis is a universal feature of aggressive tumour growth, and that OXPHOS is counterproductive to tumorigenesis still pervades the literature [146]. There is accumulating evidence that mitochondrial metabolism plays an essential role in tumour cell proliferation. Growing tumours alter their metabolic profiles to meet the bioenergetic and biosynthetic demands of increased cell growth and proliferation [147–149].

Warburg proposed that cancer could originate from the sole inhibition of respiration in human cells, but are the mitochondria of cancer cells dysfunctional? Different studies have indicated that OXPHOS is capable of synthesizing ATP in cancer cells, albeit with a low efficiency [150]. To survive under conditions of glucose limitation, tumour cells use OXPHOS to derive energy from the amino-acids, glutamine, and serine. This process (glutaminolysis) has been demonstrated to occur in multiple types of cancer cells [142,151–153]. Deregulated energetics is a hallmark of malignancy, but metabolic heterogeneity among individual tumours is unknown. A study by Caro et al. [154] demonstrates that a subset of lymphomas is defined by reliance on mitochondrial energy generation and is selectively killed when this pathway is impaired.

Collectively, these studies illustrate how differences in mitochondrial economy, bioenergetic reserve capacity, and autophagy regulate health and disease. It is now also becoming clear that physiological processes such as cell differentiation are associated with profound changes in cellular bioenergetics, including reserve capacity [155]. The challenge for us is to continue to strive to understand more fully how bioenergetics regulates cell and tissue function. Certainly, this would place us in the best position to develop better and more targeted therapies [40].

Numerous studies on cancer cell bioenergetics evidence a large variability in the relative contribution of glycolysis and OXPHOS to cellular ATP production. The corresponding differences in the capacities for glycolysis and OXPHOS demonstrate that there is a cancer-specific metabolic remodelling caused by a combination of genetic and environmental factors. The dogma that cancer cells use solely glycolysis is no longer valid; as such, a detailed bioenergetic characterization of each type of tumour must be performed in order to develop adequate treatments. The growing interest in the mitochondrion in cancer research could lead to the development of adapted metabolic therapies that might also serve to treat mitochondrial diseases [151].

The differences in mitochondrial function between normal cells and cancer cells may offer a unique potential for the design of anticancer agents that deliver mitochondrial targeting drugs to selectively kill cancer cells. The journal *Science* revealed that bioenergetics was the core of malignant transformation of tumour [156], and abnormal energy metabolism was concluded as one of the 10 most notable features of cancer cells by the journal *Cell* [157] — bioenergetics dysfunction is becoming the cornerstone for understanding the pathophysiology of mitochondrial diseases [40]. Here, we summarize the metabolic changes of cancer cells.

In cancer cells, anabolism is enhanced, both glucose and glutamine are important carbon sources which are metabolized for the generation of energy, and anabolic precursors, heavily consumed by cancer cells, are early precursors of non-essential amino acids. This process predominates in cancer cells rendering glutamine an essential amino acid and the source of tricarboxylic acid (TCA) cycle-derived anabolic metabolites. Mitochondrial dysfunction may lead to the activation of HIF-1, therefore triggering the hypoxia pathway in the tumourigenic process. The inability of mitochondria to provide enough ATP for cell survival under hypoxic conditions, results in up-regulation of the glycolytic pathway. This occurs by induction of HIF-1, which not only stimulates key steps of glycolysis but also suppresses mitochondrial respiration in cancer cells, therefore, modulating the reciprocal relationship between glycolysis and OXPHOS. The switch between glycolysis and OXPHOS is controlled by the relative activities of pyruvate dehydrogenase (PDH) and lactate dehydrogenase (LDH). HIF-1 inactivates PDH through pyruvate dehydrogenase kinase 1 (PDK1) induction, resulting in suppression of the Krebs cycle and mitochondrial respiration. In addition, HIF-1 stimulates the expression of lactate dehydrogenase A, which facilitates the conversion of pyruvate to lactate. As a result, mitochondrial contribution to ATP synthesis declines, although the mitochondria might remain functionally intact [158] (Figure 2).

Glucose is mostly phosphorylated by hexokinase II (HKII) in cancer cells, which is up-regulated as its gene promoter sensitive to typical tumour markers such as HIF-1 and has easy access to ATP being more strictly bound to the mitochondria. HKII plays a pivotal role in bioenergetic metabolism, phosphorylates glucose using ATP synthesized by OXPHOS, and releases the product ADP in close proximity of the ANT to favour ATP re-synthesis within the matrix. Its product, Glucose-6-P, is only in part oxidized to pyruvate. This, in turn, is mostly reduced to lactate being both LDH and PDK1 up-regulated. A significant part of Glucose-6-P is used to synthesize nucleotides that also require amino acids and glutamine. Glutaminolysis (breaking down glutamine into α-ketoglutarate (α-KG)) generates malate which, through the malic enzyme, will give rise to NADPH that can be used to fuel lipid biosynthesis, and oxaloacetate (OAA), which will generate citrate, which is necessary for lipid biosynthesis. Citrate in part is diverted from the TCA cycle to the cytosol, where it is a substrate of citrate lyase, which supplies acetyl-CoA for lipid and phospholipid synthesis that also requires NADPH. The reprogramming of mitochondrial metabolism in many cancer cells comprises reduced pyruvate oxidation by PDH followed by the TCA cycle, and increased anaplerotic feeding of the same cycle, mostly from glutamine. This also increases the free fatty acids' uptake, therefore β-oxidation is pushed to produce acetyl-CoA. In cancer cells, many signals can converge on the mitochondrion to decrease the mitochondria permeability transition

(MPT), with consequent enhancement of apoptosis resistance. ROS can enhance Bcl-2 and may induce mtDNA mutations. As indicated, ROS in many cancer cells are over produced. Interestingly, studies have also shown that the $\Delta\psi_m$ is approximately 60 mV higher in carcinomas as compared to their normal controls, which also contribute to the increased ROS [158] (Figure 2).

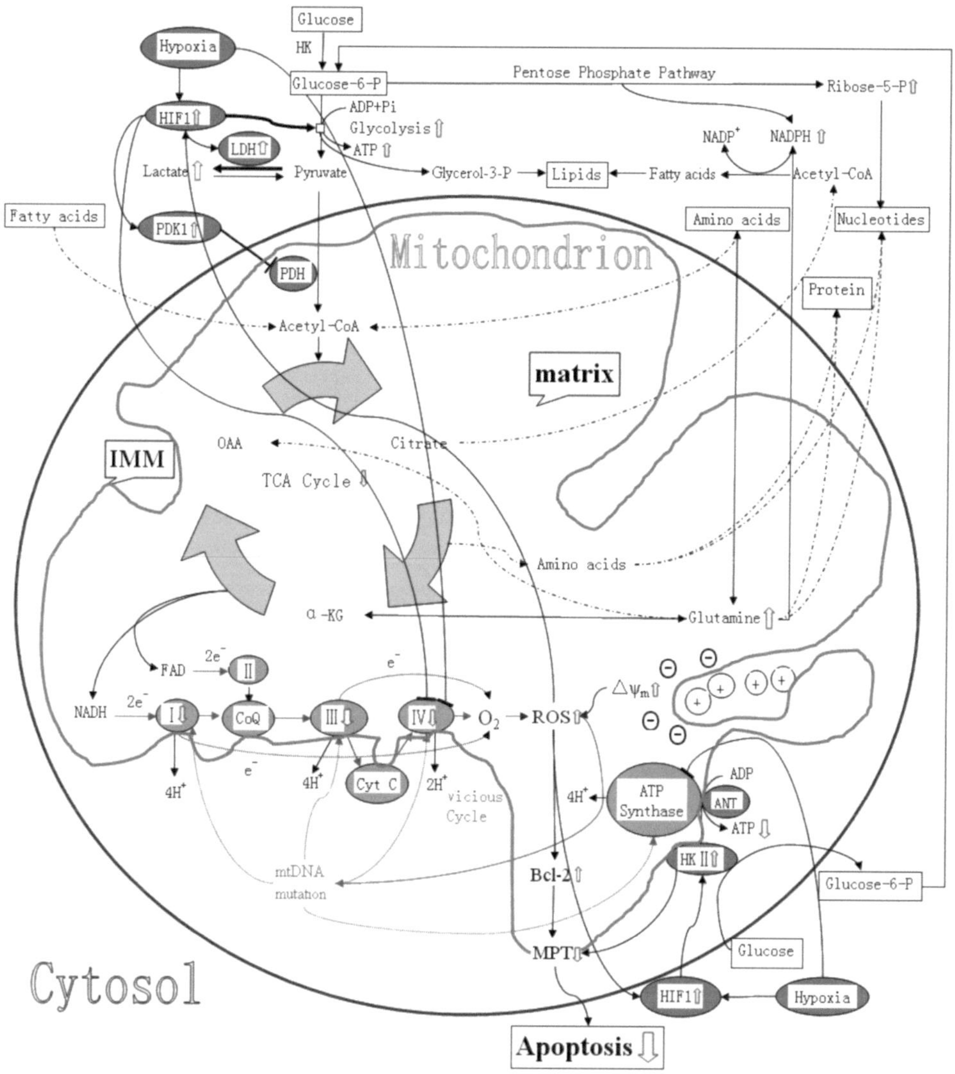

Figure 2. Schematic illustration of metabolic reprogramming frequently occurring in cancer cells, compared with mitochondrial metabolism in normal cells. Cancer cells showed increased glycolysis, pentose phosphate pathway, glutamine consumed, anabolism, $\Delta\psi_m$, and ROS generation, and reduced TCA cycle flux, respiratory complex activities, MPT, and apoptosis.

4. Qi-deficiency and mitochondrial diseases

Under normal circumstances, the body is under conditions in which the viscera are coordinated, Qi and blood are in harmony, and it is in a state of equilibrium known as "both Yin and Yang in equilibrium". If this balance is broken, the "Yin and Yang in imbalance" appears; this weakens the body's responses against disease, and the disease will later attack. Just like the Inner Canon of the Yellow Emperor says: "If the vital Qi exists in your body, the pathogenic factors won't disturb you". "If the various pathogenic factors attack the body together, Qi deficiency must occur". "wind, rain, hot or cold, will not lead to Qi deficiency alone, only the pathogenic factor won't hurt the human", these indicate the important role of the vital Qi in the fight against pathogenic factors. The so-called "vital Qi" refers to the body's primordial Qi, necessary to the body's normal functioning and ability to stay healthy; "pathogenic factors" refers to various contributing factors in illnesses. The body's vital Qi is the root cause, the pathogenic factors that cause mitochondrial diseases are symptoms.

Since Qi-deficiency is the inherent basis of mitochondrial diseases, Qi-invigorating herbal medicines and prescriptions (QIHMP), therefore, can prevent the occurrence of mitochondrial diseases according to TCM theory. Qi-invigorating herbal medicines (QIHM) are a class of herbs that can tonify the viscera and Qi of the human body, improve Qi-deficiency syndromes, enhance the body's function, improve disease resistance, have the effects of tonifying five internal organs, calming the mind, regenerating muscles, aiding resistance to cold and heat, and anti-ageing. Commonly-used QIHM include ginseng, astragalus, Codonopsis, Atractylodes, American ginseng, Chinese yam, liquorice, jujube etc., all rich in polysaccharides, which provides the material basis for improving Qi-deficiency syndrome and energy metabolism.

Studies have shown that all QIHM have the effects of improving exercise capacity, anti-fatigue, anti-oxidation, anti-hypoxia, anti-ageing, scavenging ROS, anti-apoptosis, improving immune function, and other benefits. The common regular pharmacological effects of these QIHM are closely related to the mitochondrial function; it is reasonable to assume that all QIHM invigorate Qi through the mitochondrial pathway, which provide evidence for Qi-invigorating therapy used for mitochondrial diseases.

Still, the number of therapeutic approaches for mitochondrial diseases is severely limited in Western medicine. How might we jump-start the search for treating the diseases? One promising approach might be TCM. If mitochondrial dysfunction is as important a factor in the diseases as proposed in this essay, then Qi-invigorating therapy should be as likely to target mitochondrial energetic function. If so, we might be able to modulate mitochondrial function by screening traditional Chinese therapies. These could then be applied to treating the mitochondrial diseases. If this strategy proves successful, then it may have been prescient that a major concept in the parlance of TCM is "Qi", which we propose that "Qi" is "bioenergy" [25].

According to TCM theory, all kinds of diseases and ailments are born from Qi; Qi refers to a kind of refined nutritive substance that constitutes the human body, and is the most basic motive force, maintaining life's functional activities. Qi is fundamental to our body; both life and death of humans depends on Qi. Qi is often described in the West as energy, or vital energy.

Therefore, life's activities depend on Qi. Qi underpins the basic theory of TCM and acts as its cornerstone. Qi has been used as a healing technique in China for 4000 years. Chinese people from all walks of life seek relief through a rebalancing of their Qi for ailments, from colds to cancer. From the Chinese perspective, Qi is the origin of true strength and power as well as genuine health — body, mind, and soul. In order to have good health you must have sufficient Qi. If there is not enough Qi (Qi-deficiency), one or more organs can become imbalanced and develop energy function disorders. Impaired mitochondrial ATP formation may be the key characteristic of Qi-deficiency.

The author found that Qi-deficiency led to a marked fall in cellular ATP, and a rise in cellular AMP. Qi-deficiency is the common cause of mitochondrial diseases and can lead to mitochondrial bioenergetics dysfunction, and Qi-invigoration is the basic principle for treatment of Qi-deficiency [26]. As ATP, an energy-rich biomolecule, is universally used for energizing cellular activities, the "Qi-invigorating" action may be mediated by the enhancement of mitochondrial ATP generation. In this regard, our previous studies show that all four widely used QIHM (including ginseng, astragalus root, pilose asiabell root, and white atractylodes rhizome) can increase ATP levels of liver cells *in vivo*. The concept of "Qi" in TCM is closely related to bioenergy in modern medicine; we propose a hypothesis that Qi is bioenergy according to both the ancient concept of Qi and modern bioenergetics [25]. Based on our findings, Qi-invigorating representative prescription Sijunzi decoction [26] and QIHM can enhance the mitochondrial ATP generation capacity, and they have a good effect in the treatment of Qi-deficiency syndrome. It is plausible that mitochondrial diseases involve an improvement of cellular energy status which can be accomplished by Qi-invigoration. We believed that the up-regulation of cellular activities by "Qi-invigoration" in Chinese medicine requires an increased supply of ATP, which is in turn largely supported by mitochondrial OXPHOS. Qi-invigorating prescriptions and herbal medicines have a good effect in improving energy metabolism. Mitochondrial diseases are a result of a decline in "Qi" (Qi-deficiency), and lead to deterioration in functions; therefore, Qi-invigorating therapy for mitochondrial diseases is logical.

5. Qi-invigorating therapy and prevention and treatment of mitochondrial diseases

"Qi theory" in Chinese medicine is profound. Investigation into the scientific connotations of the concept "Qi" and the mechanism of Qi-invigorating herbal medicines and prescriptions (QIHMP) by modern science over the past decade, have become a key point for the modernization of TCM.

"Qi" is closely related to "bioenergy", both "Qi" in TCM and "bioenergy" in the life sciences have played an important role. Qi-deficiency can lead to energy metabolism dysfunction, which is a common feature of mitochondrial diseases in turn, and this confirmed that Qi-deficiency is the basis of the incidence of mitochondrial diseases; Qi-invigoration is the basic principle for treating Qi-deficiency, Qi-invigoration is also able to improve mitochondrial bioenergetics. Logically, therefore, Qi-invigoration can prevent mitochondrial diseases. TCM usually interpret the properties of herbal medicines with Qi, and has become one characteristic of treating dieases, this can be understood as "regulating Qi by Qi".

Therefore, the broad and profound TCM Qi theory and the most recent research of mitochondrial diseases were integrated, the mechanism of Qi-invigorating therapy for mitochondrial diseases was clarified from the perspective of improving mitochondrial bioenergetics, and a novel perspective and new hope were provided for the prevention and treatment of mitochondrial diseases with original academic ideas.

QIHMP have a positive effect in improving the energy metabolism; for example, the Qi-invigorating representative prescriptions Sijunzi Decoction (SD) was able to improve mitochondrial function by enhancing cellular bioenergetics and had the pharmaceutical activities of mitochondrial protection [26]. *Panax ginseng* is one of the most popular QIHM and has been used to promote health, vitality, and longevity in China for millennia. *Panax ginseng* invigorates Qi by improving energy metabolism and boosting energy levels in different body parts to delay ageing [159]. QIHMP can help in boosting the level of vital energy in the body. The studies provide scientific evidence for the mechanism of Qi-invigoration in TCM, which is achieved by improving mitochondrial energy metabolism. As deficiency of Qi is thought to be the cause of mitochondrial diseases in TCM, this property is especially important for using Qi-invigorating therapy to counteract mitochondrial diseases.

The central therapeutic action of QIHMP is their ability to preserve Qi. One direction that scientists have recently explored is the mitochondrial dysfunction theory. *Astragalus membranaceus* is the most popular Qi-invigorating herbal medicine in TCM, is often used in formulas for Qi-deficiency characterized by limb weakness, fatigue, lack of appetite, and dizziness. Astragalus polysaccharides (APS), an important bioactive component of *Astragalus membranaceus*, have been applied in the prevention and treatment of cancer in TCM. APS can ameliorate vacuolar degeneration of mitochondria and fragmentation of mitochondrial cristae of hepatocytes in insulin-resistant mice, which indicates the mitochondrial dysfunction and the protective effect of APS [160]. Our preliminary studies indicate that APS can protect mitochondria by scavenging ROS, inhibiting lipid peroxidation and mitochondrial swelling, and increasing the activities of antioxidant enzymes [161]. We proposed that APS perhaps ultimately ameliorate mitochondrial dysfunction by improving energy metabolism; this may be the hypothetical anticancer and cancer-preventive mechanism of APS.

In the book *Cancer — Cares, Treatments and Preventions*, we demonstrate that APS play a role in cancer prevention by improving mitochondrial energy metabolism. We also discovered accidentally that APS could increase the levels of ATP and total adenylate pool (TAP) in hypoxic liver cells, reduce AMP levels, increase ATP/ADP, ATP/AMP ratios and adenylate energy charge (AEC) (i.e., increase cellular bioenergetics), and feedback inhibit OXPHOS by reducing the liver mitochondrial respiratory control rate (RCR), respiratory states 3, and P/O ratio, to regulate energy generation. We found that hypoxia leads to a marked fall in cellular ATP and ADP, and a rise in cellular AMP. Cellular ATP levels are closely linked to mitochondrial function, which is regulated perhaps by AEC. APS stimulated an increased output of ATP and can further decrease state 3 respiration, RCR, and P/O ratio of liver mitochondria compared to a normal group — we consider that this is the result of feedback inhibition by improving mitochondrial energy metabolism and the bioenergetic level [156]. The mitochondrial energy state can retro-regulate the nuclear-encoded energy genes. The changes in mitochondrial respiratory chain activity are followed by changes in "energy-state messengers" which include ROS (such as the diffusive H_2O_2), mitochondrial and cytosolic calcium, NADH/ NAD^+, ATP/ADP, GTP, AMP, cyclic AMP (cAMP), $\Delta\psi_m$, and ΔpH [162]. APS was able to improve mitochondrial function by enhancing cellular bioenergetics and had the pharmaceutical activities of mitochondrial protection by scavenging ROS, inhibiting lipid peroxidation, and increasing the activities of antioxidant enzymes. The study provides scientific evidence for the pathophysiological mechanism of mitochondrial diseases, which is achieved by improving mitochondrial bioenergetics.

The Mitchell theory has been unable to explain this phenomenon; in recent years, studies have shown that the Mitchell theory has limitations for OXPHOS in eukaryotic cells. The Mitchell theory implies the proton motive force (Δp) across the inner mitochondrial membrane as the energy-rich intermediate of OXPHOS. Δp is composed mainly of an electrical ($\Delta\psi_m$) and a chemical part (ΔpH) and generated by the respiratory chain complexes I, III and IV. The free energy of electron transport of the mitochondrial proton pumps is sufficient to create a Δp of 240 mV, most of which (>80%) represents the mitochondrial membrane potential ($\Delta\psi_m$) and a smaller part ΔpH. The passive proton permeability of biological membranes or the basal proton leak increases exponentially at $\Delta\psi_m$ values above 130 mV. At $\Delta\psi_m$ values above 140 mV, the formation of reactive oxygen species (ROS) increases exponentially. The rate of F_0F_1-ATP synthase is saturated and maximal at $\Delta\psi_m$ values of about 120 mV. Thus $\Delta\psi_m$ values above 140 mV are not required for maximal rates of ATP synthesis. Instead at high $\Delta\psi_m$ values, the efficiency of OXPHOS decreases due to increased basal proton leak of biological membranes. In addition, part of oxygen will be converted into harmful ROS. From both an economic and health point of view, multicellular organisms require a mechanism that does not rely on the Mitchell theory, while maintaining the $\Delta\psi_m$ at reasonably low levels (120–140 mV), thereby optimizing the efficiency of OXPHOS and can suppress the occurrence of mitochondrial diseases. Surprisingly, the German scientist Kadenbach et al. propose a new mechanism that does not rely on the Mitchell theory, in which high ATP/ADP ratio feedback inhibits CcO (complex IV), and maintains a low $\Delta\psi_m$ value, thereby preventing ROS generation and maintaining high efficiency of OXPHOS — the mechanism represents the new extension of Mitchell theory, known as the "The second mechanism of respiratory control" [163].

According to recent studies, the authors propose that QIHMP, such as *Panax ginseng, Astragalus membranaceus,* and the Sijunzi Decoction can improve mitochondrial bioenergetics, while higher levels of bioenergy will feedback inhibit OXPHOS. These studies enriched Kadenbach's "New extension of the Mitchell Theory" through multiple bioenergetic parameters; this not only provides the strongest evidence for the contention that "The second mechanism of respiratory control represents new extension of the Mitchell Theory for OXPHOS", but also proposes how to improve bioenergetic levels of cells by QIHMP intervention. A theoretical basis and novel ideas were provided for the research and development of new drugs for mitochondrial diseases, using mitochondrial bioenergetics as a target. Therefore, the authors propose that improving mitochondrial energy metabolism and bioenergetic levels are the possible biological mechanisms to prevent and treat mitochondrial diseases. Based on the current research on mitochondrial protection and improvement of energy metabolism by QIHMP, we prove that QIHMP act by improving the bioenergetic state, and have activities of making the body more energetic and dynamic. Qi-invigoration is achieved through the mitochondrial energy metabolic pathway. This provides a scientific basis to clarify why Qi-invigorating therapy in Chinese medicine is suitable for treating mitochondrial diseases from a mitochondrial bioenergetic perspective.

QIHMP have a unique advantage in the process of counteracting mitochondrial diseases; intervention can be performed by multi-level, multi-channel, and multi-target methods, focusing on increasing the vital Qi of our body, helping to improve symptoms and signs, to improve the life quality of patients, and prolong survival. This is one of the characteristics of TCM for the prevention and treatment of mitochondrial diseases, and Qi-invigorating therapy plays an important role in the comprehensive treatment of mitochondrial diseases. Qi-invigorating prescriptions (QIP), the combination of commonly used QIHM, are used for the treatment of Qi-deficiency under the guidance of Qi-invigorating therapy. If doctors can focus on pathogenesis features of Qi-deficiency at the different levels of the main symptom, accompanying symptoms, deteriorated case syndromes, and synergize with Chinese herbal medicines, such as warming Yang, nourishing Yin, calming the nerves, reducing phlegm, invigorating the circulation of blood, astringing, clearing heat medicines, and others, based on benefiting Qi and complementing deficiency, so that the monarch and ministerial drugs synergize in an orderly fashion, just match the symptoms, then QIP can be widely used in a variety of clinical disorders.

In summary, mitochondria are responsible for the generation of cellular energy and are believed to play a central role in ageing and mitochondrial diseases. *In vivo* experiments have shown that almost all QIHM could promote mitochondrial ATP generation in various types of tissue including the brain. We propose in this chapter that Qi-invigorating therapy can be used for the prevention and treatment of mitochondrial diseases for the first time in the world, and that good medical effects may thereby be attained.

6. Conclusion and perspectives

This chapter has focused on the growing body of evidence that mitochondria, although the major source of ATP, are also intimately involved in the aetiology of numerous human pathologies. Therefore, effective prevention and treatments for mitochondrial diseases has become a pressing issue. It is evident that Qi-invigorating therapy will furnish a greater efficacy and selectivity for these diseases, but will lead to fewer undesirable side effects. It has been over 50 years since the first description of a patient with a mitochondrial disease [2]; with the rapid development in mitochondrial medicine, mitochondrial disease research focused on unravelling the aetiology of mitochondrial dysfunction for the first 30 years. Currently, the most important focus is on providing a preventive method or cure for these devastating diseases.

http://dx.doi.org/10.5772/59418

A rational way to combat mitochondrial dysfunction is to correct the bioenergetic alterations seen at the cellular level. This approach is theoretically applicable in all mitochondrial diseases. Many research groups around the world have established ways to manipulate mitochondrial pathology in cellular models. Now is the time to test these therapies *in vivo*. Despite the apparent lack of therapy, the confirmation of a mitochondrial disease is important to prevent secondary mitochondrial dysfunction as seen in malnutrition or deconditioning. This chapter gives an overview of some potential breakthroughs and the hopes in pursuit of the first effective prevention and treatment for mitochondrial diseases by Qi-invigorating therapy. There seems to be light at the end of the tunnel, although currently it is difficult to predict when such treatment will become available. The primary cause of most mitochondrial diseases is a multifaceted aetiology; hence, efforts to develop effective drugs should be devoted to the design of Qi-invigorating prescriptions that work in synergy to protect the mitochondria.

TCM will provide new philosophical thinking and selective application for modern medicine. TCM is full of ancient Chinese wisdom and philosophical speculation, it advocates "preventive treatment of disease", and Chinese Preventive Medicine benefits a lot from it. Chinese medicine views the human body as a whole, focusing on the adjustment of inner balance, pays more attention to patients than to the diseases, and the systemic therapy was used for more than 2,000 years.

Developmental ideas of traditional Chinese medical philosophy and modern Western medicine are converging. The current health concepts and medical models are profoundly changed; from the perspective of developmental trends, Western medicine also began to pay attention to the disease prevention, self-care, individualized treatment and environmental influence on the disease, transition from disease-centred to patient-centred, which match the concept "disease prevention is the primacy", "man is an integral part of nature", and is consistent with the essential characteristics of "overall concept" and "treatment based on syndrome differentiation" in TCM for thousands of years. Chinese medicine believes that the health of people is interrelated with nature and is under its dominance, that people should preserve harmony with nature, that the human body is a systemic whole, that the relationship between the main viscera can be described by the five elements theory, and that health depends on the balance of Yin and Yang. TCM guides doctors in the prevention and treatment of disease through the system's theory.

However, not all clinical questions can be explained by TCM's theory; the new concepts and breakthroughs of modern Western medicine are sometimes difficult to integrate into the theoretical framework of TCM. Therefore, there is an urgent need to achieve exchanges and a convergence between the two systems, to translate the theory of TCM into the language of modern life sciences.

Qi theory is the core of the basic theory in TCM, the concept of "Qi" is complex and messy, the connotation of Qi is colourful, the extension of Qi is unlimited, and Qi has become an enigma of Chinese medicine. Since there is no concept of "Qi" in modern medicine, it is the biggest difference between Chinese and Western medicine, which leads to obstacles for the mutual communication between the two medical systems. The essence of Qi is extremely important and is an unavoidable major scientific problem to the modern development of TCM.

So the nature of "Qi" should become the key scientific issue to be resolved first. This chapter may provide a breakthrough point to reveal the essence of Qi in TCM, and to achieve further genuine integration with Western medicine.

It is not easy to do this, but it is very important for the entrance of TCM into the international academic community, and then to endow it with vitality in the future. The purpose of both Chinese and Western medicine is to maximize health protection; we should gradually break through the barriers between Chinese and Western medicine, and give full play to their respective advantages. On the one hand we want to make full use of new theoretical ideas and methods, new technologies, and multi-disciplinary cross-penetration of modern Western medicine, accelerating innovation of traditional medicine theory and technology. On the other hand, we should give full play to the characteristics and advantages of traditional medicine in the concepts of life, health, the medical model, and other aspects, provide more treatment ideas, and methods and means for modern Western medicine. The material basis and mechanism of Chinese materia medica are clarified on the basis of efficacy.

We think it is possible to build a modern medical system which fuses the advantages of both Chinese and Western medicine. This system will be inclusive and eclectic, not rest on its laurels; both based on history and look to the future; and will be superior to TCM, and possibly also superior to current Western medicine. If the challenges are shared, the challenges will be divided; if the results are shared, the results will be doubled.

With respect to the sacred cause (the maintenance and promotion of human health), let us have a broader vision, more multi-dimensional thinking, and an open mind. We believe that the convergence of traditional Chinese medicine and modern Western medicine will not only help us to achieve better health outcomes and benefit humans' well-being than are possible with the simple application of either one, but also that it will be possible to open a door leading to a wider world for us in the near future, promoting the development of the health industry.

"Qi is the root of human", Qi is the centre of TCM from basic theory to clinical practice, Qi theory is the core of the basic theory of TCM, Qi is also an enigma of Chinese medicine. The essence of "Qi" is the key scientific issue needing to be resolved first; "Qi essence, the mechanism of Qi-invigoration and Qi-invigorating therapy for the prevention and treatment of mitochondrial diseases" have been systematically studied by us in the past 20 years and had led to a series of original academic achievements. This has important scientific significance for Chinese medicine theory and its practical application. These studies may help us to find a breakthrough point to reveal the essence of Qi in TCM, in order to achieve genuine integration with Western medicine and lead the development of Western medicine. We proposed the original creative academic ideas that "Qi" and bioenergy are closely related, demonstrated that the mechanism of Qi-invigorating action was implemented by improving mitochondrial energy metabolism, and proposed a new scientific hypothesis for the prevention and treatment of mitochondrial diseases by improving mitochondrial bioenergetics with Qi-invigorating therapy.

It is hoped that the next few years will see a further convergence of Qi-invigorating therapy with mitochondrial bioenergetics function, which will provide a comprehensive view of

http://dx.doi.org/10.5772/59418

mechanisms on mitochondrial diseases. It seems likely that we are on the right track to acquire this understanding, and that it will involve mechanisms rich in novel modern medical sciences and old Qi ideas in TCM about mitochondrial diseases and how to counteract them. New perspectives, new ideas, and new hopes were proposed for mitochondrial diseases.

Acknowledgements

This work was supported by Dalian Municipal Science and Technology Project (No. 2013E15SF131) and the Talents Project of Dalian Nationalities University (No.20116126).

Author details

Xing-Tai Li[1*], Hai-Xue Kuang[2] and Jia Zhao[3]

*Address all correspondence to: xtli@dlnu.edu.cn

1 College of Life Science, Dalian Nationalities University, Dalian Economic & Technical Development Zone, Dalian, China

2 Key Laboratory of Chinese Materia Medica (Ministry of Education), Heilongjiang University of Chinese Medicine, Ministry of Education, Harbin, China

3 Basic Medical College, Jilin University, Changchun, China

References

[1] Hüttemann M, Lee I, Samavati L, et al. Regulation of mitochondrial oxidative phosphorylation through cell signaling. Biochimica et Biophysica Acta (BBA)-Molecular Cell Research, 2007; 1773(12): 1701–1720.

[2] Luft R, Ikkos D, Palmieri G, et al. A case of severe hypermetabolism of nonthyroid origin with a defect in the maintenance of mitochondrial respiratory control: a correlated clinical, biochemical, and morphological study. Journal of Clinical Investigation, 1962; 41(9): 1776–1804.

[3] López-Otín C, Blasco MA, Partridge L, et al. The hallmarks of aging. Cell, 2013; 153(6): 1194–1217.

[4] Wallace DC. Mitochondria as chi. Genetics, 2008; 179(2): 727–735.

[5] Wallace DC. A mitochondrial bioenergetic etiology of disease. The Journal of Clinical Investigation, 2013; 123(4): 1405–1412.

[6] Anderson S, Bankier AT, Barrell BG, et al. Sequence and organization of the human mitochondrial genome. Nature, 1981; 290: 457–465.

[7] Burger G, Gray MW, Lang BF. Mitochondrial genomes: anything goes. Trends in Genetics, 2003; 19(12): 709–716.

[8] Bogenhagen DF. Mitochondrial DNA nucleoid structure. Biochimica et Biophysica Acta (BBA)-Gene Regulatory Mechanisms, 2012; 1819(9): 914–920.

[9] Kukat C, Wurm CA, Spåhr H, et al. Super-resolution microscopy reveals that mammalian mitochondrial nucleoids have a uniform size and frequently contain a single copy of mtDNA. Proceedings of the National Academy of Sciences, 2011; 108(33): 13534–13539.

[10] Shoubridge EA, Wai T. Mitochondrial DNA and the mammalian oocyte. Current Topics in Developmental Biology, 2007; 77: 87–111.

[11] Meyer JN, Leung MCK, Rooney JP, et al. Mitochondria as a target of environmental toxicants. Toxicological Sciences, 2013; 134(1): 1–17.

[12] Wallace DC. Mitochondrial genetics: a paradigm for aging and degenerative diseases? Science, 1992; 256(5057): 628–632.

[13] Szeto HH. First-in-class cardiolipin-protective compound as a therapeutic agent to restore mitochondrial bioenergetics. British Journal of Pharmacology, 2014; 171(8): 2029–2050.

[14] Muravchick S, Levy RJ. Clinical implications of mitochondrial dysfunction. Anesthesiology, 2006; 105(4): 819–837.

[15] Camara AKS, Lesnefsky EJ, Stowe DF. Potential therapeutic benefits of strategies directed to mitochondria. Antioxidants & Redox Signaling, 2010; 13(3): 279–347.

[16] Liu R, Jin P, Wang Y, et al. Impaired mitochondrial dynamics and bioenergetics in diabetic skeletal muscle. PloS One, 2014; 9(3): e92810.

[17] Westermann B. Mitochondrial fusion and fission in cell life and death. Nature Reviews Molecular Cell Biology, 2010; 11(12): 872–884.

[18] Chen H, Vermulst M, Wang YE, et al. Mitochondrial fusion is required for mtDNA stability in skeletal muscle and tolerance of mtDNA mutations. Cell, 2010; 141(2): 280–289.

[19] Chen L, Knowlton AA. Mitochondrial dynamics in heart failure. Congestive Heart Failure, 2011; 17(6): 257–261.

[20] Grandemange S, Herzig S, Martinou JC. Mitochondrial dynamics and cancer. Seminars in Cancer Biology, 2009; 19(1): 50–56.

[21] Benard G, Bellance N, Jose C, et al. Relationships between mitochondrial dynamics and bioenergetics. In: Lu B, editor. Mitochondrial Dynamics and Neurodegeneration. Springer Netherlands, 2011. p. 47–68.

[22] Detmer SA, Chan DC. Functions and dysfunctions of mitochondrial dynamics. Nature Reviews Molecular Cell Biology, 2007; 8(11): 870–879.

[23] Zorzano A, Liesa M, Palacín M. Role of mitochondrial dynamics proteins in the pathophysiology of obesity and type 2 diabetes. The International Journal of Biochemistry & Cell Biology, 2009; 41(10): 1846–1854.

[24] Zorzano A, Sebastian D, Segales J, et al. The molecular machinery of mitochondrial fusion and fission: an opportunity for drug discovery? Current Opinion in Drug Discovery & Development, 2009; 12(5): 597–606.

[25] Li XT, Zhao J. An approach to the nature of Qi in TCM-Qi and bioenergy. In: Kuang H, editor. Recent Advances in Theories and Practice of Chinese Medicine. Rijeka: InTech Open Access Publisher, 2012. p. 79–108.

[26] Li XT. Investigation on the mechanism of Qi-invigoration from a perspective of effects of Sijunzi decoction on mitochondrial energy metabolism. In: Sakagami H, editor. Alternative Medicine. Rijeka: InTech Open Access Publisher, 2012. p. 247–275.

[27] Módis K, Coletta C, Erdélyi K, et al. Intramitochondrial hydrogen sulfide production by 3-mercaptopyruvate sulfurtransferase maintains mitochondrial electron flow and supports cellular bioenergetics. The FASEB Journal, 2013; 27(2): 601–611.

[28] Fisher-Wellman KH, Neufer PD. Linking mitochondrial bioenergetics to insulin resistance via redox biology. Trends in Endocrinology & Metabolism, 2012; 23(3): 142–153.

[29] Chang I, Heiske M, Letellier T, et al. Modeling of mitochondria bioenergetics using a composable chemiosmotic energy transduction rate law: theory and experimental validation. PloS One, 2011; 6(9): e14820.

[30] Demin OV, Kholodenko BN, Skulachev VP. A model of $O_2^{\,-}$ generation in the complex III of the electron transport chain. Molecular and Cellular Biochemistry, 1998; 184: 21–33.

[31] Kushnareva Y, Murphy A, Andreyev A. Complex I-mediated reactive oxygen species generation: modulation by cytochrome c and $NAD(P)^+$ oxidation–reduction state. Biochemical Journal, 2002; 368: 545–553.

[32] Brand MD. The efficiency and plasticity of mitochondrial energy transduction. Biochemical Society Transactions, 2005; 33(5): 897–904.

[33] Loeb LA, Wallace DC, Martin GM. The mitochondrial theory of aging and its relationship to reactive oxygen species damage and somatic mtDNA mutations. Proceedings of the National Academy of Sciences, 2005; 102(52): 18769–18770.

[34] Brandon M, Baldi P, Wallace DC. Mitochondrial mutations in cancer. Oncogene, 2006; 25(34): 4647–4662.

[35] Yao J, Irwin RW, Zhao L, et al. Mitochondrial bioenergetic deficit precedes Alzheimer's pathology in female mouse model of Alzheimer's disease. Proceedings of the National Academy of Sciences, 2009; 106(34): 14670–14675.

[36] Gershoni M, Templeton AR, Mishmar D. Mitochondrial bioenergetics as a major motive force of speciation. Bioessays, 2009; 31(6): 642–650.

[37] Paradies G, Paradies V, De Benedictis V, et al. Functional role of cardiolipin in mitochondrial bioenergetics. Biochimica et Biophysica Acta (BBA)-Bioenergetics, 2014; 1837(4): 408–417.

[38] Yu L, Fink BD, Herlein JA, et al. Dietary fat, fatty acid saturation and mitochondrial bioenergetics. Journal of Bioenergetics and Biomembranes, 2014; 46(1): 33–44.

[39] Paradies G, Petrosillo G, Paradies V, et al. Melatonin, cardiolipin and mitochondrial bioenergetics in health and disease. Journal of Pineal Research, 2010; 48(4): 297–310.

[40] Hill BG, Benavides GA, Lancaster JR, et al. Integration of cellular bioenergetics with mitochondrial quality control and autophagy. Biological Chemistry, 2012; 393(12): 1485–1512.

[41] Carreira RS, Lee P, Gottlieb RA. Mitochondrial therapeutics for cardioprotection. Current Pharmaceutical Design, 2011; 17(20): 2017–2035.

[42] Coskun P, Wyrembak J, Schriner SE, et al. A mitochondrial etiology of Alzheimer and Parkinson disease. Biochimica et Biophysica Acta (BBA)-General Subjects, 2012; 1820(5): 553–564.

[43] Pilsl A, Winklhofer KF. Parkin, PINK1 and mitochondrial integrity: emerging concepts of mitochondrial dysfunction in Parkinson's disease. Acta Neuropathologica, 2012; 123(2): 173–188.

[44] Karbowski M, Neutzner A. Neurodegeneration as a consequence of failed mitochondrial maintenance. Acta Neuropathologica, 2012; 123(2): 157–171.

[45] Brand M, Nicholls D. Assessing mitochondrial dysfunction in cells. Biochemical Journal, 2011; 435: 297–312.

[46] Zelickson BR, Benavides GA, Johnson MS, et al. Nitric oxide and hypoxia exacerbate alcohol-induced mitochondrial dysfunction in hepatocytes. Biochimica et Biophysica Acta (BBA)-Bioenergetics, 2011; 1807(12): 1573–1582.

[47] Higdon AN, Benavides GA, Chacko BK, et al. Hemin causes mitochondrial dysfunction in endothelial cells through promoting lipid peroxidation: the protective role of autophagy. American Journal of Physiology-Heart and Circulatory Physiology, 2012; 302(7): H1394–H1409.

[48] Wallace DC. Bioenergetics in human evolution and disease: implications for the origins of biological complexity and the missing genetic variation of common diseases. Philosophical Transactions of the Royal Society B: Biological Sciences, 2013; 368(1622): 20120267.

[49] Wallace DC. Why do we still have a maternally inherited mitochondrial DNA? Insights from evolutionary medicine. Annual Review of Biochemistry, 2007; 76: 781–821.

[50] Wallace DC. A mitochondrial paradigm of metabolic and degenerative diseases, aging, and cancer: a dawn for evolutionary medicine. Annual Review of Genetics, 2005; 39: 359–407.

[51] Wallace DC. Bioenergetic origins of complexity and disease. Cold Spring Harbor Symposia on Quantitative Biology, 2011, 76: 1–16.

[52] Bratic A, Larsson NG. The role of mitochondria in aging. The Journal of Clinical Investigation, 2013; 123 (3): 951–957.

[53] Wallace DC, Fan WW. The pathophysiology of mitochondrial disease as modeled in the mouse. Genes & Development, 2009; 23(15): 1714–1736.

[54] Schaefer AM, McFarland R, Blakely EL, et al. Prevalence of mitochondrial DNA disease in adults. Annals of Neurology, 2008; 63(1): 35–39.

[55] Rodell A, Rasmussen LJ, Bergersen LH, et al. Natural selection of mitochondria during somatic lifetime promotes healthy aging. Frontiers in Neuroenergetics, 2013; 5:1–6.

[56] Jose C, Melser S, Benard G, et al. Mitoplasticity: adaptation biology of the mitochondrion to the cellular redox state in physiology and carcinogenesis. Antioxidants & Redox Signaling, 2013; 18(7): 808–849.

[57] Desler C, Hansen TL, Frederiksen JB, et al. Is there a link between mitochondrial reserve respiratory capacity and aging? Journal of Aging Research, 2012, 2012:192503. DOI:10.1155/2012/192503

[58] He Y, Wu J, Dressman DC, et al. Heteroplasmic mitochondrial DNA mutations in normal and tumour cells. Nature, 2010; 464(7288): 610–614.

[59] Dai Y, Kiselak T, Clark J, et al. Behavioral and metabolic characterization of heterozygous and homozygous POLG mutator mice. Mitochondrion, 2013; 13(4): 282–291.

[60] Wallace DC. Diseases of the mitochondrial DNA. Annual Review of Biochemistry, 1992; 61(1): 1175–1212.

[61] Schiavi A, Ventura N. The interplay between mitochondria and autophagy and its role in the aging process. Experimental Gerontology, 2014; 56: 147–153.

[62] Wallace DC, Lott MT, Procaccio V. Mitochondrial medicine: the mitochondrial biology and genetics of metabolic and degenerative diseases, cancer, and aging. In: Ri-

moin DL, Pyeritz RE, Korf BR, editors. Emery and Rimoin's Principles and Practice of Medical Genetics. Philadelphia: Churchill Livingstone Elsevier, 2013.

[63] Wallace DC, Fan W. Energetics, epigenetics, mitochondrial genetics. Mitochondrion, 2010; 10(1): 12–31.

[64] Wallace DC, Fan W, Procaccio V. Mitochondrial energetics and therapeutics. Annual Review of Pathology, 2010; 5: 297–348.

[65] Nunnari J, Suomalainen A. Mitochondria: in sickness and in health. Cell, 2012; 148(6): 1145–1159.

[66] Kulawiec M, Ayyasamy V, Singh KK. p53 regulates mtDNA copy number and mitocheckpoint pathway. Journal of Carcinogenesis, 2009; 8(1): 8.

[67] Ballinger SW. Mitochondrial dysfunction in cardiovascular disease. Free Radical Biology and Medicine, 2005; 38(10): 1278–1295.

[68] Schon EA, DiMauro S, Hirano M. Human mitochondrial DNA: roles of inherited and somatic mutations. Nature Reviews Genetics, 2012; 13(12): 878–890.

[69] Vafai SB, Mootha VK. Mitochondrial disorders as windows into an ancient organelle. Nature, 2012; 491(7424): 374–383.

[70] Chan DC. Mitochondria: dynamic organelles in disease, aging, and development. Cell, 2006; 125(7): 1241–1252.

[71] Holt IJ, Harding AE, Morgan-Hughes JA. Deletions of muscle mitochondrial DNA in patients with mitochondrial myopathies. Nature, 1988; 331: 717–719.

[72] Wallace DC, Singh G, Lott MT, et al. Mitochondrial DNA mutation associated with Leber's hereditary optic neuropathy. Science, 1988; 242(4884): 1427–1430.

[73] Holt IJ. Zen and the art of mitochondrial DNA maintenance. Trends in Genetics, 2010; 26(3): 103–109.

[74] DiMauro S, Schon EA. Mitochondrial respiratory-chain diseases. New England Journal of Medicine, 2003; 348(26): 2656–2668.

[75] Rossignol R, Faustin B, Rocher C, et al. Mitochondrial threshold effects. Biochemical Journal, 2003; 370: 751–762.

[76] Chinnery PF, Elliott HR, Hudson G, et al. Epigenetics, epidemiology and mitochondrial DNA diseases. International Journal of Epidemiology, 2012; 41(1): 177–187.

[77] Moraes CT, DiMauro S, Zeviani M, et al. Mitochondrial DNA deletions in progressive external ophthalmoplegia and Kearns-Sayre syndrome. New England Journal of Medicine, 1989; 320(20): 1293–1299.

http://dx.doi.org/10.5772/59418

[78] Wallace DC, Zheng X, Lott MT, et al. Familial mitochondrial encephalomyopathy (MERRF): genetic, pathophysiological, and biochemical characterization of a mitochondrial DNA disease. Cell, 1988; 55(4): 601–610.

[79] Shoffner JM, Lott MT, Lezza AMS, et al. Myoclonic epilepsy and ragged-red fiber disease (MERRF) is associated with a mitochondrial DNA tRNA Lys mutation. Cell, 1990; 61(6): 931–937.

[80] Holt IJ, Harding AE, Petty RK, et al. A new mitochondrial disease associated with mitochondrial DNA heteroplasmy. American Journal of Human Genetics, 1990; 46(3): 428–433.

[81] Wallace DC, Lott MT, Procaccio V. Mitochondrial genes in degenerative diseases, cancer and aging. In: Rimoin DL, Pyeritz RE, Korf BR, editors. Emery and Rimoin's principles and practice of medical genetics. 5th ed. Philadelphia: Churchill Livingstone Elsevier, 2007. p. 194–298.

[82] Chen XJ. Mechanism of homologous recombination and implications for aging-related deletions in mitochondrial DNA. Microbiology and Molecular Biology Reviews, 2013; 77(3): 476–496.

[83] Copeland WC. Defects in mitochondrial DNA replication and human disease. Critical Reviews in Biochemistry and Molecular Biology, 2012; 47(1): 64–74.

[84] Marmolino D. Friedreich's ataxia: past, present and future. Brain Research Reviews, 2011; 67(1): 311–330.

[85] Chinnery PF, DiMauro S, Shanske S, et al. Risk of developing a mitochondrial DNA deletion disorder. The Lancet, 2004; 364(9434): 592–596.

[86] Howell N, Elson JL, Chinnery PF, et al. mtDNA mutations and common neurodegenerative disorders. Trends in Genetics, 2005; 21(11): 583–586.

[87] Mercer JR. Mitochondrial bioenergetics and therapeutic intervention in cardiovascular disease. Pharmacology & Therapeutics, 2014; 141(1): 13–20.

[88] Kohlhaas M, Maack C. Calcium release microdomains and mitochondria. Cardiovascular Research, 2013; 98(2): 259–268.

[89] Kluge MA, Fetterman JL, Vita JA. Mitochondria and endothelial function. Circulation Research, 2013; 112(8): 1171–1188. Circ. Res.

[90] Dunham-Snary KJ, Sandel MW, Westbrook DG, et al. A method for assessing mitochondrial bioenergetics in whole white adipose tissues. Redox Biology, 2014; 2: 656–660.

[91] Roger VL, Go AS, Lloyd-Jones DM, et al. Heart disease and stroke statistics — 2011 update a report from the American Heart Association. Circulation, 2011; 123(4): e18–e209.

[92] Wilson PWF, D'Agostino RB, Parise H, et al. Metabolic syndrome as a precursor of cardiovascular disease and type 2 diabetes mellitus. Circulation, 2005; 112(20): 3066–3072.

[93] Wang YC, Bleich SN, Gortmaker SL. Increasing caloric contribution from sugar-sweetened beverages and 100% fruit juices among US children and adolescents, 1988–2004. Pediatrics, 2008; 121(6): e1604–e1614.

[94] Haslam DW, James WP. Obesity. The Lancet, 2005; 366: 1197–1209.

[95] Roger VL, Go AS, Lloyd-Jones DM, et al. Heart disease and stroke statistics — 2012 update a report from the American Heart Association. Circulation, 2012; 125(1): e2–e220.

[96] Gonçalves IO, Passos E, Rocha-Rodrigues S, et al. Physical exercise prevents and mitigates non-alcoholic steatohepatitis-induced liver mitochondrial structural and bioenergetics impairments. Mitochondrion, 2014; 15: 40–51.

[97] Ascensão A, Martins MJ, Santos-Alves E, et al. Modulation of hepatic redox status and mitochondrial metabolism by exercise: therapeutic strategy for liver diseases. Mitochondrion, 2013; 13(6): 862–870.

[98] Gonçalves IO, Oliveira PJ, Ascensao A, et al. Exercise as a therapeutic tool to prevent mitochondrial degeneration in nonalcoholic steatohepatitis. European Journal of Clinical Investigation, 2013; 43(11): 1184–1194.

[99] Tseng YH, Cypess AM, Kahn CR. Cellular bioenergetics as a target for obesity therapy. Nature reviews Drug Discovery, 2010; 9(6): 465–482.

[100] Rothwell NJ, Stock MJ. Luxuskonsumption, diet-induced thermogenesis and brown fat: the case in favour. Clinical Science, 1983; 64(1): 19–23.

[101] Ferreira FM, Palmeira CM, Seiça R, et al. Diabetes and mitochondrial bioenergetics: alterations with age. Journal of Biochemical and Molecular Toxicology, 2003; 17(4): 214–222.

[102] Berdanier CD. Diabetes and nutrition: the mitochondrial part. The Journal of Nutrition, 2001; 131(2): 344S–353S.

[103] Santos RX, Correia SC, Alves MG, et al. Mitochondrial quality control systems sustain brain mitochondrial bioenergetics in early stages of type 2 diabetes. Molecular and Cellular Biochemistry, 2014; 394(1–2): 13–22.

[104] Wild S, Roglic G, Green A, et al. Global prevalence of diabetes estimates for the year 2000 and projections for 2030. Diabetes Care, 2004; 27(5): 1047–1053.

[105] Roriz-Filho JS, Sá-Roriz TM, Rosset I, et al. (Pre)diabetes, brain aging, and cognition. Biochimica et Biophysica Acta (BBA)-Molecular Basis of Disease, 2009; 1792(5): 432–443.

[106] Correia SC, Santos RX, Carvalho C, et al. Insulin signaling, glucose metabolism and mitochondria: major players in Alzheimer's disease and diabetes interrelation. Brain Research, 2012; 1441: 64–78.

[107] Santiago JA, Potashkin JA. Shared dysregulated pathways lead to Parkinson's disease and diabetes. Trends in Molecular Medicine, 2013; 19(3): 176–186.

[108] Santos RX, Correia SC, Wang X, et al. Alzheimer's disease: diverse aspects of mitochondrial malfunctioning. International Journal of Clinical and Experimental Pathology, 2010; 3(6): 570–581.

[109] Gao AW, Cantó C, Houtkooper RH. Mitochondrial response to nutrient availability and its role in metabolic disease. EMBO Molecular Medicine, 2014; 6(5): 580–589.

[110] Andreux PA, Houtkooper RH, Auwerx J. Pharmacological approaches to restore mitochondrial function. Nature Reviews Drug Discovery, 2013; 12(6): 465–483.

[111] Corpeleijn E, Saris WHM, Blaak EE. Metabolic flexibility in the development of insulin resistance and type 2 diabetes: effects of lifestyle. Obesity Reviews, 2009; 10(2): 178–193.

[112] Kelley DE. Skeletal muscle fat oxidation: timing and flexibility are everything. Journal of Clinical Investigation, 2005; 115(7): 1699–1702.

[113] Galgani JE, Moro C, Ravussin E. Metabolic flexibility and insulin resistance. American Journal of Physiology-Endocrinology and Metabolism, 2008; 295(5): E1009–E1017.

[114] Mitchell T, Johnson MS, Ouyang X, et al. Dysfunctional mitochondrial bioenergetics and oxidative stress in Akita$^{+/Ins2}$-derived β-cells. American Journal of Physiology-Endocrinology and Metabolism, 2013, 305(5): E585–E599.

[115] Nicolson GL. Metabolic syndrome and mitochondrial function: Molecular replacement and antioxidant supplements to prevent membrane peroxidation and restore mitochondrial function. Journal of Cellular Biochemistry, 2007; 100(6): 1352–1369.

[116] Gerbitz KD, Gempel K, Brdiczka D. Mitochondria and diabetes: genetic, biochemical, and clinical implications of the cellular energy circuit. Diabetes, 1996; 45(2): 113–126.

[117] Ferre T, Riu E, Bosch F, et al. Evidence from transgenic mice that glucokinase is rate limiting for glucose utilization in the liver. The FASEB Journal, 1996; 10(10): 1213–1218.

[118] Tabák AG, Herder C, Rathmann W, et al. Prediabetes: a high-risk state for diabetes development. The Lancet, 2012; 379(9833): 2279–2290.

[119] Rato L, Duarte AI, Tomás GD, et al. Pre-diabetes alters testicular PGC1-α/SIRT3 axis modulating mitochondrial bioenergetics and oxidative stress. Biochimica et Biophysica Acta (BBA)-Bioenergetics, 2014; 1837(3): 335–344.

[120] Rossignol R, Letellier T, Malgat M, et al. Tissue variation in the control of oxidative phosphorylation: implication for mitochondrial diseases. Biochemical Journal, 2000; 347: 45–53.

[121] Battersby BJ, Loredo-Osti JC, Shoubridge EA. Nuclear genetic control of mitochondrial DNA segregation. Nature Genetics, 2003; 33(2): 183–186.

[122] Smeitink JA, Zeviani M, Turnbull DM, et al. Mitochondrial medicine: a metabolic perspective on the pathology of oxidative phosphorylation disorders. Cell Metabolism, 2006; 3(1): 9–13.

[123] Duchen MR. Mitochondria in health and disease: perspectives on a new mitochondrial biology. Molecular Aspects of Medicine, 2004; 25(4): 365–451.

[124] Kwong JQ, Beal MF, Manfredi G. The role of mitochondria in inherited neurodegenerative diseases. Journal of Neurochemistry, 2006; 97(6): 1659–1675.

[125] Waldmeier PC, Zimmermann K, Qian T, et al. Cyclophilin D as a drug target. Current Medicinal Chemistry, 2003; 10(16): 1485–1506.

[126] Nicholls DG, Brand MD, Gerencser AA. Mitochondrial bioenergetics and neuronal survival modelled in primary neuronal culture and isolated nerve terminals. Journal of Bioenergetics and Biomembranes, 2015; 47: 63–74.

[127] Bozza FA, D'Avila JC, Ritter C, et al. Bioenergetics, mitochondrial dysfunction, and oxidative stress in the pathophysiology of septic encephalopathy. Shock, 2013; 39: 10–16.

[128] Petrosillo G, De Benedictis V, Ruggiero FM, et al. Decline in cytochrome c oxidase activity in rat-brain mitochondria with aging. Role of peroxidized cardiolipin and beneficial effect of melatonin. Journal of Bioenergetics and Biomembranes, 2013; 45(5): 431–440.

[129] Boveris A, Navarro A. Brain mitochondrial dysfunction in aging. IUBMB Life, 2008; 60(5): 308–314.

[130] Lin MT, Beal MF. Mitochondrial dysfunction and oxidative stress in neurodegenerative diseases. Nature, 2006; 443(7113): 787–795.

[131] Navarro A, Boveris A. The mitochondrial energy transduction system and the aging process. American Journal of Physiology-Cell Physiology, 2007; 292(2): C670–C686.

[132] Petrosillo G, Matera M, Casanova G, et al. Mitochondrial dysfunction in rat brain with aging: involvement of complex I, reactive oxygen species and cardiolipin. Neurochemistry International, 2008; 53(5): 126–131.

[133] Petrosillo G, Fattoretti P, Matera M, et al. Melatonin prevents age-related mitochondrial dysfunction in rat brain via cardiolipin protection. Rejuvenation Research, 2008; 11(5): 935–943.

[134] Gano LB, Patel M, Rho JM. Ketogenic diets, mitochondria, and neurological diseases. Journal of Lipid Research, 2014; 55(11): 2211–2228.

[135] Brinton RD. The healthy cell bias of estrogen action: mitochondrial bioenergetics and neurological implications. Trends in Neurosciences, 2008; 31(10): 529–537.

[136] Blass JP, Sheu RKF, Gibson GE. Inherent abnormalities in energy metabolism in Alzheimer disease: interaction with cerebrovascular compromise. Annals of the New York Academy of Sciences, 2000; 903(1): 204–221.

[137] Atamna H, Frey WH. Mechanisms of mitochondrial dysfunction and energy deficiency in Alzheimer's disease. Mitochondrion, 2007; 7(5): 297–310.

[138] Swerdlow RH. Mitochondria and cell bioenergetics: increasingly recognized components and a possible etiologic cause of Alzheimer's disease. Antioxidants & Redox Signaling, 2012; 16(12): 1434–1455.

[139] Siddiqui A, Rivera-Sánchez S, Castro MR, et al. Mitochondrial DNA damage is associated with reduced mitochondrial bioenergetics in Huntington's disease. Free Radical Biology and Medicine, 2012; 53(7): 1478–1488.

[140] Campbell GR, Worrall JT, Mahad DJ. The central role of mitochondria in axonal degeneration in multiple sclerosis. Multiple Sclerosis Journal, 2014; 20(14): 1806–1813.

[141] Solaini G, Sgarbi G, Baracca A. Oxidative phosphorylation in cancer cells. Biochimica et Biophysica Acta (BBA)-Bioenergetics, 2011; 1807(6): 534–542.

[142] Pollak M. Targeting oxidative phosphorylation: why, when, and how. Cancer Cell, 2013; 23(3): 263–264.

[143] Gogvadze V, Orrenius S, Zhivotovsky B. Mitochondria as targets for cancer chemotherapy. Seminars in Cancer Biology, 2009; 19(1): 57–66.

[144] Mathupala SP, Ko YH, Pedersen PL. Hexokinase-2 bound to mitochondria: cancer's stygian link to the "Warburg Effect" and a pivotal target for effective therapy. Seminars in Cancer Biology, 2009; 19(1): 17–24.

[145] Koppenol WH, Bounds PL, Dang CV. Otto Warburg's contributions to current concepts of cancer metabolism. Nature Reviews Cancer, 2011; 11(5): 325–337.

[146] DeBerardinis RJ. A mitochondrial power play in lymphoma. Cancer Cell, 2012; 22(4): 423–424.

[147] Pallotta ML. l-Proline uptake in *Saccharomyces cerevisiae* mitochondria can contribute to bioenergetics during nutrient stress as alternative mitochondrial fuel. World Journal of Microbiology and Biotechnology, 2014; 30(1): 19–31.

[148] Vander Heiden MG, Cantley LC, Thompson CB. Understanding the Warburg effect: the metabolic requirements of cell proliferation. Science, 2009; 324(5930): 1029–1033.

[149] Liu W, Le A, Hancock C, et al. Reprogramming of proline and glutamine metabolism contributes to the proliferative and metabolic responses regulated by oncogenic tran-

scription factor c-MYC. Proceedings of the National Academy of Sciences, 2012; 109(23): 8983–8988.

[150] Wu M, Neilson A, Swift AL, et al. Multiparameter metabolic analysis reveals a close link between attenuated mitochondrial bioenergetic function and enhanced glycolysis dependency in human tumor cells. American Journal of Physiology-Cell Physiology, 2007; 292(1): C125–C136.

[151] Nadege B, Patrick L, Rodrigue R. Mitochondria: from bioenergetics to the metabolic regulation of carcinogenesis. Frontiers in Bioscience, 2009; 14(11): 4015–4034.

[152] Reitzer LJ, Wice BM, Kennell D. Evidence that glutamine, not sugar, is the major energy source for cultured HeLa cells. Journal of Biological Chemistry, 1979; 254(8): 2669–2676.

[153] Young VR, Ajami AM. Glutamine: the emperor or his clothes? The Journal of Nutrition, 2001; 131(9): 2449S–2459S.

[154] Caro P, Kishan AU, Norberg E, et al. Metabolic signatures uncover distinct targets in molecular subsets of diffuse large B cell lymphoma. Cancer Cell, 2012; 22(4): 547–560.

[155] Schneider L, Giordano S, Zelickson BR, et al. Differentiation of SH-SY5Y cells to a neuronal phenotype changes cellular bioenergetics and the response to oxidative stress. Free Radical Biology and Medicine, 2011; 51(11): 2007–2017.

[156] Garber K. Energy deregulation: licensing tumors to grow. Science, 2006; 312(5777): 1158–1159.

[157] Hanahan D, Weinberg RA. Hallmarks of cancer: the next generation. Cell, 2011; 144(5): 646–674.

[158] Li XT, Zhao J. Cancer-preventive mechanism from the perspective of effects of the Astragalus polysaccharides on mitochondrial energy metabolism improvement. In: Cancer — Cares, Treatments and Preventions. Brisbane: iConcept Press; 2014. p. 141–180.

[159] Li XT, Chen R, Jin LM, et al. Regulation on energy metabolism and protection on mitochondria of *Panax ginseng* polysaccharide. The American Journal of Chinese Medicine, 2009; 37(06): 1139–1152.

[160] Mao X, Yu F, Wang N, et al. Hypoglycemic effect of polysaccharide enriched extract of *Astragalus membranaceus* in diet induced insulin resistant C57BL/6J mice and its potential mechanism. Phytomedicine, 2009; 16(5): 416–425.

[161] Li XT, Zhang YK, Kuang HX, et al. Mitochondrial protection and anti-aging activity of Astragalus polysaccharides and their potential mechanism. International Journal of Molecular Sciences, 2012; 13(2): 1747–1761.

[162] Benard G, Bellance N, Jose C, et al. Multi-site control and regulation of mitochondrial energy production. Biochimica et Biophysica Acta (BBA)-Bioenergetics, 2010; 1797(6): 698–709.

[163] Kadenbach B, Ramzan R, Wen L, et al. New extension of the Mitchell Theory for oxidative phosphorylation in mitochondria of living organisms. Biochimica et Biophysica Acta (BBA)-General Subjects, 2010; 1800(3): 205–212.